Health and Medical Aspects of Ramadan Intermittent Fasting

MoezAlIslam E. Faris • Ahmed S. BaHammam
Mohamed M Hassanein • Osama Hamdy
Hamdi Chtourou
Editors

Health and Medical Aspects of Ramadan Intermittent Fasting

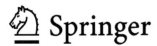 Springer

Editors
MoezAllIslam E. Faris
Department of Clinical Nutrition
and Dietetics
Faculty of Allied Medical Sciences,
Applied Science Private University
Amman, Jordan

Mohamed M Hassanein
Department of Endocrinology
Mohamed Bin Rashid University
Dubai, Dubai, United Arab Emirates

Hamdi Chtourou
High Institute of Sport and Physical
Education
University of Sfax
Sfax, Tunisia

Ahmed S. BaHammam
Department of Medicine,
College of Medicine
University Sleep Disorders Center,
King Saud University
Riyadh, Saudi Arabia

Osama Hamdy
Joslin Diabetes Center
Harvard Medical School
Bonton, MA, USA

ISBN 978-981-96-6782-6   ISBN 978-981-96-6783-3   (eBook)
https://doi.org/10.1007/978-981-96-6783-3

This Springer imprint is published by the registered company Springer Nature Singapore Pte Ltd.
The registered company address is: 152 Beach Road, #21-01/04 Gateway East, Singapore 189721,
Singapore

If disposing of this product, please recycle the paper.

Foreword

Historically, fasting has been incorporated into the rituals of monotheistic religions as a means of "cleansing the soul" and attaining a state of cognitive clarity and focus. During the past several decades, there has been a dramatic proliferation of research aimed at establishing and understanding the effects of intermittent fasting (IF) eating patterns on health and disease processes. This timely book provides a unique collection of articles on the science and practice of IF, including Ramadan fasting. In 19 chapters contributed by scientists and clinicians across the globe, this book reviews major findings emanating from research on different IF eating patterns with a focus on human studies. Collectively, this research has shown that IF can be an effective and sustainable treatment for obesity and diabetes. Moreover, IF can prevent or reverse disease processes in many different organs, including the heart, liver, lungs, intestines, and brain. Most scientific studies of Ramadan fasting have compared health indicators in the same individuals before the start of Ramadan and at the end of the one month of daytime fasting. The results of these studies are somewhat mixed but reveal improvements in cardiometabolic health as indicated by reductions in body weight, blood pressure, glucose, and atherogenic lipids. These effects of Ramadan fasting are similar to albeit considerably less pronounced than in randomized controlled trials (RCT) of daily time-restricted eating in which subjects consume all of their food within a 6–8 h time window every day.

Several interesting and important questions arise when considering the research on Ramadan fasting in light of the RCT of IF. Fasting from dawn to dusk results in different lengths of daily fasting depending upon where the person resides. For example, in 2025, Ramadan is from February 28 to March 29, during which time the fasting period during daylight hours is considerably longer in Southern latitudes than in Northern latitudes. Near the equator, the fasting period will be about 12 h. This may be important because the metabolic switch from glucose to ketones, which seems important for the health benefits of IF, occurs after 12–14 h of fasting. There are also cultural factors that may influence the results of studying people during Ramadan. For example, daily energy intake is not purposefully reduced and may even be increased during Ramadan. In addition, because Ramadan involves a major change in the timing of meals (no meals during the daytime), it may disrupt circadian rhythms, which are known to be influenced by the timing of meals. Finally, many of the effects of IF on health indicators and disease processes require 2–4 weeks to become evident. It is unclear whether daytime fasting for only 1 month each year has any long-term benefits on health.

Remarkably, information from science and religious experience converges on the same take-home message that organ systems and individuals function best with eating periods that include extended periods of fasting sufficient to cause a metabolic switch from glucose to ketone bodies. Indeed, food scarcity has been a major driver of beneficial evolutionary adaptations of the body and brain in all animals, including humans. By triggering adaptive responses of cells and organ systems, IF can help optimize health and productivity in modern societies. It is exciting to see the recent rapid increase in research on IF and its uptake as a healthy lifestyle in popular culture. There are currently more than 200 randomized controlled clinical trials of IF in progress in people with a range of medical conditions, including obesity, diabetes, heart disease, cancers, and fatty liver disease, among others. Moreover, research shows that IF can improve health indicators and physical and mental fitness in healthy individuals. This book provides a valuable collection of perspectives on the science of IF and its applications for health improvement and the treatment of chronic diseases.

Department of Neuroscience   Mark P. Mattson
Johns Hopkins University
Baltimore, MD, USA

Laboratory of Neurosciences
U.S. National Institute on Aging
Bethesda, MD, USA

Preface

Imagine a global phenomenon where over one and a half billion people simultane-ously engage in a month-long pattern of daytime fasting. This remarkable event occurs annually during Ramadan, the ninth month of the Islamic lunar calendar when Muslims worldwide observe dawn-to-dusk fasting as a fundamental act of spiritual devotion. Beyond its profound religious significance, this collective prac-tice of time-restricted eating presents scientists and healthcare researchers with an extraordinary natural experiment to understand how intermittent fasting affects human health and physiology across diverse populations and cultures.

The practice of Ramadan fasting transcends mere abstinence from food and drink—it represents a unique intersection of spiritual devotion and potential health benefits that has captured the attention of the medical community worldwide. As millions of people synchronously adjust their eating patterns, sleep schedules, and daily routines, they create an unparalleled opportunity to study the impacts of time-restricted feeding on human health. This fascinating convergence of faith and sci-ence has inspired our comprehensive exploration in *Health and Medical Aspects of Ramadan Intermittent Fasting* where we explore in depth both the physiological adaptations and health implications of this ancient practice in our modern world.

Recent studies have demonstrated significant impacts of Ramadan fasting on cardiovascular health, metabolic parameters, and mental well-being [1–3]. The daily fasting duration changes with the seasons, creating a natural experiment in chrono-biological rhythms and metabolic adaptation. Clinical evidence shows promising outcomes, with studies demonstrating reduced blood pressure in hyper-tensive patients [4], improved lipid profiles with lower total cholesterol and LDL levels [1, 2], and enhanced gut microbiota balance [5, 6]. While healthcare provid-ers must carefully manage patients with conditions such as diabetes during Ramadan, evidence-based guidelines have emerged to support clinical decision-making across different patient populations.

Our comprehensive volume addresses these challenges through carefully curated chapters that span the spectrum of health implications—from energy balance and weight management to the intricate relationships between fasting and chronic diseases. We ven-ture into emerging areas of research, examining neurocognitive function, mental health, and specific considerations for special populations such as athletes and pregnant women. The scope extends beyond individual health outcomes to consider broader societal impacts, including alignment with global health initiatives and sustainable development goals. This work represents a collaborative effort of researchers and clinicians from around the globe, bringing together diverse perspectives and experiences from leading institutions in both Muslim-majority and Western countries.

Through this international collaboration, contemporary research has yielded promising findings that extend beyond traditional metabolic studies. Careful clinical investigations have demonstrated that with proper medical supervision, many patients with chronic conditions can safely observe Ramadan fasting. This expanding knowledge base not only serves the Muslim community but also advances our understanding of intermittent fasting as a potential therapeutic tool in modern medicine.

We have designed this book to serve as an indispensable resource for healthcare professionals, researchers, and medical students seeking to understand the multifaceted health implications of Ramadan fasting. Through evidence-based insights and practical guidance, we aim to enhance healthcare delivery, inform policy decisions, and foster a more nuanced understanding of this significant religious practice in the context of modern healthcare.

As we present this comprehensive work, we acknowledge the countless researchers, clinicians, and participants who have contributed to our understanding of Ramadan fasting's health implications. Their dedication has helped bridge the gap between centuries-old religious practice and modern medical science. We invite readers to approach this volume not just as a collection of scientific findings but as a gateway to understanding how traditional practices can inform contemporary healthcare. Whether you are a healthcare provider serving Muslim communities, a researcher exploring intermittent fasting, or a student of medical sciences, we hope this book will spark new insights and inspire further investigation into this fascinating intersection of faith, health, and science. The journey of discovery in this field continues, and we are honored to contribute to this evolving body of knowledge that serves both scientific advancement and human well-being.

Amman, Jordan   MoezAlIslam E. Faris
Riyadh, Saudi Arabia   Ahmed S. BaHammam
Dubai, United Arab Emirates   Mohamed M Hassanein
Boston, MA, USA   Osama Hamdy
Sfax, Tunisia   Hamdi Chtourou

References

1. Jahrami HA, Faris ME, Janahi A, Janahi M, Abdelrahim DN, Madkour MI, et al. Does four-week consecutive, dawn-to-sunset intermittent fasting during Ramadan affect cardiometabolic risk factors in healthy adults? A systematic review, meta-analysis, and meta-regression. Nutr Metab Cardiovasc Dis. 2021.

2. Faris MAIE, Alsibai J, Jahrami HA, Obaideen AA, Obaideen AA. Impact of Ramadan diurnal intermittent fasting on the metabolic syndrome components in healthy, non-athletic Muslim people aged over 15 years: a systematic review and meta-analysis. Br J Nutr. 2020;123(1):1–22.
3. Lauche R, Fathi I, Saddat C, Klose P, Al-Abtah J, Büssing A, et al. Effects of modified ramadan fasting on mental well-being and biomarkers in healthy adult Muslims — a randomised controlled trial. Int J Behav Med. 2024.
4. Al-Jafar R, Zografou Themeli M, Zaman S, Akbar S, Lhoste V, Khamliche A, et al. Effect of religious fasting in Ramadan on blood pressure: results from LORANS (London Ramadan Study) and a meta-analysis. J Am Heart Assoc. 2021;10(20):e021560.
5. Mousavi SN, Rayyani E, Heshmati J, Tavasolian R, Rahimlou M. Effects of Ramadan and Non-Ramadan intermittent fasting on gut microbiome. Front Nutr. 2022;9.
6. Su J, Wang Y, Zhang X, Ma M, Xie Z, Pan Q, et al. Remodeling of the gut microbiome during Ramadan-associated intermittent fasting. Am J Clin Nutr. 2021;113(5):1332–42.

Acknowledgments

The completion of this book, *Health and Medical Aspects of Ramadan Intermittent Fasting*, is the culmination of significant effort and collaboration between the expert authors and the editors. We extend our deepest gratitude to the numerous individuals who contributed to its creation. First and foremost, we thank our chapter authors, whose expertise and dedication ensured the high quality and comprehensive nature of this work. Their willingness to share their insights and research findings is deeply appreciated.

We offer our sincere thanks to the publisher editors and reviewers who assisted with the production process. Their meticulous work helped ensure the book's accuracy and readability, and their efforts are invaluable.

Finally, we hope that this book will be a valuable contribution to the field and help readers better understand this important topic.

Contents

Part III Organ Systems and Disease

Part IV Special Populations

Part I
Foundational Concepts

Chapter 1
Fasting and Health: Introduction and Medical Perspective

Osama Hamdy and MoezAlIslam E. Faris

Abstract This chapter explores the historical and contemporary perspectives on fasting, encompassing its evolution from a survival mechanism to a deliberate practice for health and religious reasons. Various fasting regimens, including intermittent fasting (IF), time-restricted eating (TRE), and extended fasting (EF), are described, along with their prevalent methods and protocols. The chapter details the key metabolic and cellular mechanisms influenced by fasting, namely ketosis, autophagy, hormonal shifts, and inflammation reduction. These changes contribute to potential health benefits, such as weight loss, improved metabolic health, cardiovascular protection, enhanced cognitive function, and potentially increased longevity. However, potential risks associated with fasting, such as nutrient deficiencies and the exacerbation of eating disorders, are also discussed. The chapter concludes by emphasizing the importance of individualized approaches to fasting, guided by healthcare professionals, to maximize benefits and mitigate risks. The significance of fasting during Ramadan within a cultural and religious context is also highlighted. The chapter then introduces the subsequent chapters of the book, which explore Ramadan fasting's impact on various aspects of health (diabetes management, cardiovascular health, liver function, immunomodulation, mental health, gene expression, gut health, maternal and fetal health, and athletic performance), its socio-environmental impact, and practical considerations for medication management and dietary modifications.

Keywords Fasting · Intermittent fasting (IF) · Time-restricted eating (TRE) · Extended fasting (EF) · Ketosis · Autophagy · Metabolic health · Ramadan

O. Hamdy (✉)
Joslin Diabetes Center, Harvard Medical School, Boston, MA, USA
e-mail: osama.hamdy@joslin.harvard.edu

M. E. Faris
Department of Clinical Nutrition and Dietetics, Faculty of Allied Medical Sciences, Applied Science Private University, Amman, Jordan

© The Author(s), under exclusive license to Springer Nature Singapore Pte Ltd. 2025
M. E. Faris et al. (eds.), *Health and Medical Aspects of Ramadan Intermittent Fasting*, https://doi.org/10.1007/978-981-96-6783-3_1

3

Fasting, defined as the voluntary abstention from food and sometimes drink, evolved over centuries from a human necessity in the absence of the abundance of nutrition to a human choice as part of cultural and religious practices and, lately, a human choice to support health goals. More recently, scientific research has explored the health implications of various fasting regimes, suggesting potential benefits and risks. Both intermittent fasting (IF), time-restricted eating (TRE), and extended fasting (EF) have become popular dietary patterns. Currently, intermittent fasting (IF) is the leading nutrition trend among Americans and is practiced by approximately 10% of all adults.

IF is a pattern that involves cycling between periods of eating and fasting. Common methods include 5:2 IF (normal eating for five days and restricted intake for two nonconsecutive days), 4:3 IF (normal eating for four days and restricted intake for three nonconsecutive days), and alternate-day (AD) fasting. In general, individuals are instructed to consume only 25% of their regular eating calories on the fasting days and increase their caloric intake on non-fasting days by 25%. TRE restricts eating to a specific time frame each day, usually 4–12 h, with fasting during the remaining hours. The two most popular types of TRE are the 16:8 pattern (fasting for 16 h and eating for 8 h) and the 12:12 pattern, where the day is split into 12 h of fasting and 12 h of eating. In both methods, caloric intake is not altered. A novel method of TRE was recently introduced by the Joslin Diabetes Center of Harvard Medical School to induce diabetes remission among patients with a short duration of diabetes of <5 years. The method combines a very-low-calorie dietary pattern (VLCD) with a 16:8 TRE, where patients are instructed to fast for 16 h from their supper time but only consume between 800 and 1000 calories during the 8 h of the eating window. Extended fasting (EF) involves fasting for more than 24 h, sometimes lasting for several days. This method often requires medical supervision due to its potential for severe adverse effects. Water fasting and Fasting-mimicking diet (FMD) are the most popular methods of EF.

Fasting induces several metabolic and cellular changes that contribute to its health effects. The first is ketosis, where glycogen stores are depleted, and the body shifts to burning stored fat, producing ketones as an alternative energy source. The second is autophagy, which is the body's innate mechanism for removing worn-out intracellular components, such as mitochondria and misfolded proteins, promoting cellular repair and maintenance. Autophagy naturally slows down with age. This may play a role in some disease processes (e.g., cardiovascular disease, cancer, and neurodegenerative disorders). Supporting autophagy by downregulating nutrient-sensing pathways (NSPs) for a prolonged period can support healthy aging at the cellular level. Yoshinori Ohsumi's discovery of the mechanisms of autophagy garnered him a Nobel Prize in 2016. The third is hormonal changes, where insulin levels decrease, improving insulin sensitivity, and growth hormone levels may increase, aiding in fat metabolism and muscle preservation. The fourth is the reduction in inflammation markers, potentially lowering the risk of chronic inflammatory diseases. Moreover, EF, by suppressing NSPs, reduces insulin-like growth factor-1 (IGF-1), which is linked to several types of cancer growth.

Fasting has been shown to be associated with several health benefits. The first is weight loss and improved metabolic health, where IF and TRE lead to weight loss by reducing calorie intake and increasing metabolic rate. Studies showed that IF enhances insulin sensitivity and lowers blood glucose levels, thus reducing the risk of type 2 diabetes. The second is cardiovascular health, where fasting may lower blood pressure and triglyceride levels, with a possible increase in high-dinesty lipo-protein (HDL) cholesterol. It also reduces inflammatory markers associated with cardiovascular disease, specifically tumor necrosis factor alpha (TNF-α), interleu-kin-6 (IL-6), plasminogen activator inhibitor-1 (PAI-1), and several molecular and vascular adhesion molecules. The third is brain health, where several animal studies suggest that fasting enhances cognitive function and protects against neurodegen-erative diseases by increasing brain-derived neurotrophic factor (BDNF) and pro-moting autophagy in brain cells. The final health benefit is longevity, where experimental research indicates fasting can extend lifespan and delay age-related diseases. While human studies are limited, the findings are promising and suggest a potential for increased health span. Despite its benefits, fasting is not suitable for everyone. It can pose some risks, including nutrient deficiency, where prolonged fasting or severe calorie restriction can lead to deficiencies in essential nutrients, affecting overall health. Fasting may also trigger or exacerbate disordered eating behaviors in vulnerable individuals. Common side effects of fasting include head-aches, dizziness, fatigue, and irritability, which are usually temporary but can be severe or prolonged. EF, particularly water fasting, carries the most side effects, like hypoglycemia, hypotension, lowered immunity, malnutrition, and physical weak-ness. That is why all individuals must approach fasting with caution, considering individual health conditions and lifestyle factors. It is always recommended that individuals who would like to practice fasting consult healthcare professionals before starting a fasting regimen to ensure safety and efficacy. Future research should continue to explore the long-term effects of fasting in diverse populations to provide comprehensive recommendations and guidelines.

Ramadan, a holy month of fasting, prayer, and reflection, is a significant event for Muslims worldwide. This period of spiritual renewal also presents unique chal-lenges and opportunities for maintaining health and well-being. Understanding the physiological, dietary, and lifestyle changes that occur during Ramadan intermittent fasting (RIF) is essential for optimizing health outcomes and ensuring a meaningful spiritual experience. This book provides a comprehensive exploration of the health and medical aspects of RIF. Further, the current book delves into the physiological, dietary, and lifestyle changes experienced during this holy month. Our esteemed contributors, all leading experts in their fields, offer in-depth analyses of various topics related to the research updates on the RIF model. Prof. Osama Hamdy (Harvard Medical School, United States) and Prof. MoezAlIslam E. Faris (Applied Science Private University, Jordan) set the stage with a captivating introduction, providing a foundational understanding of fasting and its significance, with particu-lar attention to Ramadan fasting within Islamic culture in Chap. 1. In Chap. 2, Dr. Faiza Kalam (Ohio State University, United States) and colleagues explore the simi-larities and differences between Ramadan fasting and other intermittent fasting regimens, offering valuable insights into the unique aspects of the Ramadan model. Navigating research challenges specific to Ramadan fasting is addressed in this book by Prof. Ahmed S. BaHammam (King Saud University, Saudi Arabia) and Prof. MoezAlIslam E. Faris (Applied Science Private University, Jordan) in Chap. 3. Dr. Nader Lessan (Imperial College London/Abu Dhabi, UAE) sheds light on energy metabolism and its complex relationship with fasting in Chap. 4, discussing the physiological adaptations that occur during the month of Ramadan. Gene expression and autophagy are explored by a consortium of experts led by Dr. Nabil Eid (Islamic Medical University, Malaysia) in Chap. 5. The intricate connection between meal timing, circadian rhythms, and sleep during Ramadan is unraveled by Prof. Ahmed BaHammam (King Saud University, Saudi Arabia) in Chap. 6. The book continues with dedicated chapters addressing various aspects of health and Ramadan, including cardiovascular health (Chap. 7) by Dr. Iftikhar Alam (Pacha Khan University, Pakistan) and coauthors; liver diseases (Chap. 8) by Prof. Mohamed Emara (Kafrelsheikh University, Egypt) and colleagues; gut health and the gut microbiome (Chap. 9) by Dr. Falak Zeb (University of Sharjah, UAE) and colleagues; and, lastly, in this section on organ systems and disease, mental health and neurocognitive functions (Chap. 10) by Dr. Hamid AlHaj (University of Sharjah, UAE) and coauthors. Prof. Mohamed Labib Salem (Tanta University, Egypt) delves into the fascinating world of immunomodulation and its connection to intermittent fasting, including Ramadan fasting, exploring potential benefits and implications for overall health, cancer prevention, and management, particularly in Chap. 11. In Chap. 12, Prof. Mohamed M. Hassanein (Dubai Health Authority, UAE) addresses the challenges and opportunities of managing diabetes during Ramadan, offering practical guidance for healthcare professionals and individuals with diabetes. Prof. Leen Al-Kassab (Harvard Medical School, United States) and her colleagues explore maternal and fetal health during Ramadan in Chap. 13. Prof. Hamdi Chtourou (University of Sfax, Tunisia) and co-authors examine the interplay between physical activity and athletic performance during Ramadan (Chap. 14), followed by strategies to mitigate physiological and psychological challenges during Ramadan (Chap. 15). Dietary and lifestyle modifications during Ramadan are discussed by Dr. Maha Alhussain (King Saud University, Saudi Arabia) and Dr. Boumediene Khaled (University of Sidi-Bel-Abbès, Algeria) in Chap. 16. Food safety practices, foodborne illnesses, and food waste reduction are addressed by Prof. Morad AlHoly and Prof. Amin Olaimat (Hashemite University, Jordan) in Chap. 17. Prof. Yasser Bustanji (University of Sharjah, UAE) tackles the crucial issue of medication management during Ramadan in Chap. 18. Finally, extending beyond health, the book explores the environmental and social impacts of Ramadan with a focus on the Sustainable Development Goals (SDGs), authored by Dr. Khaled Obaideen (University of Sharjah, UAE) and coauthors in Chap. 19.

Throughout this journey, we aim to provide a comprehensive and informative resource for healthcare professionals, researchers, and anyone interested in understanding the complexities of Ramadan fasting and its impact on health and well-being.

Further Reading

1. Varady KA, Hellerstein MK. Alternate-day fasting and chronic disease prevention: a review of human and animal trials. Am J Clin Nutr. 2007;86(1):7–13.
2. Patterson RE, Sears DD. Metabolic effects of intermittent fasting. Annu Rev Nutr. 2017;37:371–93.
3. Gill S, Panda S. A smartphone app reveals erratic diurnal eating patterns in humans that can be modulated for health benefits. Cell Metab. 2015;22(5):789–98.
4. Cahill GF. Fuel metabolism in starvation. Annu Rev Nutr. 2006;26:1–22.
5. Longo VD, Mattson MP. Fasting: molecular mechanisms and clinical applications. Cell Metab. 2014;19(2):181–92.
6. Madeo F, Pietrocola F, Eisenberg T. Caloric restriction mimetics: towards a molecular definition. Nat Rev Drug Discov. 2015;14(6):450–60.
7. Ho KY, Veldhuis JD, Johnson ML, Furlanetto R, Evans WS, Alberti KG, Thorner MO. Fasting enhances growth hormone secretion and amplifies the complex rhythms of growth hormone secretion in men. J Clin Invest. 1988;81(4):968–75.
8. Fontana L, Partridge L. Promoting health and longevity through diet: from model organisms to humans. Cell. 2015;161(1):106–18.
9. Harvie M, Howell A. Could intermittent energy restriction and intermittent fasting reduce rates of cancer in obese, overweight, and normal-weight subjects? A summary of evidence. Adv Nutr. 2017;8(5):707–19.
10. Tinsley GM, La Bounty PM. Effects of intermittent on body composition and clinical health markers in humans. Nutr Rev. 2015;73(10):661–74.
11. Antoni R, Johnston KL, Collins AL, Robertson MD. Effects of intermittent fasting on glucose and lipid metabolism. Proc Nutr Soc. 2017;76(3):361–8.
12. Mattson MP, Wan R. Beneficial effects of intermittent fasting and caloric restriction on the cardiovascular and cerebrovascular systems. J Nutr Biochem. 2005;16(3):129–37.
13. Witte AV, Fobker M, Gellner R, Knecht S, Floel A. Caloric restriction improves memory in elderly humans. Proc Natl Acad Sci. 2009;106(4):1255–60.
14. Anson RM, Guo Z, de Cabo R, Iyun T, Rios M, Hagepanos A, et al. Intermittent fasting dissociates the beneficial effects of dietary restriction on glucose metabolism and neuronal resistance to injury from calorie intake. Proc Natl Acad Sci. 2003;100(10):6216–20.
15. Mitchell SJ, Bernier M. Daily fasting improves health and survival in male mice independent of diet composition and calories. Cell Metab. 2019;29(1):221–8.
16. Harrop EN, Moser C. Unintended consequences of restrictive dieting in adolescent athletes. Curr Sports Med Rep. 2020;19(6):210–5.
17. Halberg N, Henriksen M, Soderhamn N, Stallknecht B, Ploug T, Schjerling P, Dela F. Effect of intermittent fasting and refeeding on insulin action in healthy men. J Appl Physiol. 2005;99(6):2128–36.
18. Maughan RJ, Shirreffs SM. Development of hydration strategies to optimize performance for athletes in high-intensity sports and sports with repeated, intense efforts. Scand J Med Sci Sports. 2010;20:59–69.
19. Alkurd R, Mahrous L, Zeb F, Khan MA, Alhaj H, Khraiwesh HM, Faris ME. Effect of calorie restriction and intermittent fasting regimens on brain-derived neurotrophic factor levels and cognitive function in humans: a systematic review. Medicina (Kaunas). 2024;60(1):191. https://doi.org/10.3390/medicina60010191. PMID: 38276070; PMCID: PMC10819730
20. MoezAlIslam E. Faris, Haitham A. Jahrami, Asma A. Obaideen, Mohamed I. Madkour. Impact of diurnal intermittent fasting during Ramadan on inflammatory and oxidative stress markers in healthy people: systematic review and meta-analysis. J Nutr Intermediary Metabolism. 2019;15:18–26.

Chapter 2
Classification and Health Implications of Different Intermittent Fasting Regimens

Faiza Kalam, Maria Hafez, Tolulope Ilori, Dana Nabeel Abdel-rahim, and Rand Talal Akasheh

Abstract In this chapter, we provide an overview of different fasting approaches, with a focus on intermittent fasting (IF) and highlight how Ramadan fasting differs from other IF regimens. Intermittent fasting involves alternating periods of eating and fasting, which may occur within a day or across specific days in a week. Intermittent fasting has demonstrated effects on metabolic health, weight regulation, and disease prevention. This chapter examines the scientific evidence supporting these benefits, focusing on glucose and insulin regulation, lipid profiles, blood pressure, inflammatory markers, oxidative stress, nonalcoholic fatty liver disease (NAFLD), and cancer. The chapter aims to provide a nuanced understanding of different fasting protocols and how fasting can be utilized to improve health outcomes.

Keywords Ramadan fasting · Intermittent fasting · Fasting models · Metabolic changes · Fasting · Cancer

F. Kalam (✉) · R. T. Akasheh
Division of Cancer Prevention and Control, Department of Internal Medicine, College of Medicine, The Ohio State University, Columbus, OH, USA
e-mail: Faiza.Kalam@osumc.edu; Rand.Akasheh@osumc.edu

M. Hafez
Clinical Breast Cancer Research, Department of Medical Oncology, Sidney Kimmel Comprehensive Cancer Center, Thomas Jefferson University, Philadelphia, PA, USA
e-mail: Maria.hafez@jefferson.edu

T. Ilori
Clinical Breast Cancer Research, Department of Medical Oncology, Sidney Kimmel Comprehensive Cancer Center, Thomas Jefferson University, Philadelphia, PA, USA

Cooper Medical School of Rowan University, Cooper University Health Care, Camden, NJ, USA
e-mail: Tolulope.Ilori@jefferson.edu

D. N. Abdel-rahim
Research Institute for Medical and Health Sciences, University of Sharjah, Sharjah, UAE

M. E. Faris et al. (eds.), *Health and Medical Aspects of Ramadan Intermittent Fasting*, https://doi.org/10.1007/978-981-96-6783-3_2

2.1 Introduction

Intermittent fasting (IF) involves alternating between eating periods and fasting. Depending on the type, fasting may occur during specific hours each day, be repeated daily, or involve fasting on selected days throughout the week.

IF has been extensively studied over the past few decades, and growing evidence supports its potential benefits. Although many questions remain about its long-term effects on human health, fasting has gained significant public interest, reflected in the popularity of commercial books and wellness trends. However, more high quality clinical, basic, and translational research is needed to better understand its mechanisms and optimize its use.

2.2 Types of Fasting

Fasting can be broadly divided into intermittent fasting and periodic fasting. Intermittent fasting typically involves fasting for specific hours each day or on certain days throughout the week. In contrast, periodic fasting refers to consuming very low calories – often between 0–800 kcal- for several consecutive days each month (Fig. 2.1).

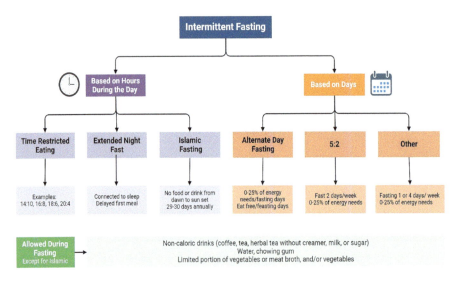

Fig. 2.1 Types of intermittent fasting

2.2.1   Fasting Based on Specific Hours During the Day

2.2.1.1   Time-Restricted Eating (TRE)

Time-restricted eating (TRE) involves consuming food within a specific number of hours each day, typically between 4 and 10 h, and fasting for the rest of the day. This pattern is usually followed on a daily basis. Some people adopt this regimen temporarily, while others incorporate it as a long-term lifestyle. Human clinical research have examined a range of fasting windows, including 14, 16, 18, and 20 hs. Additionally, some researchers have explored different timing strategies. Early time-restricted eating (e-TRE) refers to restricting food intake to earlier hours of the day (e.g., 8 AM to 2 PM), while late time-restricted eating (l-TRE) shifts the eating window to later hours (e.g., after 4 PM).

2.2.1.2   Prolonged Night Fasting (PNF)

Prolonged night fasting is another form of time-restricted eating in which the fasting period is aligned with nighttime sleep. In this method, the fasting period during the night continues into the morning, delaying the first meal to achieve the desired fasting duration. Some researchers also define this type of fasting as a form of late time-restricted eating (l-TRE).

2.2.1.3   Islamic Fasting

One of the most popular forms of fasting in Islam is Ramadan intermittent fasting (RIF), also referred to as intermittent dry fasting (IDF). During the holy month of Ramadan Muslims refrain from all food and drinks (including water) from dawn to sunset. This type of fasting is often described as a dry fast because nothing is ingested during the fasting hours. Ramadan fasting lasts for 29 or 30 consecutive days each year, and is observed annually by Muslims. Additionally, some Muslims practice this fasting on other religious occasions, such as every Monday and Thursday, the ten days preceding Eid Al-Adha, or during the three "white days" of each lunar month (13th–15th).

2.2.2   Fasting Based on Specific Days

2.2.2.1   Alternate-Day Fasting (ADF)

Alternate-day fasting (ADF) involves alternating between fasting and non-fasting (or feasting) days. On fasting days, caloric intake may be as low as zero, although noncaloric drinks and water are typically allowed. On non-fasting days, individuals can eat freely. Given the challanges of consuming zero calories on fasting days, a modified version of ADF was developed, which allows up to 25% of daily caloric needs on fasting days.

2.2.2.2   The 5:2 Diet

The 5:2 diet involves fasting for two nonconsecutive days each week, repeated weekly as a temporary plan or a long-term lifestyle. On non-fasting days, individuals eat freely, while on fasting days, energy intake is restricted to 0–25% of daily energy needs. This fasting pattern corresponds to the voluntary Islamic fasting on Mondays and Thursdays though it can be followed regardless of caloric restriction.

2.2.2.3   The 4:3 or 6:1 Diet

Similar to the 5:2 diet, some people might choose to fast more frequently such as 3 days per week (4:3 diet) or less frequently such as 1 day per week (6:1 diet). On non-fasting days, eating is ad libitum, while fasting days involve restricting intake to 0–25% of daily energy needs.

2.2.3   Periodic Fasting

Periodic fasting involves fasting for a specific number of consecutive days each month, typically repeated every month. One of the most well-known form is the fasting-mimicking diet (FMD), in which energy intake is restricted for 3–5 days per month. During these fasting days, individuals consume approximately 0–800 kcal per day.

2.3   What Is Typically Allowed During Fasting?

Noncaloric drinks are typically allowed. These include water, black coffee, tea, and herbal tea, without added sugar or creamer. Sugar-free chewing gum is also allowed. Occasionally, individuals might consume small portions of meat or vegetable broth, or raw vegetables, depending on the fasting protocol. During Ramadan fasting, however, no food or drink is allowed during the fasting hours.

2.4   Benefits of Intermittent Fasting

Intermittent fasting has been associated with benefits such as improved weight management, enhanced cardiometabolic health, reduced inflammation and oxidative stress, and potential role in cancer prevention and control (Fig. 2.2).

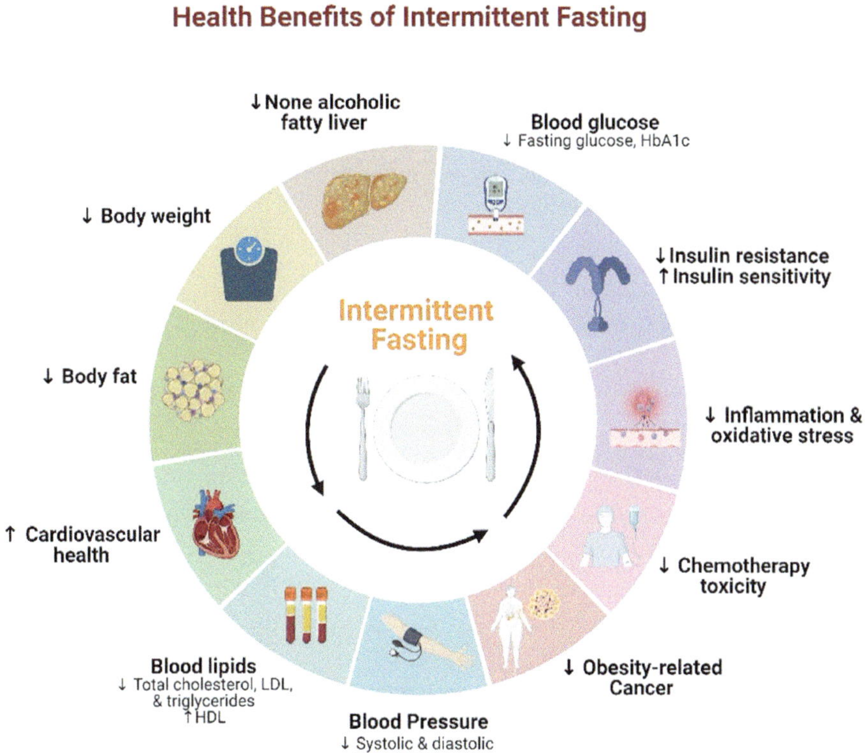

Health Benefits of Intermittent Fasting

Fig. 2.2 Health benefits of intermittent fasting

2.4.1 Weight and Body Fat Regulation

Intermittent fasting (IF) has been shown to support weight management, particularly for achiving weight loss [1–19] and body fat reduction [6, 11, 14, 17–20], as well as weight maintenance. The degree of weight loss varies depending on the type, duration, and intensity of the fasting protocol with reduction ranging from approximately 1–13% over 2–26 weeks. The primary mechanism behind weight loss in intermittent fasting is an unintentional caloric deficit that occurs created by the restricted eating window. Reducing the hours of eating during the day can lead to a significant reduction in daily caloric intake. For instance, time-restricted eating often results in skipping meals, which can decrease overall caloric consumption by approximately 350–550 kcal per day [2–4, 9, 21].

Additionally, modified alternate-day fasting, where individuals consume 0–25% of their daily caloric needs on fasting days, can produce an average weekly caloric deficit of 4500–6000 kcal with 3 fasting days and 6000–8000 kcal for a 4-day fasting week, assuming a baseline daily requirement of ~2000 kcal. This substantial caloric deficit contributes to weight loss and reductions in body fat [1, 9, 14].

Importantly, IF may help preserve lean muscle mass while promoting fat loss. This benefit is partly linked to favorable hormonal adaptations, such as increases in human growth hormone (HGH) and reductions in insulin levels, which together enhances fat metabolism and protects muscle tissue [17, 19].

Taken together, clinical evidence suggests that intermittent fasting is an effective and evidence-based strategy for improving body weight, reducing adiposity, and supporting metabolic health.

2.4.2   The Effect on Cardiometabolic Disease Risk

2.4.2.1   Diabetes-Related Markers and Risks

Intermittent fasting improves glucoregulatory markers, including fasting glucose [1, 2, 7, 11, 19, 22, 23], fasting insulin [2, 6, 19, 22, 24], and insulin sensitivity [2, 6], resulting in improved glycemic control [1, 2] and glycated hemoglobin (HbA1c) [2, 4, 15]. Moreover, individuals with type 2 diabetes may experience significant improvements in their glycemic control [4, 12] when fasting under medical supervision.

2.4.2.2   Blood Lipids

Intermittent fasting improves blood lipids, including reductions in total cholesterol [1, 19], Low-Density Lipoprotein (LDL) cholesterol [1, 2, 6, 7, 12, 14, 15, 19], and triglycerides [6, 7, 9, 12, 15, 16] and increases in High-Density Lipoprotein (HDL) cholesterol [8, 9, 12]. Together, these changes may help reduce the risk of atherosclerosis and cardiovascular disease. Blood lipid levels can vary based on the type and duration of fasting, but overall, intermittent fasting shows promise in managing blood lipid levels.

2.4.2.3   Blood Pressure

Intermittent fasting might lead to improvements in blood pressure, which is a critical factor in preventing cardiovascular diseases. The mechanism behind this effect is thought to be related to weight loss and improved insulin sensitivity, both of which can contribute to lower blood pressure levels. However, whether it is the fasting itself or its effects that lead to this improvement remains under investigation. Studies reported significant decreases in systolic [2, 6, 10, 11, 13–15, 19, 24] and diastolic [2, 6, 13–15, 19, 24] blood pressure among individuals participating in intermittent fasting trials.

2.4.3 The Effect on Nonalcoholic Fatty Liver Disease (NAFLD)

Intermittent fasting has been shown to be effective in reducing hepatic steatosis and improving liver function supporting its potential as a therapeutic strategy for managing nonalcoholic fatty liver disease (NAFLD). The reduction in caloric intake and the metabolic changes induced by fasting can help decrease liver fat accumulation and improve markers of liver function. Clinical studies suggest that intermittent fasting can reduce liver enzyme levels and improve liver histology in individuals with NAFLD [25–28]. See Chap. 8 for more details on fasting and liver disease.

2.4.4 The Effect on Inflammation and Oxidative Stress

Intermittent fasting reduces inflammation markers and oxidative stress. Studies on intermittent fasting showed a significant reduction in inflammation markers, including C-reactive protein (CRP) [14, 29, 30] and oxidative stress [18], which are linked to an increased risk of many chronic diseases. Fasting can help mitigate the inflammatory processes that contribute to conditions like cardiovascular disease, diabetes, and cancer [31].

2.4.5 Intermittent Fasting and Cancer

Intermittent fasting (IF) has garnered increasing attention for its potential role in cancer prevention. Multiple studies suggest that IF can influence cancer risk factors such as insulin sensitivity, oxidative stress, and inflammation [32]. A study found that a 5:2 fasting regimen improved metabolic markers linked to cancer risk in obese women [6]. However, further research is required to determine the long-term effects of IF on cancer development and progression.

2.4.5.1 The Mechanisms of Intermittent Fasting in Cancer

The anticancer effects of IF can be attributed to various biological mechanisms. IF has been shown to induce a metabolic shift from glucose to ketone bodies, potentially hindering cancer cell growth by reducing their energy sources [33]. IF may stimulate autophagy, a process that removes dysfunctional cells, maintains cellular balance, and prevents tumor growth [34]. Additionally, IF can modulate the immune system, enhancing the body's ability to detect and destroy cancer cells. It may also improve the efficacy of chemotherapy and radiotherapy by increasing cancer cell sensitivity to treatments while protecting healthy cells [35].

2.4.5.2 Fasting as a Potential Cancer Treatment

Prolonged fasting periods have been explored as a supplementary approach to traditional cancer treatments. Preclinical studies indicate that short-term fasting cycles can protect healthy cells from chemotherapy's adverse effects while making cancer cells more susceptible to treatment [36]. A preliminary human study found that fasting before chemotherapy reduced the side effects of treatment and improved the overall well-being of breast cancer patients. However, larger, well-designed studies are still needed to confirm these benefits and develop standardized fasting protocols for clinical use [37].

2.4.5.3 Impact of Prolonged Fasting and Fasting-Mimicking Diet on Cancer Treatment Toxicities in Humans

Prolonged fasting periods and fasting-mimicking diets (FMDs), which provide essential nutrients while promoting beneficial metabolic changes, have shown promise in reducing the toxic effects of cancer therapies. Preclinical studies indicate that FMD may enhance chemotherapy efficacy in preclinical models by limiting glucose availability to cancer cells, thereby inhibiting their growth [38]. A clinical trial in patients undergoing chemotherapy reduced treatment-related toxicities and improved tumor response rate [39]. These findings suggest that dietary interventions such as FMD could improve the tolerability and effectiveness of cancer treatments.

References

1. Catenacci VA, et al. A randomized pilot study comparing zero-calorie alternate-day fasting to daily caloric restriction in adults with obesity. Obesity. 2016;24(9):1874–83.
2. Wilkinson MJ, et al. Ten-hour time-restricted eating reduces weight, blood pressure, and atherogenic lipids in patients with metabolic syndrome. Cell Metab. 2020;31(1):92–104.e5.
3. Gabel K, et al. Effect of time-restricted feeding on the gut microbiome in adults with obesity: a pilot study. Nutr Health. 2020;26(2):79–85.
4. Carter S, Clifton P, Keogh J. The effects of intermittent compared to continuous energy restriction on glycaemic control in type 2 diabetes; a pragmatic pilot trial. Diabetes Res Clin Pract. 2016;122:106–12.
5. Schübel R, et al. Effects of intermittent and continuous calorie restriction on body weight and metabolism over 50 wk: a randomized controlled trial. Am J Clin Nutr. 2018;108(5):933–45.
6. Harvie MN, et al. The effects of intermittent or continuous energy restriction on weight loss and metabolic disease risk markers: a randomized trial in young overweight women. Int J Obes. 2011;35(5):714.
7. Kahleova H, et al. Eating two larger meals a day (breakfast and lunch) is more effective than six smaller meals in a reduced-energy regimen for patients with type 2 diabetes: a randomized crossover study. Diabetologia. 2014;57:1552–60.

8. McAllister MJ, et al. Time-restricted feeding improves markers of cardiometabolic health in physically active college-age men: a 4-week randomized pre-post pilot study. Nutr Res. 2020;75:32–43.
9. Hua C, et al. Intermittent fasting in weight loss and cardiometabolic risk reduction: a randomized controlled trial. J Nurs Res. 2022;30(1):e185.
10. Antoni R, et al. Intermittent v. continuous energy restriction: differential effects on postprandial glucose and lipid metabolism following matched weight loss in overweight/obese participants. Br J Nutr. 2018;119(5):507–16.
11. Bhutani S, et al. Alternate day fasting and endurance exercise combine to reduce body weight and favorably alter plasma lipids in obese humans. Obesity. 2013;21(7):1370–9.
12. Carter S, Clifton PM, Keogh JB. Effect of intermittent compared with continuous energy-restricted diet on glycemic control in patients with type 2 diabetes: a randomized noninferiority trial. JAMA Netw Open. 2018;1(3):e180756.
13. Gabel K, et al. Effects of 8-hour time restricted feeding on body weight and metabolic disease risk factors in obese adults: a pilot study. Nutr Healthy Aging. 2018;4(4):345–53.
14. Varady KA, et al. Alternate day fasting for weight loss in normal weight and overweight subjects: a randomized controlled trial. Nutr J. 2013;12:1–8.
15. Kunduraci YE, Ozbek H. Does the energy restriction intermittent fasting diet alleviate metabolic syndrome biomarkers? A randomized controlled trial. Nutrients. 2020;12(10):3213.
16. Gu L, et al. Effects of intermittent fasting in humans compared to a non-intervention diet and caloric restriction: a meta-analysis of randomized controlled trials. Front Nutr. 2022;9:871682.
17. Li C, et al. Eight-hour time-restricted feeding improves endocrine and metabolic profiles in women with anovulatory polycystic ovary syndrome. J Transl Med. 2021;19:1–9.
18. Cienfuegos S, et al. Effects of 4-and 6-h time-restricted feeding on weight and cardiometabolic health: a randomized controlled trial in adults with obesity. Cell Metab. 2020;32(3):366–78.e3.
19. Kalam F, et al. Alternate day fasting combined with a low-carbohydrate diet for weight loss, weight maintenance, and metabolic disease risk reduction. Obes Sci Pract. 2019;5(6):531–9.
20. Moro T, et al. Time-restricted eating effects on performance, immune function, and body composition in elite cyclists: a randomized controlled trial. J Int Soc Sports Nutr. 2020;17:1–11.
21. Moro T, et al. Effects of eight weeks of time-restricted feeding (16/8) on basal metabolism, maximal strength, body composition, inflammation, and cardiovascular risk factors in resistance-trained males. J Transl Med. 2016;14:1–10.
22. Hutchison AT, et al. Time-restricted feeding improves glucose tolerance in men at risk for type 2 diabetes: a randomized crossover trial. Obesity. 2019;27(5):724–32.
23. Pureza IROM, et al. Effect of early time-restricted feeding on the metabolic profile of adults with excess weight: a systematic review with meta-analysis. Clin Nutr. 2021;40(4):1788–99.
24. Sutton EF, et al. Early time-restricted feeding improves insulin sensitivity, blood pressure, and oxidative stress even without weight loss in men with prediabetes. Cell Metab. 2018;27(6):1212–21.e3.
25. Milgrom Y, et al. Ten-hour intermittent fasting plus mediterranean diet versus mediterranean diet alone for treatment of nonalcoholic fatty liver disease (NAFLD). Harefuah. 2024;163(2):93–6.
26. Ezpeleta M, et al. Effect of alternate day fasting combined with aerobic exercise on non-alcoholic fatty liver disease: a randomized controlled trial. Cell Metab. 2023;35(1):56–70.e3.
27. Feehan J, et al. Time-restricted fasting improves liver steatosis in non-alcoholic fatty liver disease—a single blinded crossover trial. Nutrients. 2023;15(23):4870.
28. Kord-Varkaneh H, et al. Effects of time-restricted feeding (16/8) combined with a low-sugar diet on the management of non-alcoholic fatty liver disease: a randomized controlled trial. Nutrition. 2023;105:111847.
29. Razavi R, et al. The alternate-day fasting diet is a more effective approach than a calorie restriction diet on weight loss and hs-CRP levels. Int J Vitam Nutr Res. 2020;91(3-4):242–50.

30. Bowen J, et al. Randomized trial of a high protein, partial meal replacement program with or without alternate day fasting: similar effects on weight loss, retention status, nutritional, metabolic, and behavioral outcomes. Nutrients. 2018;10(9):1145.
31. Kalam F, et al. Intermittent fasting interventions to leverage metabolic and circadian mechanisms for cancer treatment and supportive care outcomes. JNCI Monogr. 2023;2023(61):84–103.
32. Harvie M, Howell A. Energy restriction and the prevention of breast cancer. Proc Nutr Soc. 2012;71(2):263–75.
33. Longo VD, Mattson MP. Fasting: molecular mechanisms and clinical applications. Cell Metab. 2014;19(2):181–92.
34. Shabkhizan R, Haiaty S, Moslehian MS, Bazmani A, Sadeghsoltani F, Bagheri HS, et al. The beneficial and adverse effects of autophagic response to caloric restriction and fasting. Adv Nutr. 2023;14(5):1211–25.
35. Lee C, Raffaghello L, Brandhorst S, Safdie FM, Bianchi G, Martin-Montalvo A, et al. Fasting cycles retard growth of tumors and sensitize a range of cancer cell types to chemotherapy. Sci Transl Med. 2012;4(124):124ra27.
36. Raffaghello L, Lee C, Safdie FM, Wei M, Madia F, Bianchi G, Longo VD. Starvation-dependent differential stress resistance protects normal but not cancer cells against high-dose chemotherapy. Proc Natl Acad Sci. 2008;105(24):8215–20.
37. de Groot S, Pijl H, van der Hoeven JJ, Kroep JR. Effects of short-term fasting on cancer treatment. J Exp Clin Cancer Res. 2019;38:1–14.
38. Cohen CW, Fontaine KR, Arend RC, Alvarez RD, Leath CA III, Huh WK, et al. A ketogenic diet reduces central obesity and serum insulin in women with ovarian or endometrial cancer. J Nutr. 2018;148(8):1253–60.
39. Dorff TB, Groshen S, Garcia A, Shah M, Tsao-Wei D, Pham H, et al. Safety and feasibility of fasting in combination with platinum-based chemotherapy. BMC Cancer. 2016;16:1–9.

Chapter 3
Methodological Challenges in Researching the Health Impacts of Ramadan Fasting

Ahmed S. BaHammam and MoezAlIslam E. Faris

Abstract Researching the health impacts of Ramadan fasting presents a complex challenge due to the unique and varied nature of the observance. This chapter addresses these complexities by critically examining the methodological difficulties inherent in studying Ramadan's health effects. Central to the discussion is the need for precise research methods that account for the cultural, geographical, and seasonal differences affecting fasting practices. The chapter points out the importance of understanding changes in dietary habits, sleep patterns, and physical activities during Ramadan and how fasting duration varies across different geographical locations. It also emphasizes the significance of ethical considerations, primarily cultural and religious sensitivity, in conducting this research. Strategies for selecting diverse participants, using control groups, and implementing comprehensive data collection methods are explored. The impact of these methodological approaches on the generalizability and reliability of research findings is a key focus. This chapter is a valuable guide for researchers engaged in Ramadan fasting studies. It offers insights that help understand its health implications more deeply and informs public health guidelines and clinical practices related to this culturally and religiously significant observance.

Keywords Fasting physiology · Research design · Circadian pattern · Behavioral adaptations · Mealtime

A. S. BaHammam (✉)
Department of Medicine, College of Medicine, University Sleep Disorders Center, King Saud University, Riyadh, Saudi Arabia

The Strategic Technologies Program of the National Plan for Sciences and Technology and Innovation in the Kingdom of Saudi Arabia (08-MED511-02), Riyadh, Saudi Arabia
e-mail: ashammam@ksu.edu.sa

M. E. Faris
Department of Clinical Nutrition and Dietetics, Faculty of Allied Medical Sciences, Applied Science Private University, Amman, Jordan

© The Author(s), under exclusive license to Springer Nature Singapore Pte Ltd. 2025
M. E. Faris et al. (eds.), *Health and Medical Aspects of Ramadan Intermittent Fasting*, https://doi.org/10.1007/978-981-96-6783-3_3

3.1   Introduction

Ramadan fasting, a globally observed principal Islamic ritual, has garnered increasing attention in health research due to its varied health benefits, including cardiometabolic improvements and psychological well-being [1–3]. However, the diverse and expanding literature on this subject presents unique methodological and interpretative challenges, especially given the profound cultural and lifestyle variations among Ramadan fasting observers. These changes, deeply rooted in culture, significantly impact health research, encompassing shifts in eating and sleep patterns, social behaviors, and spiritual practices [4].

Research has shown that fasting during Ramadan can influence physical activity levels [5, 6], sleep quantity and quality [7–11], and dietary habits and nutritional composition [12–14], all of which play critical roles in health outcomes. Additionally, the duration of fasting varies with geographical location, ranging from 10 to 21 h, and is influenced by seasonal changes due to the Islamic (Hijri) lunar calendar [4, 15–17]. These variations necessitate careful consideration in research design to ensure accurate and generalizable findings.

This chapter outlines the methodological challenges and considerations for conducting effective and culturally sensitive health research during Ramadan. It provides an overview of the factors influencing health outcomes, including physical activity, sleep patterns, dietary habits, and the impacts of geographical and seasonal variations. The goal is to guide researchers in designing studies that reflect the unique aspects of Ramadan fasting, thereby enhancing the validity and generalizability of their findings.

3.2   Common Methodological Pitfalls in Ramadan Fasting Research

3.2.1   Sleep Duration and Timing

Ramadan fasting, observed in the ninth month of the Islamic calendar, is uniquely influenced by its lunar basis, leading to a yearly shift in timing. This shift, typically moving the month by about 11 days earlier in the Gregorian calendar each year, results in Ramadan occurring in different seasons approximately every 9 years. Consequently, the duration of daily fasts varies—they extend in the summer with longer days (reaching 17–19 h) and shorten in the winter (about 12 h). These changes directly affect sleep patterns; for example, shorter nights and earlier summer dawn disrupt normal sleep cycles and affect the nighttime allowed for eating, thus impacting the food quantity consumed and the subsequent body weight change. Additionally, geographical factors like latitude influence fasting durations, longer in summer and shorter in winter, particularly away from the equator. This leads to variations in day length and environmental conditions, affecting not only the fasting hours but also sleep duration and patterns [8, 11, 15, 18] and food quantity and quality consumed during the night hours and, hence, the consequent health implications [17]. In hotter months, the tendency to take midday naps due to extended fasting hours can further impact nighttime sleep, demonstrating the intricate relationship between fasting practices and circadian rhythms.

Fasting duration or time length is pivotal in moderating the different dietary and lifestyle changes accompanying Ramadan fasting and, hence, the health consequences of fasting. Faris et al. [17] developed an easy way to estimate the fasting duration using reference websites that provide sunrise and sunset times for any city or location, with the addition of 80 min on average to correct for the abstinence time between the dawn and the sunrise time points for the corresponding lunar days. This average fasting time duration per day showed a profound effect as a main moderator in explaining the resulting changes in metabolic syndrome components among people observing Ramadan fasting, especially fasting glucose and triglycerides [17]. Further, fasting duration is a main moderator in shaping the effect of ramadan fasting (RF) on body weight changes, with longer fasting duration during Ramadan related to a more substantial reduction in body weight at the end of Ramadan [19]. Last, in a most recent and most comprehensive meta-analysis on the cardiometabolic risk factors, using 91 studies comprising 4431 adults aged 18–85 years, fasting duration was the only significant moderator for the high-density lipoprotein cholesterol (HDL-C) ($P = 0.001$) change at the end of Ramadan. The longer the duration, the more the increase in the HDL-C observed [20].

Furthermore, lifestyle modifications during Ramadan often include heightened nighttime activities, such as religious observances, social gatherings, and entertainment, which lead to a delay in bedtime and reduced sleep duration [11, 13, 15, 21]. Insufficient sleep or inconsistent sleep patterns are linked to higher rates of illness and morbidity [22–24]. For example, a lack of sleep or reduced sleep duration is associated with an elevated risk of heart disease [25], stroke [26], type 2 diabetes [27], hyperlipidemia [28], hypertension [29], cancer [30], systemic inflammation [31], and obesity [32, 33]. Consequently, insufficient sleep during Ramadan may counteract the beneficial effects of fasting and compromise the measured health biomarkers. A lack of adequate nocturnal sleep over the 30 days of Ramadan could confound the potential positive effects of fasting on various health parameters. Typically, fasting observers are expected to rise around dawn for the predawn meal, *Suhoor*, a practice believed to promote early waking and sleeping [15]. However, real-world observations indicate a tendency toward later bedtimes and shorter sleep durations during Ramadan. Several studies have consistently observed a notable shift to later bedtimes and wake times during Ramadan [7, 34–36]. This shift in sleep patterns is not limited to Muslims; non-Muslim residents in Saudi Arabia also experience delayed bedtimes during Ramadan, indicating that these changes are linked to the lifestyle alteration characteristic of this period [36]. Additionally, there is a documented decrease in nighttime sleep duration during Ramadan [7]. A comprehensive meta-analysis encompassing 24 studies highlighted an average reduction of 1 h in total sleep time, with adolescents experiencing the most significant decrease.

This variability in sleep patterns and duration requires careful consideration in study design to ensure that findings are representative, applicable, and minimally affected by changes in sleep.

3.2.2 Circadian Rhythm

Central and peripheral biological clocks regulate body functions following a circadian rhythm, and their desynchrony can lead to various health problems, including cardiometabolic dysfunctions [37]. While the central biological clock is controlled mainly by light exposure, peripheral clocks are affected by mealtimes [37]. Studies have demonstrated that disruptions in circadian rhythm, especially when combined with altered mealtimes or sleep patterns, can significantly impact cardiometabolic health, increasing the risk of disorders like obesity, diabetes, and cardiovascular diseases [37].

During Ramadan fasting, mealtimes shift from day to night, raising questions about its impact on the body's circadian rhythm and, consequently, on health outcomes. Recent research indicates a close interaction between mealtimes and circadian rhythms, with eating during the night phase leading to a misalignment between the peripheral and central biological clocks, increasing the risk of cardiometabolic disorders [37]. A systematic review and meta-analysis (SRMA) of ten studies found that late meal timing adversely affects weight and metabolism [10]. Moreover, the practice of staying awake and eating at night, followed by daytime sleep, does not compensate for the loss of nocturnal sleep, as evidenced by the high incidence of "shift work disorder" among night shift workers, characterized by sleep disturbances and excessive sleepiness [11, 12].

A recent practice guideline statement for maintaining optimal health during Ramadan advises ensuring adequate nighttime sleep (4–6 h), supplemented by 1.5–2 h of daytime sleep, to preserve the circadian rhythm and sleep quality [21]. Additionally, it is recommended to confine eating during Ramadan to two primary meals at night—one at sunset and another before dawn—with an optional snack if necessary [21]. However, real-world studies indicate that some fasting individuals consume multiple meals at night, accompanied by shorter sleep durations and later bedtimes [8, 13, 38]. Theoretically, these lifestyle changes could disrupt the circadian rhythm and negate the potential health benefits of Ramadan fasting.

Research on circadian rhythms during Ramadan can be divided into two main categories. The first encompasses studies conducted in noncontrolled, free-living environments, which identified significant delays in bedtime and waking times and the delayed peak of melatonin levels [35, 39]. The second category, comprising more recent controlled studies, accounted for variables such as sleep schedules, light exposure, and meal timings and observed no changes in circadian rhythms [8].

Research designs must consider these factors thoroughly in light of the complex relationship between meal timing, sleep patterns, and circadian rhythm, particularly during Ramadan fasting. This approach is essential to evaluate the health impacts of fasting during Ramadan accurately. Understanding the intricate interplay between these elements will clarify the potential health effects of Ramadan fasting and inform guidelines to mitigate risks associated with circadian rhythm disruptions, especially in altered meal and sleep schedules.

3.2.3 Dietary Modifications During Ramadan

Understanding the nuances of dietary changes during Ramadan is pivotal for accurate health impact research. Globally, studies consistently reveal substantial shifts in dietary habits throughout Ramadan. For example, research in Nigeria highlighted an uptick in fruit and vegetable consumption and a decline in sugary drinks, correlating with weight loss and enhanced health [40]. In Saudi Arabia, Alzhrani et al. observed increased calorie and carbohydrate intake during Ramadan, coupled with sleep pattern and chronotype shifts and minor weight reduction [13]. This underscores the intricate link between diet, sleep, and weight during Ramadan [38]. Additionally, Shatila et al., in Lebanon, reported substantial dietary intake variations during Ramadan, necessitating tailored dietary guidelines that reflect these unique patterns [12].

A recent meta-analysis of 85 studies encompassing 4594 fasting participants examining the total calorie and macronutrient (carbohydrates, protein, fats, fibers, and water) intakes upon Ramadan fasting suggests variable changes in these dietary components, with high heterogeneity reported among the recruited studies [14]. The study showed significant reductions in energy, carbohydrate, and protein intakes during Ramadan. Further, age was one of the considerable moderators for the intake of the six dietary components, while physical activity was the main moderator for water intake during Ramadan. The remarkable rising role of age and physical activity in this study necessitates considering these two variables in designing and executing Ramadan fasting research.

Another important variable that should be considered in assessing changes in dietary intakes upon Ramadan fasting is the dietary assessment tool. While different assessment tools have been utilized, such as three-day 24-food recall, food record, and food frequency questionnaire (FFQ), various tools have been shown to elicit differences in the total macro- and micronutrient intake during Ramadan. Relying on less memory-based techniques in assessing the nutritional composition and dietary intake of fasting people would result in a more accurate estimate and, hence, in drawing a more precise picture concerning the effect of dietary intakes on the health outcomes of fasting. This is more emphasized in the recent meta-analysis on macronutrient and caloric intakes for fasting people, where different assessment tools showed various levels of total calories, carbohydrates, and water intake [14].

These findings highlight the critical need to account for dietary modifications in research methodologies assessing Ramadan fasting's health effects [9, 41]. They illustrate the complex interplay among diet, sleep, and health, which is essential for understanding the true impact of Ramadan fasting on health outcomes.

3.2.4   Physical Activity Variations During Ramadan

Addressing changes in physical activity during Ramadan is fundamental for designing and interpreting health-related studies. Research consistently indicates significant variations in physical activity patterns during Ramadan, which may impact the health outcomes of those who observe fasting. Farooq et al. observed a marked decrease in daily physical activity among fasting Muslims, contrasting with increased activity in non-fasting individuals, underscoring the importance of considering these changes in health impact assessments of Ramadan fasting [5]. Similarly, another study found a high prevalence of low physical activity and reduced sleep durations in individuals with type 2 diabetes during Ramadan [42]. Supporting these findings, our research demonstrates that energy expenditure and metabolic equivalent of tasks (METs) significantly decrease during Ramadan, accompanied by shifts in the circadian pattern of body temperature and delays in the acrophase of energy expenditure [43].

In contrast, Alotaibi et al. associated Ramadan diurnal intermittent fasting with a healthier lifestyle, including increased physical activity and adherence to a Mediterranean diet [44]. These results highlight the need for health studies on Ramadan fasting to account for physical activity changes, as these variations can profoundly affect the health outcomes of fasting observants [41]. Hence, integrating these factors into the study design and analysis is vital to accurately evaluating the health impacts of fasting during Ramadan.

3.2.5   Medication Management During Ramadan

Ramadan diurnal fasting is distinct from time-restricted eating, primarily because, during Ramadan, observers are not allowed to take oral medications during the fasting hours [45]. This unique aspect introduces significant methodological challenges in researching the health impacts of Ramadan fasting. The necessity for Muslims to adjust medication schedules during fasting, often opting for long-acting formulations or altering dosing times to non-fasting hours, might influence health outcomes [46, 47]. There is a lack of high-quality research on medication use and dosing during Ramadan, with most studies being retrospective and observational, with small sample sizes [47]. A notable research pitfall is the current lack of specific data on how these changes in medication timing affect health outcomes, particularly for chronic conditions like cardiovascular diseases, where medication adherence is crucial [47]. The arbitrary alteration in medication intake without proper guidance can affect the pharmacokinetics and pharmacodynamics of drugs, thus influencing their efficacy and safety [47]. Therefore, there is an urgent need to develop well-defined guidelines for adjusting or switching medications to maintain effectiveness and safety during fasting [47]. Researchers must account for these factors when designing studies to accurately attribute health outcomes to fasting practices rather than medication mismanagement. This necessitates a thorough understanding of the adjustments in dose, timing, or medication type during Ramadan and their direct impact on health outcomes. Addressing these challenges in future research will provide a more accurate understanding of the effects of fasting during Ramadan on health, filling a significant gap in the current literature.

3.2.6 Participant Diversity

The wide-ranging observance of Ramadan across various cultural, ethnic, and socioeconomic groups demands a research approach incorporating a diverse participant pool. This is fundamental for ensuring that the findings are unbiased and representative and for understanding the differential impacts of fasting. Diverse participant inclusion is necessary when considering geographical, seasonal, and cultural variations. Such variability necessitates research that captures a wide range of fasting experiences across different regions.

Furthermore, lifestyle changes during Ramadan, such as altered work and school schedules, increased nocturnal activities, and variations in social and religious practices, can influence individuals' health and well-being. These factors can vary significantly among socioeconomic groups, underscoring the importance of including diverse participants to capture the full spectrum of Ramadan experiences [15].

Therefore, studies with a large sample of a diverse participant pool are essential to understanding the health implications of fasting during Ramadan. This approach ensures more accurate, representative, and generalizable findings, providing a holistic view of the impact of Ramadan fasting on health across the globe.

3.2.7 Control Groups and Comparisons

In Ramadan fasting research, the prevalent use of observational studies brings inherent weaknesses that affect their validity and reliability. These studies often lack stringent control over various variables, complicating the task of isolating the specific effects of fasting from other factors, such as lifestyle changes, cultural practices, or environmental conditions. The concurrent changes in sleep patterns, physical activity, and diet during Ramadan further blur the distinction, making it challenging to attribute any observed changes solely to fasting. Moreover, observational studies are susceptible to biases, such as selection bias, where the study population might not accurately represent the general fasting community, and recall bias, which is particularly relevant in dietary studies. This leads to potential inaccuracies in data interpretation, and such studies cannot conclusively establish causality, only suggesting associations between Ramadan fasting and specific health outcomes.

While repeated measures for the same group do not equate to having a control group, the pre–post design for the same cohort may be the most suitable approach, given the practical constraints. Recruiting a non-fasting control group from the same ethnic background during Ramadan can be difficult in most Muslim countries. Moreover, including a non-fasting control group from a different ethnicity may lead to inaccurate results, particularly when studying metabolic and physiological health outcomes, due to potential confounding factors.

In contrast, controlled studies employing well-designed control groups are fundamental in accurately determining the effects of fasting. As highlighted in nutrition education intervention research, well-designed trials with control or comparison groups are essential for assessing the efficacy and effectiveness of interventions, including those in Ramadan fasting studies [48]. These control groups act as a necessary benchmark, enabling researchers to differentiate the specific impacts of fasting from other confounding factors like seasonal changes, dietary habits, or lifestyle modifications often associated with Ramadan. This approach, imperative for attributing changes to the intervention itself, has been historically underemphasized in research literature but is critical to enhancing study validity.

Control groups are vital for several reasons:

1. *Isolating the Effect of Fasting:* They allow for the isolation of fasting effects from other confounding variables.
2. *Accounting for Seasonal Variations:* Control groups fasting outside Ramadan or not fasting provide a baseline for understanding these seasonal effects on health outcomes [41, 49].
3. *Understanding Dietary and Lifestyle Changes:* Control groups help differentiate the effects of dietary and lifestyle changes from fasting, such as nocturnal eating and reduced physical activity during Ramadan, which might independently affect health.
4. *Enhancing Study Validity:* Including control groups enhances the study's overall validity, ensuring that the effects observed can be confidently attributed to fasting rather than other factors.
5. *Facilitating Comparative Analysis:* They provide a standard for comparison, enabling a more meaningful analysis of the specific impacts of Ramadan fasting.

Given these factors, while observational studies offer valuable data in natural settings, their limitations highlight the need for more rigorous, controlled experimental research for a deeper and more accurate understanding of the health impacts of Ramadan fasting. Addressing these methodological challenges is essential to advancing the field and providing reliable, evidence-based recommendations for health professionals and individuals observing Ramadan fasting.

3.2.8 Self-Reporting and Measurement Bias

In dietary research, particularly studies focusing on Ramadan fasting, the reliance on self-reporting for data collection is prevalent. However, this method is susceptible to various biases and inaccuracies, which can significantly impact the validity of the research findings. The challenges associated with self-reporting in dietary studies, especially during Ramadan, can be categorized and addressed as follows:

1. *Recall Bias:* This occurs when participants fail to remember their dietary habits accurately. The unique eating patterns during Ramadan, characterized by significant alterations, exacerbate this issue, leading to potential underreporting or excessive food intake [50].
2. *Social Desirability Bias:* Participants may report dietary intake that they perceive as socially acceptable or desirable rather than their actual consumption. This bias is particularly pertinent during Ramadan, when fasting holds religious and cultural importance, potentially influencing participants' reporting [51].
3. *Altered Perception of Hunger and Satiety:* The changes in hunger and satiety perception during Ramadan fasting can influence how participants perceive and report their food intake. The fasting process may alter an individual's perception of consumption during non-fasting hours [52].

Suggested strategies to address these include:

1. *Food Diaries:* Encouraging participants to maintain detailed food diaries can yield more accurate information about dietary intake. The effectiveness of this method hinges on the participants' commitment to accuracy and honesty in recording their intake [53].
2. *Digital Tracking Applications:* The advent of digital technology has introduced tracking tools that aid in more precise and convenient recording of food intake. These applications can enhance the accuracy of self-reported data [54].
3. *Cross-Verification with Biomarkers:* Utilizing biomarkers offers an objective approach to measuring dietary intake. For example, blood tests can indicate nutrient levels that correlate with food consumption, thereby providing a means to validate self-reported data [55].
4. *Combining Multiple Methods:* Employing a multifaceted approach that integrates self-reported data, food diaries, digital tracking, and biomarkers can offer a more comprehensive and accurate assessment of dietary intake [56].

While self-reporting is a fundamental method in dietary studies, including those on Ramadan fasting, it is not without biases, such as recall bias, social desirability bias, and altered perceptions of hunger and satiety. Employing a combination of methods, including food diaries, digital tracking applications, and biomarkers, along with cross-verifying self-reported data, can significantly enhance the accuracy and reliability of these studies.

3.2.9   Timing and Sample Collection in Ramadan Health Research

Several studies that assessed hormonal or health biomarker changes during Ramadan used a single daily sample to determine the impact of Ramadan fasting. In the context of health research during Ramadan, measuring specific health parameters or biomarkers once daily presents significant methodological pitfalls, mainly due to neglecting circadian rhythms and their potential alteration [4, 57]. Several hormones and biomarkers are known to follow circadian rhythms, and these rhythms can be significantly impacted by changes in sleep patterns and eating schedules, which are common during Ramadan [4, 57]. For instance, cortisol levels, which typically peak in the morning, may exhibit altered secretion patterns due to changes in sleep–wake cycles during Ramadan [58]. Similarly, the melatonin hormone has been shown to present a shift delay when studied in the free-living environment during Ramadan [39, 59]. Likewise, the timing of food intake, which is drastically altered during Ramadan, can influence the diurnal variation of blood glucose levels, lipid profiles, and other metabolic markers [60]. Neglecting these factors can lead to misinterpretation of data, as the biomarker levels may not solely reflect the impact of fasting but also the changes in circadian rhythms and meal timings [9, 41, 61, 62]. Therefore, to accurately assess the impact of Ramadan fasting on health parameters, it is crucial to document the timing of the last meal, consider multiple daily measurements, and possibly consider a cosinor analysis, which is a method used to examine cyclical data, such as biomarkers showing circadian rhythm changes [43]. This approach would provide a more comprehensive understanding of the physiological changes occurring during Ramadan and their implications for health and disease.

Fixing the time point of blood sampling before and during Ramadan is crucial in eliminating the effect of timing on the targeted biomarkers. This is confirmed by ensuring that blood samples are collected after 8–12 h of complete fasting for the two time points (before and after). This dictates having clear information about the last meal during the eating night hours of Ramadan and asking the recruited patient/subject to visit the clinic for blood sampling directly after this minimum interval.

3.2.10   Physiological Adaptations and Methodological Considerations in Ramadan Fasting Research

In the context of Ramadan and health research, the duration of the fasting period, which spans an entire month, introduces a significant methodological consideration: the potential for physiological adaptation. Research indicates that the body may adapt to the fasting and altered eating patterns over the course of the month, leading to different physiological responses at the beginning compared to the end of Ramadan [63]. This phenomenon necessitates a careful approach to study design, as experiments conducted at the beginning of Ramadan might yield different results from those performed at the end of the month.

Additionally, some studies have shown that bedtime and rise time get delayed in some cultures as Ramadan progresses [7, 34–36, 43]. Our team's work assessing hormones and several biomarkers during Ramadan under controlled conditions has demonstrated the potential for physiological adaptation over fasting [9, 41, 62, 64]. These studies show that various physiological parameters, including hormonal levels, inflammation markers, and oxidative stress indicators, can change in response to fasting itself and as part of an adaptive process over the weeks of Ramadan. This suggests that the body gradually adjusts to the altered eating and sleeping patterns during the fasting month, leading to different physiological states at the beginning, middle, and end of Ramadan. These potential adaptations could influence a wide range of health parameters, including metabolic markers, physical endurance, and cognitive function, potentially leading to varying results, depending on the timing of the experiment within the month of Ramadan. This underscores the importance of considering these adaptive changes in health research related to Ramadan fasting, as they can significantly influence study outcomes and interpretations.

3.3 Challenges and Considerations in Systematic Reviews for Ramadan Health Research

Systematic reviews and meta-analyses (SRMAs) in Ramadan health research are essential for deriving evidence-based conclusions. However, the high heterogeneity of the retrieved studies, secondary to the inherent diversity in cultural and lifestyle practices associated with Ramadan fasting, introduces unique challenges. First, the global heterogeneity in Ramadan observance results in a wide range of study designs and outcomes, complicating the process of aggregating and analyzing data in SRMAs due to the difficulty in comparing and synthesizing findings from studies with varied methodologies. Second, accurately interpreting data from diverse cultural contexts is essential. SRMAs must consider these variations to prevent misinterpretation or overgeneralization, often requiring a detailed examination of each study's cultural background and, possibly, subgroup analyses. Third, the diverse experiences of participants from different backgrounds can lead to varied health outcomes, impacting data interpretation and SRMA conclusions' generalizability. Fourth, assessing the methodological quality of studies becomes more complex in the context of cultural diversity, as SRMAs need to consider how cultural factors might influence study quality and potential biases. Finally, SRMAs can offer valuable recommendations for future research, identifying gaps in the current literature, particularly regarding cultural and lifestyle variations, and suggesting areas for further investigation.

Subgroup analyses, as part of conducting SRMAs, are essential in elaborating on the effect of different moderators mediating RF's impact on variable health outcomes. Age, sex, health/disease condition of the fasting participants, and fasting duration and seasons are essential moderators that help improve our understanding of the effect of different inherent variables that shape the fasting health outcomes [14, 17, 19, 20, 65]. In summary, while SRMAs are indispensable in Ramadan health research, navigating the challenges posed by methodological diversity and cultural variations is crucial. Careful consideration of these factors is essential to ensure that reviews are comprehensive, accurate, and relevant to diverse populations.

3.4 Enhancing Research Methodologies in Ramadan Health Research

The advancement of research methodologies in Ramadan fasting studies is pivotal for a deeper understanding of its health impacts [66]. While specific studies on this topic are scarce, applying general research principles can significantly elevate the quality of such research.

1. *Diverse Participant Selection:* It is imperative to include a broad spectrum of participants, encompassing various ethnicities, geographical locations, and socioeconomic and cultural backgrounds. This inclusivity is essential for generalizing findings across the global Muslim community, which is disseminated worldwide across continents and countries.
2. *Longitudinal Study Design:* Implementing longitudinal studies will provide valuable insights into the long-term health effects of Ramadan fasting, offering a more comprehensive understanding of its impacts over time, even after the end of Ramadan.
3. *Interdisciplinary Collaboration:* A collaborative approach involving experts from nutrition, medicine, psychology, and sociology is essential for a holistic understanding of Ramadan fasting's multifaceted impacts.
4. *Standardization of Research Tools:* Employing standardized and validated measurement tools and protocols is vital for ensuring data consistency and comparability across various studies, enhancing the reliability of research findings.

3.4.1 Leveraging Technological Innovations

Integrating modern technology can significantly enhance objective assessment, data accuracy, and analysis in Ramadan fasting research.

1. *Wearable Technology:* Utilizing wearable devices for real-time monitoring of physiological parameters like heart rate, sleep patterns, and physical activity can provide invaluable insights during Ramadan.
2. *Mobile Dietary Tracking, Physical Activity Tracking, and Sleep Monitoring Applications:* Mobile applications for tracking diet, physical activity, and sleep can facilitate more precise and comprehensive data collection, contributing to more accurate research outcomes.
3. *Advanced Data Analysis:* Implementing sophisticated data analytics, deep machine learning algorithms, and other AI techniques can reveal intricate patterns and deep correlations in large datasets, offering a deeper understanding of the data.

3.4.2   Ethical Considerations in Fasting Research

Maintaining high ethical standards is mandatory in fasting research to safeguard participants' well-being and uphold their dignity and autonomy.

1. *Cultural and Religious Sensitivity:* Researchers must be sensitive to Ramadan's cultural and religious aspects and ensure that all practices and beliefs are respected throughout the study.
2. *Participant Health and Safety:* The health and safety of participants, particularly those with preexisting conditions, such as diabetes, hypertension, or cardiovascular diseases, should be paramount. Provisions should be in place for participants to safely withdraw or break their fast if necessary.

Incorporating these guidelines and technological advancements will lead to more robust, accurate, and ethically sound Ramadan fasting studies. This comprehensive approach is essential for unraveling the complex interplay between fasting, health, and sociocultural dynamics.

3.5   Animal Models in Studying Health Impacts of Ramadan Fasting

Utilizing animal models, mainly rodents, in Ramadan fasting and health research offers a unique opportunity to explore the physiological and metabolic effects of fasting. We recently used rats to exemplify this approach [67]. Applying the Ramadan fasting model, rats were subjected to a fasting regime during the active phase that mimicked the human fasting schedule during Ramadan, followed by assessments of health parameters to evaluate the health impacts of the fasting model [67].

In designing such studies, researchers must consider several key factors:

1. *Animal Selection:* Rodents are a practical, feasible choice due to their metabolic and physiological similarities to humans. The specific health outcomes of interest can guide whether mice or rats are more suitable.
2. *Fasting Protocol:* It is crucial to adapt the fasting period to reflect the rodents' faster metabolism. Typically, a 12-hour fasting period for rodents mimics the longer fasting duration in humans.
3. *Dietary Control and Monitoring:* Standardizing the diet and closely monitoring food and water intake are essential to minimize variability and replicate the nutritional changes observed during Ramadan.
4. *Health Outcome Measurement:* To evaluate the effects of fasting, regular assessments of various health parameters, such as organ function, metabolic markers, and behavioral changes, are necessary.

5. *Chronobiological Aspects:* Considering rodents are nocturnal, aligning the fasting windows with their natural active and feeding periods is essential for the study's validity.
6. *Environmental Conditions:* Standardizing environmental factors, such as temperature and humidity, is crucial to minimize variability and ensure that the observed effects are primarily due to fasting. Maintaining consistent ecological conditions throughout the study helps control for potential confounding factors.
7. *Ethical Compliance:* Following ethical guidelines and ensuring animal welfare throughout the study are paramount.

As demonstrated in our study, this research approach provides valuable insights into the potential health benefits and mechanisms of Ramadan fasting [67]. However, it is important to acknowledge the limitations in directly translating findings from animal models to humans due to inherent physiological differences. Therefore, while animal models are a powerful tool in Ramadan fasting research, their results should be carefully interpreted and cautiously extrapolated to human health. Thus, human studies should complement the animal model of Ramadan fasting research to understand Ramadan fasting's health impacts comprehensively.

3.6 Conclusion

This chapter has provided an in-depth exploration of the various methodological challenges inherent in researching the health impacts of Ramadan fasting. It is evident that the unique nature of Ramadan, characterized by changes in dietary habits, sleep patterns, and physical activity, and its occurrence across different seasons and geographical locations present complex variables that must be methodically accounted for in research designs. The impact of fasting during Ramadan on health is many-sided, influencing physical, psychological, and metabolic outcomes. This complexity necessitates a detailed approach to research methodologies to ensure the accuracy and reliability of findings. Researchers must consider the cultural, geographical, and seasonal variations in fasting practices, alongside the physiological and psychological adaptations during Ramadan.

The chapter highlights the need for diverse participant selection, control groups, and comprehensive data collection methods, including technology in tracking physiological and dietary changes. These strategies are essential to overcome the methodological pitfalls discussed and enhance the research findings' validity and generalizability. Furthermore, ethical considerations, particularly cultural and religious sensitivity, are pivotal in conducting Ramadan fasting research. Ensuring participant safety and respecting their beliefs and practices are fundamental to obtaining meaningful and ethically sound results.

In conclusion, advancing research methodologies in Ramadan fasting studies is imperative for a deeper and more accurate understanding of its impacts on health. Addressing the methodological challenges outlined in this chapter is critical to generating robust research findings, which can inform public health guidelines and clinical practices related to Ramadan fasting. As the practice continues to gather global interest, continued efforts in refining research methodologies will undoubtedly contribute to a more comprehensive understanding of this significant cultural and religious observance and its implications for health and well-being.

References

1. Karasneh RA, Al-Azzam SI, Alzoubi KH, Hawamdeh SS, Sweileh WM. Global research trends of health-related publications on Ramadan fasting from 1999 to 2021: a bibliometric analysis. J Relig Health. 2022;61(5):3777–94. https://doi.org/10.1007/s10943-022-01573-x.
2. AbuShihab K, Obaideen K, Alameddine M, Alkurd RAF, Khraiwesh HM, Mohammad Y et al. Reflection on Ramadan fasting research related to sustainable development goal 3 (good health and well-being): a bibliometric analysis. J Relig Health. 2023. https://doi.org/10.1007/s10943-023-01955-9.
3. Obaideen K, Abu Shihab KH, Madkour MI, Faris ME. Seven decades of Ramadan intermittent fasting research: bibliometrics analysis, global trends, and future directions. Diabetes Metab Syndr Clin Res Rev. 2022;16(8):102566. https://doi.org/10.1016/j.dsx.2022.102566.
4. BaHammam AS, Almeneessier AS. Recent evidence on the impact of Ramadan diurnal intermittent fasting, mealtime, and circadian rhythm on cardiometabolic risk: a review. Front Nutr. 2020;7:28. https://doi.org/10.3389/fnut.2020.00028.
5. Farooq A, Chamari K, Sayegh S, El Akoum M, Al-Mohannadi AS. Ramadan daily intermittent fasting reduces objectively assessed habitual physical activity among adults. BMC Public Health. 2021;21(1):1912. https://doi.org/10.1186/s12889-021-11961-9.
6. Khan MAB, BaHammam AS, Amanatullah A, Obaideen K, Arora T, Ali H, et al. Examination of sleep in relation to dietary and lifestyle behaviors during Ramadan: a multi-national study using structural equation modeling among 24,500 adults amid COVID-19. Front Nutr. 2023;10:1040355. https://doi.org/10.3389/fnut.2023.1040355.
7. Bahammam AS, Alaseem AM, Alzakri AA, Sharif MM. The effects of Ramadan fasting on sleep patterns and daytime sleepiness: an objective assessment. J Res Med Sci. 2013;18(2):127–31.
8. Almeneessier AS, BaHammam AS. How does diurnal intermittent fasting impact sleep, daytime sleepiness, and markers of the biological clock? Current insights. Nat Sci Sleep. 2018;10:439–52. https://doi.org/10.2147/NSS.S165637.
9. Almeneessier AS, Bahammam AS, Sharif MM, Bahammam SA, Nashwan SZ, Pandi Perumal SR, et al. The influence of intermittent fasting on the circadian pattern of melatonin while controlling for caloric intake, energy expenditure, light exposure, and sleep schedules: a preliminary report. Ann Thorac Med. 2017;12(3):183–90. https://doi.org/10.4103/atm.ATM_15_17.
10. Bahammam AS, Almushailhi K, Pandi-Perumal SR, Sharif MM. Intermittent fasting during Ramadan: does it affect sleep? J Sleep Res. 2014;23(1):35–43. https://doi.org/10.1111/jsr.12076.
11. Faris MAE, Jahrami HA, Alhayki FA, Alkhawaja NA, Ali AM, Aljeeb SH, et al. Effect of diurnal fasting on sleep during Ramadan: a systematic review and meta-analysis. Sleep Breath. 2020;24(2):771–82. https://doi.org/10.1007/s11325-019-01986-1.
12. Shatila H, Baroudi M, El Sayed AR, Chehab R, Forman MR, Abbas N, et al. Impact of Ramadan fasting on dietary intakes among healthy adults: a year-round comparative study. Front Nutr. 2021;8:689788. https://doi.org/10.3389/fnut.2021.689788.

13. Alzhrani A, Alhussain MH, BaHammam AS. Changes in dietary intake, chronotype, and sleep pattern upon Ramadan among healthy adults in Jeddah, Saudi Arabia: a prospective study. Front Nutr. 2022;9:966861. https://doi.org/10.3389/fnut.2022.966861.

14. Abdelrahim DN, El Herrag SE, Khaled MB, Radwan H, Naja F, Alkurd R et al. Changes in energy and macronutrient intake during Ramadan fasting: a systematic review, meta-analysis, and meta-regression. Nutr Rev. 2023. https://doi.org/10.1093/nutrit/nuad141.

15. BaHammam AS, Alghannam AF, Aljaloud KS, Aljuraiban GS, AlMarzooqi MA, Dobia AM, et al. Joint consensus statement of the Saudi Public Health Authority on the recommended amount of physical activity, sedentary behavior, and sleep duration for healthy Saudis: background, methodology, and discussion. Ann Thorac Med. 2021;16(3):225–38. https://doi.org/10.4103/atm.atm_32_21.

16. Faris ME, Laher I, Khaled MB, Zouhal H. Editorial: the model of Ramadan diurnal intermittent fasting: unraveling the health implications, volume II. Front Nutr. 2023;10:1247771. https://doi.org/10.3389/fnut.2023.1247771.

17. Faris MA-IE, Jahrami HA, Alsibai J, Obaideen AA. Impact of Ramadan diurnal intermittent fasting on the metabolic syndrome components in healthy, non-athletic Muslim people aged over 15 years: a systematic review and meta-analysis. Br J Nutr. 2020;123(1):1–22. https://doi.org/10.1017/S000711451900254X.

18. Bahammam A. Does Ramadan fasting affect sleep? Int J Clin Pract. 2006;60(12):1631–7. https://doi.org/10.1111/j.1742-1241.2005.00811.x.

19. Jahrami HA, Alsibai J, Clark CCT, Faris MAE. A systematic review, meta-analysis, and meta-regression of the impact of diurnal intermittent fasting during Ramadan on body weight in healthy subjects aged 16 years and above. Eur J Nutr. 2020;59(6):2291–316. https://doi.org/10.1007/s00394-020-02216-1.

20. Jahrami HA, Faris ME, Janahi AI, Janahi MI, Abdelrahim DN, Madkour MI, et al. Does four-week consecutive, dawn-to-sunset intermittent fasting during Ramadan affect cardiometabolic risk factors in healthy adults? A systematic review, meta-analysis, and meta-regression. Nutr Metab Cardiovasc Dis. 2021;31(8):2273–301.

21. Alfawaz RA, Aljuraiban GS, AlMarzooqi MA, Alghannam AF, BaHammam AS, Dobia AM, et al. The recommended amount of physical activity, sedentary behavior, and sleep duration for healthy Saudis: a joint consensus statement of the Saudi Public Health Authority. Ann Thorac Med. 2021;16(3):239–44. https://doi.org/10.4103/atm.atm_33_21.

22. Consensus Conference P, Watson NF, Badr MS, Belenky G, Bliwise DL, Buxton OM, et al. Joint consensus statement of the American Academy of Sleep Medicine and Sleep Research Society on the recommended amount of sleep for a healthy adult: methodology and discussion. J Clin Sleep Med. 2015;11(8):931–52. https://doi.org/10.5664/jcsm.4950.

23. Cappuccio FP, D'Elia L, Strazzullo P, Miller MA. Sleep duration and all-cause mortality: a systematic review and meta-analysis of prospective studies. Sleep. 2010;33(5):585–92.

24. Aurora RN, Kim JS, Crainiceanu C, O'Hearn D, Punjabi NM. Habitual sleep duration and all-cause mortality in a general community sample. Sleep. 2016;39(11):1903–9. https://doi.org/10.5665/sleep.6212.

25. Liu Y, Wheaton AG, Chapman DP, Cunningham TJ, Lu H, Croft JB. Prevalence of healthy sleep duration among adults—United States, 2014. MMWR Morb Mortal Wkly Rep. 2016;65(6):137–41. https://doi.org/10.15585/mmwr.mm6506a1.

26. Li W, Wang D, Cao S, Yin X, Gong Y, Gan Y, et al. Sleep duration and risk of stroke events and stroke mortality: a systematic review and meta-analysis of prospective cohort studies. Int J Cardiol. 2016;223:870–6. https://doi.org/10.1016/j.ijcard.2016.08.302.

27. Zizi F, Pandey A, Murrray-Bachmann R, Vincent M, McFarlane S, Ogedegbe G, et al. Race/ethnicity, sleep duration, and diabetes mellitus: analysis of the National Health Interview Survey. Am J Med. 2012;125(2):162–7. https://doi.org/10.1016/j.amjmed.2011.08.020.

28. Zhan Y, Chen R, Yu J. Sleep duration and abnormal serum lipids: the China Health and Nutrition Survey. Sleep Med. 2014;15(7):833–9. https://doi.org/10.1016/j.sleep.2014.02.006.

29. Wang Y, Mei H, Jiang YR, Sun WQ, Song YJ, Liu SJ, et al. Relationship between duration of sleep and hypertension in adults: a meta-analysis. J Clin Sleep Med. 2015;11(9):1047–56. https://doi.org/10.5664/jcsm.5024.
30. Markt SC, Grotta A, Nyren O, Adami HO, Mucci LA, Valdimarsdottir UA, et al. Insufficient sleep and risk of prostate cancer in a large Swedish cohort. Sleep. 2015;38(9):1405–10. https://doi.org/10.5665/sleep.4978.
31. Irwin MR, Olmstead R, Carroll JE. Sleep disturbance, sleep duration, and inflammation: a systematic review and meta-analysis of cohort studies and experimental sleep deprivation. Biol Psychiatry. 2016;80(1):40–52. https://doi.org/10.1016/j.biopsych.2015.05.014.
32. Miller MA, Kruisbrink M, Wallace J, Ji C, Cappuccio FP. Sleep duration and incidence of obesity in infants, children, and adolescents: a systematic review and meta-analysis of prospective studies. Sleep. 2018;41(4). https://doi.org/10.1093/sleep/zsy018.
33. Magee L, Hale L. Longitudinal associations between sleep duration and subsequent weight gain: a systematic review. Sleep Med Rev. 2012;16(3):231–41. https://doi.org/10.1016/j.smrv.2011.05.005.
34. Bahammam. Sleep patterns, daytime sleepiness, and eating habits during the month of Ramadan. Sleep Hypnosis. 2003;5:165–74.
35. BaHammam A. Effect of fasting during Ramadan on sleep architecture, daytime sleepiness and sleep pattern. Sleep Biol Rhythm. 2004;2:135–43.
36. BaHammam A. Assessment of sleep patterns, daytime sleepiness, and chronotype during Ramadan in fasting and nonfasting individuals. Saudi Med J. 2005;26(4):616–22.
37. BaHammam AS, Pirzada A. Timing matters: the interplay between early mealtime, circadian rhythms, gene expression, circadian hormones, and metabolism—a narrative review. Clocks Sleep. 2023;5(3):507–35. https://doi.org/10.3390/clockssleep5030034.
38. Almeneessier AS, Pandi-Perumal SR, BaHammam AS. Intermittent fasting, insufficient sleep, and circadian rhythm: interaction and effects on the cardiometabolic system. Curr Sleep Med Rep. 2018;4(3):179–95. https://doi.org/10.1007/s40675-018-0124-5.
39. Bogdan A, Bouchareb B, Touitou Y. Ramadan fasting alters endocrine and neuroendocrine circadian patterns. Meal time as a synchronizer in humans? Life Sci. 2001;68(14):1607–15. https://doi.org/10.1016/s0024-3205(01)00966-3.
40. Sulaiman SK, Tsiga-Ahmed FI, Faris ME, Musa MS, Akpan UA-O, Umar AM, et al. Nigerian Muslim's perceptions of changes in diet, weight, and health status during Ramadan: a Nationwide cross-sectional study. Int J Environ Res Public Health. 2022;19(21):14340.
41. Almeneessier AS, BaHammam AA, Alzoghaibi M, Olaish AH, Nashwan SZ, BaHammam AS. The effects of diurnal intermittent fasting on proinflammatory cytokine levels while controlling for sleep/wake pattern, meal composition, and energy expenditure. PLoS One. 2019;14(12):e0226034. https://doi.org/10.1371/journal.pone.0226034.
42. Alghamdi AS, Alghamdi KA, Jenkins RO, Alghamdi MN, Haris PI. Impact of Ramadan on physical activity and sleeping patterns in individuals with type 2 diabetes: the first study using Fitbit device. Diabetes Ther. 2020;11(6):1331–46. https://doi.org/10.1007/s13300-020-00825-x.
43. BaHammam A, Alrajeh M, Albabtain M, Bahammam S, Sharif M. Circadian pattern of sleep, energy expenditure, and body temperature of young, healthy men during the intermittent fasting of Ramadan. Appetite. 2010;54(2):426–9. https://doi.org/10.1016/j.appet.2010.01.011.
44. Alotaibi MI, Elsamad G, Aljardahi AN, Alghamdi AN, Alotaibi AI, Alorabi HM, et al. Changes in dietary and lifestyle behaviors and mental stress among medical students upon Ramadan diurnal intermittent fasting: a prospective cohort study from Taif/Saudi Arabia. BMC Public Health. 2023;23(1):1462. https://doi.org/10.1186/s12889-023-16385-1.
45. Jaber D, Albsoul-Younes A, Wazaify M. Physicians' knowledge, attitude and practices regarding management of medications in Ramadan. East Mediterr Health J. 2014;20(1):56–62.
46. Grindrod K, Alsabbagh W. Managing medications during Ramadan fasting. Can Pharm J (Ott). 2017;150(3):146–9. https://doi.org/10.1177/1715163517700840.

47. Yousef Ahmed A, Sultan Mohammed A-J, Aljohara Abdullah A, Meshael Ibrahim A. Medication therapy during the holy month of Ramadan. Pharmacol Toxicol Biomed Rep. 2019;5(2):56–64.
48. Byrd-Bredbenner C, Wu F, Spaccarotella K, Quick V, Martin-Biggers J, Zhang Y. Systematic review of control groups in nutrition education intervention research. Int J Behav Nutr Phys Act. 2017;14(1):91. https://doi.org/10.1186/s12966-017-0546-3.
49. Almeneessier AS, BaHammam AA, Olaish AH, Pandi-Perumal SR, Manzar MD, BaHammam AS. Effects of diurnal intermittent fasting on daytime sleepiness reflected by EEG absolute power. J Clin Neurophysiol. 2019;36(3):213–9. https://doi.org/10.1097/WNP.0000000000000569.
50. Althubaiti A. Information bias in health research: definition, pitfalls, and adjustment methods. J Multidiscip Healthc. 2016;9:211–7. https://doi.org/10.2147/jmdh.S104807.
51. Hebert JR, Clemow L, Pbert L, Ockene IS, Ockene JK. Social desirability bias in dietary self-report may compromise the validity of dietary intake measures. Int J Epidemiol. 1995;24(2):389–98. https://doi.org/10.1093/ije/24.2.389.
52. Papies E, Stroebe W, Aarts H. Pleasure in the mind: restrained eating and spontaneous hedonic thoughts about food. J Exp Soc Psychol. 2007;43(5):810–7. https://doi.org/10.1016/j.jesp.2006.08.001.
53. Thompson FE, Subar AF. Dietary assessment methodology. In: Coulston AM, Boushey CJ, Ferruzzi MG, editors. Nutrition in the prevention and treatment of disease. Cambridge: Academic Press; 2013. p. 5–46.
54. Illner AK, Freisling H, Boeing H, Huybrechts I, Crispim SP, Slimani N. Review and evaluation of innovative technologies for measuring diet in nutritional epidemiology. Int J Epidemiol. 2012;41(4):1187–203. https://doi.org/10.1093/ije/dys105.
55. Freedman LS, Commins JM, Moler JE, Arab L, Baer DJ, Kipnis V, et al. Pooled results from 5 validation studies of dietary self-report instruments using recovery biomarkers for energy and protein intake. Am J Epidemiol. 2014;180(2):172–88. https://doi.org/10.1093/aje/kwu116.
56. Burrows TL, Martin RJ, Collins CE. A systematic review of the validity of dietary assessment methods in children when compared with the method of doubly labeled water. J Am Diet Assoc. 2010;110(10):1501–10. https://doi.org/10.1016/j.jada.2010.07.008.
57. Qasrawi SO, Pandi-Perumal SR, BaHammam AS. The effect of intermittent fasting during Ramadan on sleep, sleepiness, cognitive function, and circadian rhythm. Sleep Breath. 2017;21(3):577–86. https://doi.org/10.1007/s11325-017-1473-x.
58. Roky R, Iraki L, HajKhlifa R, Lakhdar Ghazal N, Hakkou F. Daytime alertness, mood, psychomotor performances, and oral temperature during Ramadan intermittent fasting. Ann Nutr Metab. 2000;44(3):101–7. https://doi.org/10.1159/000012830.
59. BaHammam A. Effect of fasting during Ramadan on sleep architecture, daytime sleepiness and sleep pattern. Sleep Biol Rhythms. 2004;2(2):135–43.
60. Lessan N, Ali T. Energy metabolism and intermittent fasting: the Ramadan perspective. Nutrients 2019;11(5). https://doi.org/10.3390/nu11051192.
61. Almeneessier AS, Alzoghaibi M, BaHammam AA, Ibrahim MG, Olaish AH, Nashwan SZ, et al. The effects of diurnal intermittent fasting on the wake-promoting neurotransmitter orexin-A. Ann Thorac Med. 2018;13(1):48–54. https://doi.org/10.4103/atm.ATM_181_17.
62. Alzoghaibi MA, Pandi-Perumal SR, Sharif MM, BaHammam AS. Diurnal intermittent fasting during Ramadan: the effects on leptin and ghrelin levels. PLoS One. 2014;9(3):e92214. https://doi.org/10.1371/journal.pone.0092214.
63. Leiper JB, Molla AM, Molla AM. Effects on health of fluid restriction during fasting in Ramadan. Eur J Clin Nutr. 2003;57(Suppl 2):S30–8. https://doi.org/10.1038/sj.ejcn.1601899.
64. BaHammam AS, Pandi-Perumal SR, Alzoghaibi MA. The effect of Ramadan intermittent fasting on lipid peroxidation in healthy young men while controlling for diet and sleep: a pilot study. Ann Thorac Med. 2016;11(1):43–8. https://doi.org/10.4103/1817-1737.172296.

65. Faris M, Jahrami H, Abdelrahim D, Bragazzi N, BaHammam A. The effects of Ramadan intermittent fasting on liver function in healthy adults: a systematic review, meta-analysis, and meta-regression. Diabetes Res Clin Pract. 2021;178:108951.
66. Shadman Z, Hedayati M, Larijani B, Akhoundan M, Khoshniat M. Recommended guideline for designing and interpreting of Ramadan fasting studies in medical research. J Nutr Fasting Health. 2015;3(4):156–65.
67. Alasmari AA, Al-Khalifah AS, BaHammam AS, Alshiban NMS, Almnaizel AT, Alodah HS, et al. Ramadan fasting model exerts hepatoprotective, anti-obesity, and anti-hyperlipidemic effects in an experimentally-induced nonalcoholic fatty liver in rats. Saudi J Gastroenterol. 2024;30(1):53–62. https://doi.org/10.4103/sjg.sjg_204_23.

Part II
Metabolic and Physiological Effects

Chapter 4
Ramadan Fasting and Energy Balance: Relevance to Weight Loss Strategies

Nader Lessan

Abstract Ramadan fasting (RF) is mandatory for all healthy adult Muslims and is practiced by Muslims globally once a year. Changes in sleeping patterns and circadian rhythms accompany the dawn-to-sunset abstention from all food and drink. There are also changes in food intake and appetite, with an increasing desire for food reaching a peak by iftar time; there are variable changes in weight, with an average weight loss of around 1–2 kg reported in various studies, including meta-analyses. There is, therefore, no doubt that energy balance is altered during Ramadan fasting. In effect, there is gradual glycogen depletion during the day, followed by replenishment in the evening. As the Ramadan fasting day progresses, there is a gradual shift in fuel utilization from carbohydrate to fat. Whether and how different components of energy expenditure (EE) change during Ramadan is a question of interest and has important implications. There is much inter-individual variability in changes in various aspects of energy metabolism in the context of Ramadan fasting. The handful of studies on energy expenditure during Ramadan fasting seem to point to overall insignificant changes to resting metabolic rate (RMR) and total energy expenditure (TEE). However, activity energy expenditure (AEE) is altered in timing and duration and is, on average, reduced. Sleeping pattern, time, and quality change with a net overall, mostly modest reduction in duration. To date, no direct studies of the thermic effect of food (TEF) have been performed during Ramadan fasting. This review examines the existing evidence on energy balance in the context of Ramadan and will discuss the possible implications not just for Ramadan but beyond.

Keywords Energy expenditure · Resting metabolic rate (RMR) · Total energy expenditure (TEE) · Activity energy expenditure (AEE) · Thermic effect of food (TEF) · Ramadan fasting

N. Lessan (✉)
Imperial College London Diabetes Centre, Abu Dhabi, United Arab Emirates

Imperial College London, London, UK

© The Author(s), under exclusive license to Springer Nature Singapore Pte Ltd. 2025
M. E. Faris et al. (eds.), *Health and Medical Aspects of Ramadan Intermittent Fasting*, https://doi.org/10.1007/978-981-96-6783-3_4

4.1 Introduction

Ramadan fasting (RF) entails complete abstinence from eating and drinking between dawn and sunset for a whole month every year. It is an obligatory practice for all healthy adult Muslims [Holy Quran, Chapter 1, verse 185].

Ramadan is a lunar month lasting 29 or 30 consecutive days, depending on the sighting of the new moon. The lunar year has 12 months but is 10 (or 11) days shorter than the Gregorian calendar.

The primary change in Ramadan energy balance is a major shift in the time of meals and pattern of eating. Other changes can be considered secondary and include alterations in appetite [1], food content [2–4], sleeping times [4–7], and activity patterns [6, 8, 9]. The "normal" pattern of eating with three main meals in the morning, midday, and evening is replaced. During Ramadan fasting, the midday meal is completely skipped. An early breakfast is taken just before dawn. No food or drink is allowed until sunset. Between sunset and the next dawn, the person is free to eat and drink. In most Muslim countries and temperate climates, depending on the season, there is a prolonged gap between the early morning and evening meals. The gap between the evening meal and the predawn meal is much shorter and different as there is no need for fasting, and most people get some sleep before waking up predawn.

Important secondary changes of Ramadan fasting include changes in appetite [1]. On "normal" non-Ramadan days, there are three main peaks in appetite corresponding to main meals. Appetite scores go up before meals to moderately high levels. In Ramadan fasting, this changes; from a low level after waking up, there is a progressive rise until sunset, when the appetite gets quite intense [1].

There are also changes in food content and energy intake. The iftar meal is often rich in carbohydrates and starts with some dates or sweets. The meal also tends to be bigger in size and variety [3, 10, 11]. Depending on culture and personal preferences, the evening meals may be one or two. The predawn meal can also have quite varied content but is usually lighter than the iftar meal.

There is wide inter- and intraindividual variation in food and its components during Ramadan. Factors determining food composition and timing include hunger, as well as psychological, social, cultural, and financial aspects. In most cultures, typically, three main meals are consumed: breakfast, lunch, and dinner, and these are accompanied by varied snacks (Fig. 4.1). Under weight-stable conditions, energy intake and expenditure are similar. Alterations in this "normal" pattern can have important implications for energy balance, with a negative energy balance leading to weight loss. This would be the case in fasting states if energy intake is less than energy expenditure (EE).

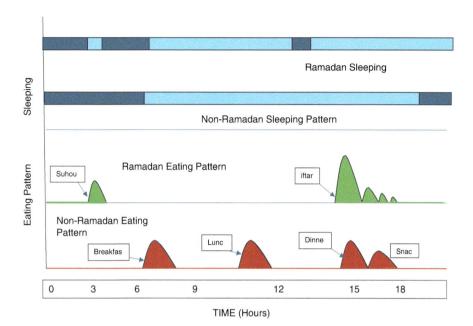

Fig. 4.1 Changes in sleeping and eating patterns during Ramadan. (After Tomader Ali and Nader Lessan, Diabetes Met Res Rev 2023, e3728)

4.2 Different Stages of Fasting

There are three different stages of fasting as hours and days pass from the last meal (Fig. 4.2). The postabsorptive phase lasts 6–24 h. During this stage, the central nervous system (CNS) depends on glucose from glycogen breakdown. At this stage, there is an increase in lipolysis, ketogenesis, and to a lesser extent, gluconeogenesis. The second stage, the gluconeogenesis stage, occurs on days 1–10; protein breakdown is used to generate glucose for use by the CNS. Other tissues use ketones and fat as metabolic fuel. Lipogenesis and ketogenesis increase and then plateau. Gluconeogenesis begins to decrease, and glycogenolysis ceases. After 10 days of fasting, the body goes into stage 3, the protein conservation phase. There is a further drop in protein breakdown to a minimum. At this stage, fatty acids are used by the body, but the CNS depends on ketone as fuel [12, 13].

Several interesting examples of prolonged fasting have been reported in the literature. A 31-day fast in a human subject was studied and reported by Francis Benedict in 1915. Among other findings, a drop in body weight was reported in different phases. The initial rate of weight loss of around 0.85 kg/day declined to around 0.3 kg/day by day 31 [14, 15]. A 44-day fast in a man in 2006 led to an overall weight loss of 24.5 kg, equivalent to 25% of body weight. Between a quarter to a third of this was due to body fat loss. The rest was a result of the loss of fat-free mass, mostly muscle, accounting for 20% of total body protein [16].

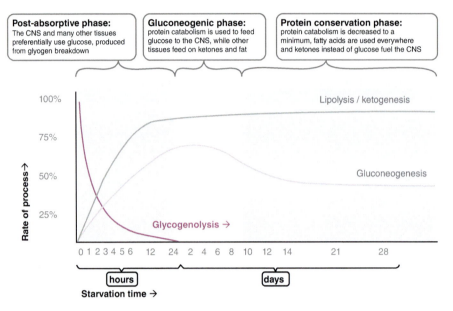

Fig. 4.2 Stages of fasting from onset to several weeks. (After Alex Yartsev, https://derangedphysi-ology.com/main/required-reading/endocrinology-metabolism-and-nutrition/Chapter%20318/physiological-adaptation-prolonged-starvation)

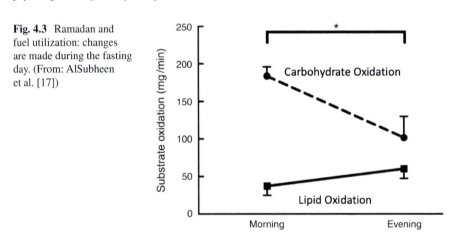

Fig. 4.3 Ramadan and fuel utilization: changes are made during the fasting day. (From: AlSubheen et al. [17])

Ramadan fasting is quite distinct from such prolonged fasting. It is an intermittent form of dry fasting synchronized with day/night cycles. It is a dry form of fasting where no food or drink is allowed during daylight hours. Furthermore, the same schedule is followed for a full lunar month. As such, in terms of fuel utilization, there is intermittent, probably partial, glycogen depletion and repletion. There is, therefore, a gradual shift from the preferred source of fuel from carbohydrate to fat stores as the fasting day progresses (Fig. 4.3). By implication, the body never enters a protein catabolism/gluconeogenesis stage. In contrast, body fat stores are employed on a daily basis.

4.3   Energy Expenditure and Its Components

Energy spent over 24 h (total energy expenditure (TEE)) has three components: resting metabolic rate (RMR), activity energy expenditure (AEE), and thermic effect of food (TEF) (Fig. 4.4) [18, 19]. Here, we give a brief account of energy expenditure as a concept relevant to Ramadan. For a more detailed discussion of energy expenditure in humans, the reader is referred to the excellent review by Fernandez-Verdejo et al. [18].

Energy expenditure changes in four phases in life; the highest total energy expenditure and resting energy expenditure (REE) per body weight occur in infancy and childhood, dropping to adult levels by the early 20 s, and then remaining stable until the sixth decade, declining rapidly thereafter [20].

RMR, or REE, is the energy needed to sustain life in a resting state. This includes maintaining body temperature and ionic gradients across cells, repairing internal organs, and supporting cardiac function and respiration. On average, and depending on how active a person is, RMR accounts for about two-thirds of the total energy expenditure and is influenced by age, sex, body weight, physiological states such as pregnancy and lactation, and hormonal status. Men generally have a higher energy expenditure per body weight [18, 19, 21].

Thyroid dysfunction is a typical and good example where RMR is altered [21]. As an example, a 30-year-old female patient with an RMR of 1450 kcal/24 h may have an RMR of 1250 if she were moderately hypothyroid. The same patient could have her RMR rise to 2000 kcal/24 h in moderate/gross thyrotoxicosis [author's unpublished data].

AEE is the second largest (and the most variable) component of energy expenditure. AEE is the energy required for physical work and is related directly to body

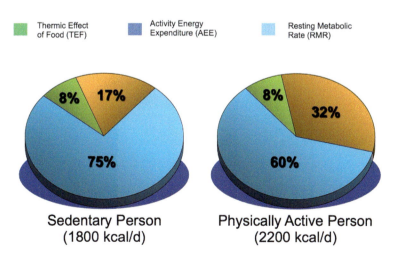

Fig. 4.4 Components of total daily energy expenditure. (After Segal KR et al. Am J Clin Nutr. 1984;40:995–1000)

weight, the distance that weight is moved, and the state of physical fitness [18]. With increasing activity, energy expenditure rises. A sedentary person may expend as little as 100–300 kcal/day in activity, whereas a very active individual may reach 3000 kcal/day.

TEF is the increase in energy expenditure that occurs with food intake. It is, in effect, the energy cost of digesting food and typically lasts several hours. Different macronutrients have different thermic effects; protein causes a greater rise in EE than fat; for instance, [21], TEF is normally a small component of TEE, representing around 10% of total daily energy expenditure. However, it is an important component and is relevant in states with energy imbalance.

4.4 Changes in Appetite During Ramadan Fasting

As the hours of fasting increase, there is a rise in hunger scores (Fig. 4.5). Appetite reaches quite intense levels by the evening and goes down again after the iftar meal is consumed. This daily pattern continues until the end of Ramadan. However, in females, there is some adaptation as Ramadan progresses. By the end of Ramadan, total and evening appetite and hunger scores are lower in females, compared to males and also in comparison to early Ramadan [1, 22].

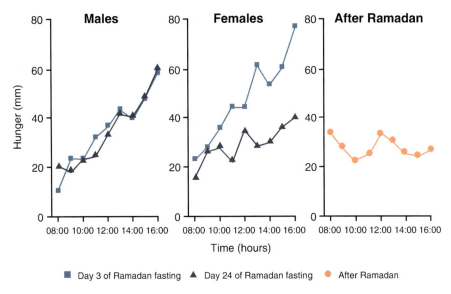

Fig. 4.5 Changes in hunger–satiety cycles during Ramadan (Finch GM et al. Appetite. 1998;31(2):159–70)

4.5   Weight Changes in Ramadan Fasting

One of the more readily measurable outcomes of fasting during Ramadan is the change in body weight. The drastic changes to meal timings, the longer daytime gap between the main meals, the changes in appetite and satiety, and the alterations in sleeping times and patterns lead to changes in eating behaviors and weight changes in most individuals who practice Ramadan fasting. This is subject to great inter-individual variability, which is influenced by social, cultural, geographic, and religious factors [3, 23–26].

On average, there is a net modest weight loss of 1–2 kg, as shown in several mostly small studies [27–30] and also demonstrated in meta-analyses [24, 26, 31]. Some others have reported weight gain [23, 25, 31, 32]. A study of 202 participants recruited at mosques in East London showed a net weight loss of around 0.8 kg by the end of Ramadan. The lost weight was regained by 4–5 weeks after Ramadan [31]. A meta-analysis by Kul et al. showed a small weight loss of around 0.7 kg in fasting men but no significant change in women [33]. Another meta-analysis by Fernando and colleagues [24] showed that the mean weight loss with Ramadan fasting was 1.34 kg. Ramadan weight loss seems to be greater among Asian populations, compared with Africans and Europeans [32]. Still, there seems to be no significant sex difference in the absolute magnitude of weight loss with Ramadan fasting.

4.6   Energy Expenditure During Ramadan Fasting

Studies of energy expenditure during Ramadan are very few (Table 4.1). The question is whether, how, and to what extent different aspects of energy expenditure change with Ramadan fasting. Should energy expenditure change? Before looking at the evidence base for this, the answer to this question is probably yes. After all, the pattern of activity and sleep obviously changes. With that alone, one might expect changes with the immediate transition from a "normal" pattern of eating to the Ramadan eating pattern on the very first day of Ramadan.

Furthermore, as the month of Ramadan progresses and with adaptations to the new patterns, one might expect further changes. One must also bear in mind that with different day lengths in various latitudes and seasons and with other cultures and dietary habits, there is an expected variability in these changes. Studies of energy dynamics during Ramadan are on a small number of subjects by nature, and generalizing the findings has to be done with some caution.

Resting metabolic rate (RMR): Most studies (except the study by BaHammam et al.) used indirect calorimetry.

Activity energy expenditure (AEE): AEE was measured by accelerometry/activity monitors in most studies (except the study by Agagunduz et al., which was questionnaire-based; El Ati et al. did not measure AEE). Total energy expenditure

Table 4.1 Summary of studies on energy expenditure and Ramadan fasting

Year	First author	References	Country	N	F/M	Age	BMI (kg/m^2)	RMR change during Ramadan	AEE change during Ramadan	TEE change during Ramadan	Energy intake	Other comments
1995	Jalila El Ati	[34]	Tunisia	16	16/0	25–39	22.7 +/- 0.3	Not significant at 8 AM	Not measured	Not measured	No significant change	Multiple time points (x6) during daytime
2010	Ahmed BaHammam	[35]	Saudi Arabia	7	0/7	18–24 (20.5 +/- 2.9)	22.6 +/- 2.7	Not measured	Lower METS and EE in Ramadan	Lower METS and EE in Ramadan	No record	The main focus is on circadian rhythm and sleep. SenseWear armband
2014	Jessica McNeil	[36]	Canada	Ten normal weight, ten obese	0/10 + 10	25, 37	24.4, 34.8	Not significant	Not significant	Not measured	Not assessed	Comparisons between lean and obese
2017	Sana'a Alsubheen	[17]	Canada	Nine fasting, eight control	0/9 + 8	32.2 +/- 7.8	26.5 +/- 5.0	Not reported	Reduced	Not measured	No significant differences	Main focus on anthropometry and substrate oxidation
2021	Duygu Agagunduz	[37]	Turkey	27	16/11	27.6 +/- 1.69	NK	A decrease of about 100 kcal/day	No difference	Reduction of 300 kcal/day	No significant difference	Reduction in RMR and TEE in Ramadan is greater in females
2018	Nader Lessan	[9]	UAE	29	16/13	33 0.3 +/- 8.7	24.6 +/- 2.9	No significant change	Lower in Ramadan	No significant change	Not assessed	No significant change in RMR and TEE Lower AEE in Ramadan. Change in activity patterns

EE energy expenditure, *AEE* activity energy expenditure, *RMR* resting metabolic rate, *TEE* total energy expenditure, *METS* metabolic equivalent of tasks

(TEE): The only research measuring TEE was the one by Lessan et al. (doubly labeled water technique). El Ati et al. used direct calorimetry to look at different aspects of energy expenditure. BaHammam et al. used accelerometry/armbands and reported metabolic equivalents. Thermic effect of food (TEF): No study has measured TEF during Ramadan. TEF before and after Ramadan was measured in the study by McNeil et al.

4.7 Does Resting Metabolic Rate Change During Ramadan Fasting?

Several changes relevant to fasting can affect resting metabolic rate:

1. During the first 4 days of continuous fasting, heart rate increases by around 100%, driven by a rise in norepinephrine release. This can be associated with an increase in resting metabolic rate.
2. With prolonged fasting, RMR is known to decrease. This may be a counterregulatory way to reduce energy loss [19, 38, 39].
3. Resting metabolic rate is related to body mass. A significant weight gain can lead to a rise in RMR, and conversely, a reduction in weight can lead to a drop in metabolic rate [19]. On average, fasting during Ramadan leads to a net weight loss of around 1.34 kg, as indicated by a meta-analysis [24]. However, the effect of fasting during Ramadan on weight is highly variable. As such, one might expect the resulting change in RMR to be subject to similar variability.
4. The resting metabolic rate is influenced by circadian rhythmicity since these rhythms also influence the hormones that affect metabolism. Changes in the sleep/wakefulness cycle during Ramadan have been shown to affect circadian rhythms [4, 40, 41].
5. There is a change in substrate oxidation with fasting [17]. Ramadan results in a shift in fuel oxidation from morning to evening, with an increase in fat oxidation and a decrease in carbohydrate oxidation. As the hours of fasting pass, glycogen stores are gradually consumed, and the fasting individual resorts to body fat stores for fuel.

In practice, the RMR change with Ramadan fasting seems to be modest or insignificant. Only a few studies have investigated resting metabolism in the context of fasting during Ramadan [9, 17, 34, 36, 42]. Of these, only three have used the gold standard indirect calorimetry for measuring RMR.

El Ati (1995) and colleagues investigated different aspects of energy expenditure in the context of Ramadan fasting in 16 female participants [34]. They explored RMR at four different time points around Ramadan (before Ramadan, the first week of Ramadan, the last week of Ramadan, and the week after Ramadan) and also looked at daily RMR trends [34]. The study found no difference in 8-AM RMR between pre-Ramadan, Ramadan, and post-Ramadan days. On pre- and post-Ramadan days, energy expenditure was much higher in the morning, presumably due to the thermic effect of food at breakfast time. This effect was absent during Ramadan days.

In contrast, there was a marked rise in energy expenditure in the evening on Ramadan days. This was probably also due to the thermic effect of food at the iftar meal, which was a higher peak compared to non-Ramadan times. Unfortunately, the authors give no information on the relationship between each of the time points and the last meal. Interestingly, metabolic rate increases throughout the day and into the evening, particularly during Ramadan.

BaHammam and colleagues (2010) conducted a study focusing mainly on circadian rhythms and sleep changes with fasting during Ramadan [35]. The study also used armbands to examine energy expenditure in this context. It reported lower METS and energy expenditure in Ramadan, as estimated by armband accelerometry and other parameters.

Alsubheen and colleagues (2017) investigated nine men (aged 32 years, BMI 26.5 kg/m^2) who observed Ramadan fasting and compared them with eight non-fasting control subjects [17]. The study used indirect calorimetry to assess substrate oxidation, but no RMR data were reported. The study beautifully demonstrated a shift in fuel utilization from carbohydrates to lipids as the fasting day progresses. The main focus of the study was the changes in anthropometry and substrate oxidation. Notably, the study was conducted in Canada, where the fasting window was around 18 h.

In our Ramadan and Energy Expenditure (RAMEE) study [9], we investigated energy expenditure (measured by indirect calorimetry) in 29 healthy nonobese individuals (13 men and 16 women aged 19–52 years). We found no significant change in RMR (Fig. 4.7) between Ramadan fasting and the outside-Ramadan period. The mean RMR was 1365.7 ± 230.2 kcal/d for Ramadan and 1362.9 ± 273.6 kcal/d for the post-Ramadan period ($P = 0.713$). RMR per fat-free mass also showed no difference between Ramadan and post-Ramadan periods. However, respiratory quotient (RQ) during and after Ramadan was significantly different ($n = 29$; $P < 0.0001$) with a lower value of 0.80 ± 0.06 during Ramadan, compared to 0.88 ± 0.05 after Ramadan, indicating an increased fat vs. carbohydrate utilization during Ramadan. There was no significant difference in RMR when comparing pre-Ramadan to week 1, week 2, and post-Ramadan values in a small subgroup of participants on whom multiple time point data were available (Fig. 4.6). The study also showed inter-individual variation in the direction and magnitude of RMR change during Ramadan with a rise of up to 23% in some individuals and a reduction of up to 16% in others. Controlling for the effects of sex, age, weight, and number of hours since *Suhoor*, RMR was significantly lower in the second, third, and fourth weeks of Ramadan than in the first week of Ramadan. As expected, male sex and weight were positively associated with resting metabolic rate.

4.7.1 Activity Energy Expenditure During Ramadan Fasting

With the longer gap between the main meals of the day and changes in sleeping times, activity patterns during Ramadan change. Much activity occurs in the evening hours and after iftar, although there is great inter-individual variability in the

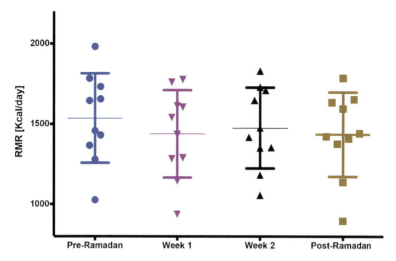

Fig. 4.6 RMR change with Ramadan. Pre-Ramadan, Ramadan week 1, Ramadan week 2, and post-Ramadan compared. There was a significant difference between the RMR before Ramadan vs. the first week of Ramadan ($P = 0.008$). (Lessan and Saadane, RAMEE study, unpublished data)

Activity: Ramadan vs post-Ramadan

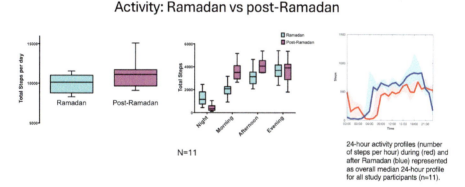

Fig. 4.7 Activity and activity patterns during Ramadan fasting

type, amount, and timing of activity. The latter is not surprising, as AEE is mostly voluntary and is the most highly variable component of energy expenditure.

Agagunduz and colleagues investigated activity energy expenditure pre-Ramadan, during Ramadan, and post-Ramadan but found no overall significant difference [37]. Activity was assessed through questionnaires, and there was no direct measurement.

The RAMEE study reported some of these activity patterns (Fig. 4.7) [9]. There was no overall change in activity energy expenditure between Ramadan and

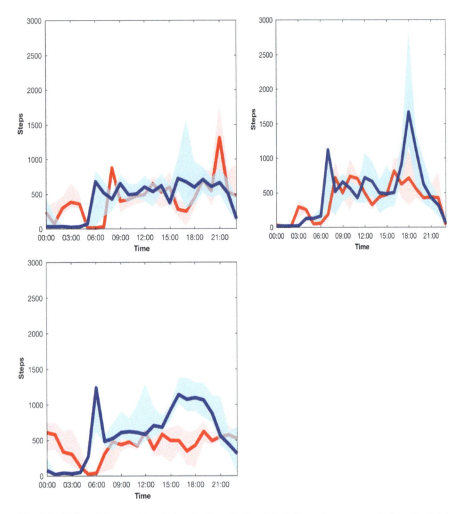

Fig. 4.8 24-h activity profiles during (red) and after (blue) Ramadan, represented as the total number of steps per hour for three different subjects. Times of no activity are indicative of sleep and are different in different individuals. (Lessan N, Saadane I, RAMEE study, unpublished data)

non-Ramadan periods. However, activity levels had a unique pattern through different timings of the day during Ramadan compared to after Ramadan (Fig. 4.8). At night (00:00–06:00), activity levels were higher in Ramadan compared to the non-Ramadan period ($P = 0.001$). Morning (06:00–12:00) and afternoon (12:00–18:00) activity levels were lower during Ramadan compared to 2 months after Ramadan ($P = 0.001$ and $P = 0.002$, respectively). Unlike other timings of the day, differences in activity levels in the evening (18:00–00:00) during Ramadan compared to after Ramadan were not observed ($P = 0.70$).

4.7.2 Thermic Effect of Food and Ramadan Fasting

A study by McNeil and colleagues (2014) compared different aspects of energy expenditure between lean ($n = 10$) and obese ($n = 10$) men before and after Ramadan [36]. As expected, the study found differences between the two groups, but there were no significant changes when comparing pre- and post-Ramadan time points. The study was not designed to look at energy expenditure during Ramadan itself, though, and as such, there was no TEF measurement during Ramadan.

There have been no studies specifically investigating the thermic effect of food during Ramadan fasting. However, there are a number of considerations in speculating what changes to TEF might be expected with the Ramadan fast. First, TEF is related to serum insulin and insulin resistance. Insulin resistance and plasma insulin levels are known to be higher during the Ramadan fast, especially in the evening and around the iftar period. This may lead to a reduction in TEF. Second, dietary fat has a lower thermic effect than protein. Several studies of diet during Ramadan have, indeed, reported a higher fat content; this can also cause a reduction in TEF during Ramadan. Finally, a major meal is skipped during Ramadan, and although this can, in part, be compensated by over-snacking at night, a net reduction in TEF may be expected. Well-conducted studies of TEF during Ramadan can provide a better insight into energy dynamics during Ramadan and help with weight management around the Ramadan period.

4.7.3 Does Total Energy Expenditure Change During Ramadan Fasting?

To date, only two published studies have investigated and reported total energy expenditure changes with Ramadan fasting. The RAMEE study conducted by our group (2018) examined different aspects of energy expenditure in the context of Ramadan fasting [9]. TEE was measured in a subgroup of individuals ($n = 10$) during and after the Ramadan fasting period using the gold standard doubly labeled water technique. The technique makes it possible to measure TEE in free-living conditions and, as such, has major advantages. RAMEE found no significant difference in TEE between Ramadan and post-Ramadan periods (Fig. 4.7). However, definite changes were observed in activity and activity energy expenditure at different times of the day, with a reduction in AEE during fasting daylight hours during Ramadan (Fig. 4.8). After iftar, activity increased. It is also noteworthy that there was a lot of inter-individual variability in the magnitude and direction of change in TEE with Ramadan fasting. The TEE of some participants did not differ in Ramadan, compared to after Ramadan. In contrast, others had up to 500-kcal/day higher or 1400-kcal/day lower TEE in Ramadan, compared to after Ramadan.

In contrast, a study by Agagunduz and colleagues (2021) reported an overall reduction of around 300 kcal/day during Ramadan fasting, compared to the baseline

Fig. 4.9 Total energy expenditure (TEE) and resting metabolic rate (RMR) during and after Ramadan fasting. (From: Lessan N et al. Am J Clin Nutr 2018;107:54–71)

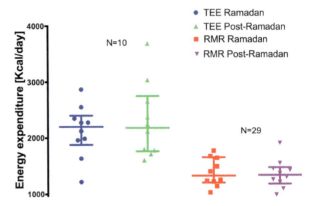

value before Ramadan [37]. However, this study did not directly measure TEE. Rather, TEE was estimated from the resting metabolic rate using physical activity level (PAL) derived from activity questionnaires.

4.7.4   Energy Intake in Ramadan

A primary, dramatic, and major change in Ramadan fasting is the alteration in mealtimes. The midday meal, lunch, is skipped completely. There is complete abstinence from any form of food or drink between dawn and sunset. After sunset, the main evening meal is eaten, and there is an ad libitum allowance for food until dawn. With such a dramatic change, there are also inevitable changes in food content. The pattern of food intake [3] and the overall energy content of food [43] also change. A small study of 16 healthy fasting female volunteers during Ramadan reported that 84% of total energy intake was taken at the evening meal (Fig. 4.9).

In contrast, in non-fasting periods, 9.4%, 41.6%, and 21.8% of total energy intake were taken at breakfast, lunch, and dinner, respectively [34]. The study reported no significant change in energy intake between Ramadan and non-Ramadan periods. A more recent study of 62 women showed a significant mean reduction of 136 and 210 kcal/day in total energy intake in early Ramadan, compared to after Ramadan in pre- and post-menopausal women, respectively [43]. Another study conducted in Algeria ($n = 276$, all women) showed a bigger reduction (335 kcal/day) in energy intake during Ramadan, compared to the non-Ramadan period [2]. Dietary and lifestyle changes of Ramadan are discussed in further detail in another chapter of this book.

4.8   Sleeping Patterns in Ramadan

Another important change in Ramadan is sleeping and wakefulness times; most will wake up about an hour before dawn to eat. At dawn, prayers are offered. Depending on local and family culture, most individuals get a few hours of work before starting daily activities. There is often a mid-/late- afternoon nap as well. So, sleeping in Ramadan follows a completely different and broken pattern.

A meta-analysis by Faris and colleagues showed a reduction of total sleeping duration of around 1 h during Ramadan fasting [7]. The RAMEE study showed different sleeping patterns in other subjects, with some individuals managing with very little sleep [9]. Changes in sleep during Ramadan fasting are important and are dealt with in detail elsewhere in this book.

4.9 Discussion: What Does All This Mean?

Ramadan fasting is accompanied by remarkable and sudden changes in lifestyle, affecting a global Muslim population of over two billion. A synchronous meal pattern replaces the liberal pattern of eating and drinking, with none in daylight hours and the main meals at sunset and before dawn. There is an inevitable change in sleep and activity patterns and energy balance. Although main mealtimes are quite rigid, there is major inter-individual variability in the content and amount of food consumed, the degree of snacking in the evening and nighttime, activity, rest, sleeping time, and quality of sleep.

These changes have an impact on different aspects of energy expenditure, although other components are affected to various extents. The effect on resting metabolism seems to be quite modest and indeed minimal on average. However, resting metabolism is altered at different times of the fasting day; one study reported a rise in RMR from morning to afternoon and evening [34].

Fasting during Ramadan affects activity and energy expenditure to a much greater extent. In particular, the pattern, type, duration, and distribution of activity and exercise are altered, resulting in an overall significant reduction in activity energy expenditure during Ramadan. Importantly, there is great inter-individual variability in different aspects of AEE and how it changes during Ramadan fasting. As much of the activity is under voluntary control, addressing AEE, together with dietary advice, can be used to promote health during Ramadan [9].

To what extent the thermic effect of food changes during Ramadan is currently unclear due to a lack of direct evidence. Investigating TEF during Ramadan/Ramadan-type fasting is quite challenging and needs quite carefully designed and implemented studies.

Total daily energy expenditure during Ramadan seems to be minimally affected by fasting. However, the impact of Ramadan on TEE is subject to inter-individual variability, as it is for AEE [9].

An important aspect of energy balance dynamics in the context of Ramadan fasting is inter-individual variability. The TEE, RMR, and AEE changes with Ramadan fasting vary greatly in different individuals. Although at a population level, the overall change in RMR and TEE seems minimal, in some individuals, there is an increase, whereas in others, there is a reduction. In many, the change is indeed insignificant [9].

The end markers of energy balance, namely weight and body fat, also demonstrate this inter-individual variability. However, an overall weight reduction of around 1.5 kg has been shown in meta-analyses. It is also known that in most individuals, this reverts to the pre-Ramadan weight within a few weeks. The Ramadan model is a unique model for examining the concepts of energy balance. It is now accepted that there is a "coupling" of energy intake and output such that a similar change follows in energy expenditure to that of the energy intake side of the equation. This does not necessarily happen immediately and may take some time [19]. The modest weight loss during Ramadan is therefore not surprising, as is the weight gain post-Ramadan. These phenomena are not universal, though, and do not apply to all individuals. Ramadan studies are generally small in participant numbers; much of this is due to the difficulty in finding suitable and willing participants. Ramadan research highlights the overall findings, such as mean weight loss. Variability in different aspects of energy balance warrants further exploration as there is much to learn from the smaller group of people who gain the greatest benefit in health, specifically weight loss that can be sustained.

Acknowledgments The author wishes to thank the Research Team at the Imperial College London Diabetes Centre for their work on the RAMEE study reported in this manuscript. In particular, the author wishes to thank Miss Ilham Saadane for her work in RAMEE study and the figures quoted in this chapter.

References

1. Finch GM, Day JE, Razak, Welch DA, Rogers PJ. Appetite changes under free-living conditions during Ramadan fasting. Appetite. 1998;31(2):159–70. https://doi.org/10.1006/appe.1998.0164.
2. Khaled BM, Belbraouet S. Effect of Ramadan fasting on anthropometric parameters and food consumption in 276 type 2 diabetic obese women. Int J Diabetes Dev Ctries. 2009;29(2):62–8. https://doi.org/10.4103/0973-3930.53122.
3. Ali Z, Abizari AR. Ramadan fasting alters food patterns, dietary diversity, and body weight among Ghanaian adolescents. Nutr J. 2018;17(1):75. https://doi.org/10.1186/s12937-018-0386-2.
4. Reilly T, Waterhouse J. Altered sleep-wake cycles and food intake: the Ramadan model. Physiol Behav. 2007;90(2–3):219–28. https://doi.org/10.1016/j.physbeh.2006.09.004.
5. Alzhrani A, Alhussain MH, BaHammam AS. Changes in dietary intake, chronotype, and sleep pattern upon Ramadan among healthy adults in Jeddah, Saudi Arabia: a prospective study. Front Nutr. 2022;9:966861. https://doi.org/10.3389/fnut.2022.966861.
6. Alghamdi AS, Alghamdi KA, Jenkins RO, Alghamdi MN, Haris PI. Impact of Ramadan on physical activity and sleeping patterns in individuals with type 2 diabetes: the first study using Fitbit device. Diabetes Ther. 2020;11(6):1331–46. https://doi.org/10.1007/s13300-020-00825-x.
7. Faris ME, Jahrami HA, Alhayki FA, Alkhawaja NA, Ali AM, Aljeeb SH, et al. Effect of diurnal fasting on sleep during Ramadan: a systematic review and meta-analysis. Sleep Breath. 2020;24(2):771–82. https://doi.org/10.1007/s11325-019-01986-1.
8. Al-Hourani HM, Atoum MF. Body composition, nutrient intake and physical activity patterns in young women during Ramadan. Singapore Med J. 2007;48(10):906–10.

9. Lessan N, Saadane I, Alkaf B, Hambly C, Buckley AJ, Finer N, et al. The effects of Ramadan fasting on activity and energy expenditure. Am J Clin Nutr. 2018;107(1):54–61. https://doi.org/10.1093/ajcn/nqx016.

10. Nachvak SM, Pasdar Y, Pirsaheb S, Darbandi M, Niazi P, Mostafai R, et al. Effects of Ramadan on food intake, glucose homeostasis, lipid profiles, and body composition. Eur J Clin Nutr. 2019;73(4):594–600. https://doi.org/10.1038/s41430-018-0189-8.

11. Waterhouse J, Alkib L, Reilly T. Effects of Ramadan upon fluid and food intake, fatigue, and physical, mental, and social activities: a comparison between the UK and Libya. Chronobiol Int. 2008;25(5):697–724. https://doi.org/10.1080/07420520802397301.

12. Cahill GF Jr. Starvation in man. N Engl J Med. 1970;282(12):668–75. https://doi.org/10.1056/NEJM197003192821209.

13. Cahill GF Jr. Fuel metabolism in starvation. Annu Rev Nutr. 2006;26:1–22. https://doi.org/10.1146/annurev.nutr.26.061505.111258.

14. Benedict FG. Chemical and physiological studies of a man fasting thirtyone days. Proc Natl Acad Sci USA. 1915;1(4):228–31. https://doi.org/10.1073/pnas.1.4.228.

15. Kerndt PR, Naughton JL, Driscoll CE, Loxterkamp DA. Fasting: the history, pathophysiology and complications. West J Med. 1982;137(5):379–99.

16. Korbonits M, Blaine D, Elia M, Powell-Tuck J. Refeeding David Blaine—studies after a 44-day fast. N Engl J Med. 2005;353(21):2306–7. https://doi.org/10.1056/NEJM200511243532124.

17. Alsubheen SA, Ismail M, Baker A, Blair J, Adebayo A, Kelly L, et al. The effects of diurnal Ramadan fasting on energy expenditure and substrate oxidation in healthy men. Br J Nutr. 2017;118(12):1023–30. https://doi.org/10.1017/S0007114517003221.

18. Fernandez-Verdejo R, Sanchez-Delgado G, Ravussin E. Energy expenditure in humans: principles, methods, and changes throughout the life course. Annu Rev Nutr. 2024; https://doi.org/10.1146/annurev-nutr-062122-031443.

19. Rosenbaum M. Appetite, energy expenditure, and the regulation of energy balance. Gastroenterol Clin N Am. 2023;52(2):311–22. https://doi.org/10.1016/j.gtc.2023.03.004.

20. Westerterp KR, Yamada Y, Sagayama H, Ainslie PN, Andersen LF, Anderson LJ, et al. Physical activity and fat-free mass during growth and in later life. Am J Clin Nutr. 2021;114(5):1583–9. https://doi.org/10.1093/ajcn/nqab260.

21. Yavuz S, Salgado Nunez Del Prado S, Celi FS. Thyroid hormone action and energy expenditure. J Endocr Soc. 2019;3(7):1345–56. https://doi.org/10.1210/js.2018-00423.

22. Lamri-Senhadji MY, El Kebir B, Belleville J, Bouchenak M. Assessment of dietary consumption and time-course of changes in serum lipids and lipoproteins before, during and after Ramadan in young Algerian adults. Singapore Med J. 2009;50(3):288–94.

23. Bakhotmah BA. The puzzle of self-reported weight gain in a month of fasting (Ramadan) among a cohort of Saudi families in Jeddah, Western Saudi Arabia. Nutr J. 2011;10:84. https://doi.org/10.1186/1475-2891-10-84.

24. Fernando HA, Zibellini J, Harris RA, Seimon RV, Sainsbury A. Effect of Ramadan fasting on weight and body composition in healthy non-athlete adults: a systematic review and meta-analysis. Nutrients. 2019;11(2). https://doi.org/10.3390/nu11020478.

25. Hajek P, Myers K, Dhanji AR, West O, McRobbie H. Weight change during and after Ramadan fasting. J Public Health (Oxf). 2012;34(3):377–81. https://doi.org/10.1093/pubmed/fdr087.

26. Jahrami HA, Alsibai J, Clark CCT, Faris ME. A systematic review, meta-analysis, and meta-regression of the impact of diurnal intermittent fasting during Ramadan on body weight in healthy subjects aged 16 years and above. Eur J Nutr. 2020;59(6):2291–316. https://doi.org/10.1007/s00394-020-02216-1.

27. Nomani MZ, Hallak MH, Siddiqui IP. Effects of Ramadan fasting on plasma uric acid and body weight in healthy men. J Am Diet Assoc. 1990;90(10):1435–6.

28. Poh B, Zawiah H, Ismail M, Henry C. Changes in body weight, dietary intake and activity pattern of adolescents during Ramadan. Malays J Nutr. 1996;2(1):1–10.

29. Ziaee V, Razaei M, Ahmadinejad Z, Shaikh H, Yousefi R, Yarmohammadi L, et al. The changes of metabolic profile and weight during Ramadan fasting. Singapore Med J. 2006;47(5):409–14.

30. Haouari M, Haouari-Oukerro F, Sfaxi A, Ben Rayana MC, Kaabachi N, Mbazaa A. How Ramadan fasting affects caloric consumption, body weight, and circadian evolution of cortisol serum levels in young, healthy male volunteers. Horm Metab Res. 2008;40(8):575–7. https://doi.org/10.1055/s-2008-1065321.

31. Kul S, Savas E, Ozturk ZA, Karadag G. Does Ramadan fasting alter body weight and blood lipids and fasting blood glucose in a healthy population? A meta-analysis. J Relig Health. 2014;53(3):929–42. https://doi.org/10.1007/s10943-013-9687-0.

32. Sadeghirad B, Motaghipisheh S, Kolahdooz F, Zahedi MJ, Haghdoost AA. Islamic fasting and weight loss: a systematic review and meta-analysis. Public Health Nutr. 2014;17(2):396–406. https://doi.org/10.1017/s1368980012005046.

33. Kul S, Savas E, Ozturk ZA, Karadag G. Does Ramadan fasting alter body weight and blood lipids and fasting blood glucose in a healthy population? A meta-analysis. J Relig Health. 2013; https://doi.org/10.1007/s10943-013-9687-0.

34. el Ati J, Beji C, Danguir J. Increased fat oxidation during Ramadan fasting in healthy women: an adaptative mechanism for body-weight maintenance. Am J Clin Nutr. 1995;62(2):302–7.

35. BaHammam A, Alrajeh M, Albabtain M, Bahammam S, Sharif M. Circadian pattern of sleep, energy expenditure, and body temperature of young healthy men during the intermittent fasting of Ramadan. Appetite. 2010;54(2):426–9. https://doi.org/10.1016/j.appet.2010.01.011.

36. McNeil J, Mamlouk MM, Duval K, Schwartz A, Nardo Junior N, Doucet E. Alterations in metabolic profile occur in normal-weight and obese men during the Ramadan fast despite no changes in anthropometry. J Obes. 2014;2014:482547. https://doi.org/10.1155/2014/482547.

37. Agagunduz D, Acar-Tek N, Bozkurt O. Effect of intermittent fasting (18/6) on energy expenditure, nutritional status, and body composition in healthy adults. Evid Based Complement Alternat Med. 2021;2021:7809611. https://doi.org/10.1155/2021/7809611.

38. National Research Council. Diet and health: implications for reducing chronic disease risk. Washington, DC: The National Academies Press; 1989.

39. Forbes GB. Lean body mass-body fat interrelationships in humans. Nutr Rev. 1987;45(8):225–31. https://doi.org/10.1111/j.1753-4887.1987.tb02684.x.

40. Bahammam A. Does Ramadan fasting affect sleep? Int J Clin Pract. 2006;60(12):1631–7. https://doi.org/10.1111/j.1742-1241.2005.00811.x.

41. BaHammam A. Assessment of sleep patterns, daytime sleepiness, and chronotype during Ramadan in fasting and nonfasting individuals. Saudi Med J. 2005;26(4):616–22.

42. Karaagaoglu N, Yucecan S. Some behavioural changes observed among fasting subjects, their nutritional habits and energy expenditure in Ramadan. Int J Food Sci Nutr. 2000;51(2):125–34.

43. AlZunaidy NA, Al-Khalifa AS, Alhussain MH, Mohammed MA, Alfheeaid HA, Althwab SA, et al. The effect of Ramadan intermittent fasting on food intake, anthropometric indices, and metabolic markers among premenopausal and postmenopausal women: a cross-sectional study. Medicina (Kaunas). 2023;59(7). https://doi.org/10.3390/medicina59071191.

Chapter 5
Effect of Ramadan Intermittent Fasting on Autophagy and Gene Expression

A. Alim Al Bari, Mohamed Ibrahim Madkour, Maha M. Saber-Ayad, and Nabil Eid

Abstract Intermittent fasting (IF), encompassing various regimens, garners attention for its multifaceted health benefits, which span metabolic improvements and the attenuation of age-related inflammation. Ramadan intermittent fasting (RIF), a prominent IF model, yields favorable outcomes in body composition, glucose regulation, lipid profiles, and liver function tests. Notably, RIF's alteration of diurnal eating patterns underscores its role in chrono-nutrition interventions, which modulate nutritional metabolism via circadian rhythms. Targeting overnutrition through IF represents a pivotal strategy for mitigating these public health challenges. Fasting and caloric restriction represent effective interventions for disease prevention and aging delay. RIF affects the expression of different genes related to metabolism, inflammation, autophagy, oxidative stress, and other biological processes. This chapter discusses the impact of IF in general and RIF in particular on gene expression and signaling pathways involved in various metabolic, inflammatory, and other processes. A special focus on autophagy and the impact of gene variants on response to RIF is provided. A summary is provided for the clinical trials exploring the clini-

A. A. Al Bari
Faculty of Science, Department of Pharmacy, University of Rajshahi, Rajshahi, Bangladesh
e-mail: alimalbari347@ru.ac.bd

M. I. Madkour
Department of Medical Laboratory Sciences, College of Health Sciences, University of Sharjah, Sharjah, United Arab Emirates
e-mail: mmadkour@sharjah.ac.ae

M. M. Saber-Ayad
Department of Clinical Sciences, College of Medicine, University of Sharjah, Sharjah, United Arab Emirates
e-mail: msaber@sharjah.ac.ae

N. Eid (✉)
Department of Human Biology, Anatomy Division, School of Medicine, IMU University, Kuala Lumpur, Malaysia
e-mail: nabilsaleheid@imu.edu.my

cal and molecular underpinnings of fasting. It holds promise in elucidating its diverse biological effects and informing personalized health interventions. Finally, future perspectives and research opportunities are discussed.

Keywords Intermittent fasting · Ramadan intermittent fasting · Autophagy · Gene expression · Circadian rhythms · Metabolic health · Inflammation · Oxidative stress · Chrono-nutrition · Disease prevention

5.1 Introduction

Overnutrition has been recognized as one of the major health risk factors for a broad range of human diseases, especially metabolic disorders such as diabetes and non-alcoholic fatty liver disease (NAFLD), neurodegenerative diseases, and cancers [1]. Moreover, maternal overnutrition leads to the development of obesity in subsequent generations and cognitive deficits in adulthood [2, 3]. Therefore, targeting overnutrition represents a straightforward yet effective strategy for addressing these public health challenges. Fasting and caloric/dietary restriction as dietary interventions for fighting overnutrition have been widely investigated and bridged from religious and philosophical aspects to medical treatment [4] because of their potential roles in protecting against multiple human diseases and delaying aging in most species [5].

Over the years, various forms of intermittent fasting (IF) have gained popularity in scientific circles and among the general public worldwide due to their numerous health benefits. IF is a safe and costless intervention that offers health benefits and disease prevention, particularly chronic metabolic and aging-related diseases [6] (Fig. 5.1). IF is also shown to reduce inflammatory and cellular senescence markers and counteract age-associated chronic inflammation (often referred to as "inflammaging") [7–9].

Several systematic reviews and meta-analyses demonstrate the numerous beneficial health impacts of Ramadan intermittent fasting (RIF), including improvements in body composition, glucose homeostasis (blood sugar level), lipid profiles (by regulating "bad" cholesterol), and other cardiometabolic risk factors (by reducing hypertension) [10–13] and liver function tests [14]. In addition, RIF reduces low-grade systemic inflammation and oxidative stress, thus preventing subsequent adverse health effects [15]. Interestingly, in individuals with overweight or obesity, RIF lowers visceral adiposity [16].

One of the most commonly practiced models of IF is RIF, which has received continuous attention [17]. RIF, distinct from caloric restriction (CR), represents a dramatic shift from normal diurnal eating to nocturnal patterns, representing an emerging model for exploring chrono-nutrition interventions that impact nutritional metabolism via circadian rhythms [17]. Circadian rhythms have a significant influence on various essential bodily functions, including sleep patterns, hormone release, appetite, digestion, and body temperature. For example, in overweight and obese individuals, RIF can significantly reduce the level of the hunger hormone,

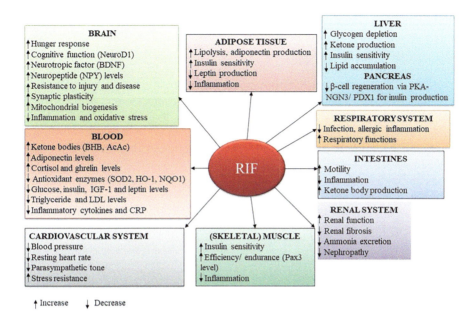

Fig. 5.1 Functional effects and pervasive benefits of Ramadan diurnal intermittent fasting in different organ systems of the body
The effects on the brain and cardiovascular, respiratory, and renal systems, as well as the liver, intestine, blood, adipose tissue, and skeletal muscles, are outlined

ghrelin [18]. This is important because fasting aids in weight loss without making one feel excessively hungry, unlike many other diets. Although diets and calorie restriction have positive effects on brain health, such strategies are notoriously hard to sustain over time for many people. They can have detrimental impacts on lean people [19]. Interestingly, several observational and clinical studies suggest that RIF boosts brain health and cognitive function [19]. Ramadan fasting also increases endorphins, the body's natural painkillers and "feel-good" chemicals. This fosters a sense of positivity, enhances well-being, and promotes better mental health [20, 21]. Interestingly, adolescent tennis players who fast during Ramadan reported increased self-confidence and reduced somatic and cognitive anxiety as a result of mental imagery training [20].

5.2   Cell-Signaling Pathways of RIF

Several nutrigenomic studies examine the relationship between the effect of RIF and the associated dietary and lifestyle changes on the expression of specific genes related to human health and diseases. RIF entails a protective impact against oxidative stress and its adverse metabolic-related derangements in patients with overweight and obesity by significantly enhancing the anti-oxidative stress genes (*TFAM, Nrf2,* and *SOD2*) and highly downregulating metabolism-controlling genes, *sirtuin 1–3 (SIRT1-3)* [22]. Table 5.1 summarizes the conclusions of various studies on the impact of RIF on inflammation, oxidative stress, autophagy, and the gut microbiome. Figure 5.2 describes the molecular mechanisms of RIF as a potential intervention tool. Intriguingly, a previous overview suggested IF as an approach to combat severe acute respiratory syndrome coronavirus 2 (SARS-CoV-2) infection through a dietary regimen composed of a ketogenic breakfast, supplemented by two doses of lauric acid–rich medium-chain triglycerides (TGs) at breakfast and lunch times, followed by 8–12-h IF, and a fruit- and vegetable-rich dinner [38].

Neurotransmitters and neurotrophic factors are signaling molecules that play a crucial role in cell proliferation, differentiation, survival, and the functions of neurons. The plasma levels of serotonin, brain-derived neurotrophic factor (BDNF), and nerve growth factor (NGF) are significantly increased during the fasting month of Ramadan [39]. Higher levels of NGF protein help regulate the growth, maintenance, proliferation, and survival of neurons. Fasting also increases the expression of BDNF, a protein that supports the growth and survival of brain cells. The increased production of BDNF enhances memory, learning, and mental clarity. Low levels of BDNF have been attributed to an increased risk of Alzheimer's disease (AD) [40]. However, several studies have shown a significant reduction in BDNF levels and an improvement in mood-related symptoms after RIF [41]. BDNF, a neurotrophin, has been studied in relation to mental health disorders, cognition, physical activity, and nutrition [42]. Cortisol is a glucocorticoid hormone released in a circadian rhythm to regulate the hypothalamic–pituitary–adrenal axis, particularly in stress-related disorders. BDNF and cortisol levels significantly decreased in the last days of RIF compared to 1 week prior to RIF. These effects of RIF have been shown to benefit mood-related symptoms and health-related quality of life [42].

In the case of reduction of body weight (BW) and visceral fat content, as well as regulation of satiety and eating-controlling hormones (leptin, adiponectin, and ghrelin) [18, 43], RIF shows a positive impact on the interaction between body genes and environmental factors that shape human susceptibility to develop obesity. The fat mass and obesity-associated (*FTO*) gene has metabolic effects related to energy metabolism and body fat deposition. The expressions of *FTO* significantly decreased at the end of Ramadan. RIF is also associated with downregulating the *FTO* gene expression in subjects with obesity. Thus, RIF presumably entails a protective effect against body weight gain and its adverse metabolic-related derangements in subjects with obesity [11]. Ramadan fasting is associated with improvements in some cardiometabolic risk factors, such as circulating γ-glutamyl transferase (GGT) and high-sensitivity C-reactive protein (*hs*-CRP); serum lipid profile; atherogenic index; and leukocyte expression of IL-1α [11].

Circadian rhythms regulate numerous physiological processes, including energy metabolism, hormone synthesis, and immune responses. Shift work, including the fasting month of Ramadan, causes severe disturbance in sleeping patterns by inducing alterations in core *circadian locomotor output cycles kaput (CLOCK)* genes to

Table 5.1 Several non-randomized, within-subject designs provide the impact of fasting for 1 month of Ramadan (dawn to sunset) on inflammation, oxidative stress, autophagy, and the gut microbiome

	Study population	Summary of study outcomes Cytokines/parameters	Level change	References
Inflammation	50 healthy subjects, 21 M and 29 F, mean age: 32.7 Y	IL-6, IL-1β, and tumor necrosis factor alpha (TNF-α) levels decreased	↓	[23]
	12 healthy M subjects, mean age: 25.1 years	IL-6, IL-8, and IL-1β levels reduced	↓	[24]
	57 subjects with BMI $\geq$ 25 kg/m², 35 M and 22 F, mean age: 36.2 Y	IL-6, TNF-α, and IGF 1 levels reduced	↓	[16]
	34 healthy M subjects, mean age: 35 Y	IGF 1 and IL-2 levels reduced	↓	[25]
	56 subjects with BMI $\geq$ 25 kg/m², 34 M and 22 F, mean age: 35.72 Y	IGF 1 levels reduced	↓	[22]
	42 subjects with NAFLD, mean age: 37.59 Y	IL-6 and *hs*-CRP reduced	↓	[26]
	58 healthy M subjects, age: 20–40 Y	CXCL1, CXCL10, and CXCL12 decreased	↓	[27]
	74 subjects with NAFLD, 39 M and 35 F, mean age: 51.8 Y	CRP reduced	↓	[28]
	14 M subjects with obesity with BMI $\geq$ 30–40, mean age: 24 Y	IL-6 level lowered	↓	[29]
Oxidative stress	14 healthy subjects, 13 M and 1 F, mean age: 32 Y	Upregulating NR1D1 protein, which is the inhibitor of NLRP3 inflammasome	↑ (11-fold)	[30]
	56 subjects with BMI $\geq$ 25 kg/m², 34 M and 22 F, mean age: 35.72 Y	Antioxidant gene, including TFAM, SOD2, and Nrf2, expression increased	↑	[22]
	40 subjects with hypertension, mean age: 55 Y	Glutathione increased, and malondialdehyde levels decreased	↓	[31]

(continued)

Table 5.1 (continued)

	Study population	Summary of study outcomes		References
		Cytokines/parameters	Level change	
Autophagy	14 subjects with metabolic syndrome, 8 M and 6 F, mean age: 59 Y	Autophagy, oxidative stress, and inflammation biomarkers including PRKCSH	↑ Autophagy ↓ oxidative stress	[32]
Immune function	50 healthy subjects, 21 M and 29 F, mean age: 32.7 Y	Total leukocytes, granulocytes, lymphocytes, and monocytes IL-1β, IL-6, and TNFα	→ →	[23]
	14 subjects with metabolic syndrome, 8 M and 6 F, mean age: 59 Y	Calreticulin (CALR) gene protein products	↑ (16-fold)	[32]
	14 subjects with metabolic syndrome, 8 M and 6 F, mean age: 59 Y	Insulin resistance	→	[32]
Obesity, metabolic syndrome	57 subjects with BMI ≥ 25 kg/m², 35 M and 22 F, mean age: 36.2 Y	Total cholesterol, triacylglycerol, visceral fat, BMI, and systolic blood pressure	→	[16]
	40 subjects with hypertension, mean age: 55 Y	Blood pressure and lipid profiles in hypertensive patients	→	[31]
	Subjects with type 2 diabetes mellitus (DM), age: 48.0–60.1 Y	Fasting glucose level and lipid profiles in diabetic patients	→	[33]
	82 subjects with metabolic syndrome, coronary artery disease, 38 M and 44 F, age: 54 Y	Body weight and BMI	→	[34]
Gut microbiome	30 healthy M subjects, age: 18.63 Y, 27 healthy M subjects, age: 39.9 Y	Gut microbiome diversity in the young cohort. Upregulation of *Lachnospiraceae* and *Ruminococcaceae* in the middle-aged cohort	↑ ↑	[35]
	Nine healthy subjects, 2 M and 7 F, age: 45 Y	*Bacteroidetes* phylum	↑ Beta diversity	[36]
	34 healthy subjects, age range 18–40 Y	*Bacteroidetes* and *Proteobacteria*. *Firmicutes* and *Bacteroidetes*	↑ →	[37]

BMI body mass index, *M* male, *F* female, *Y* years, *NAFLD* nonalcoholic fatty liver disease, *CRP* C-reactive protein, *NR1D1* nuclear receptor subfamily 1 group D member 1, *TFAM* transcription factor A, mitochondrial, *SOD2* superoxide dismutase 2, *Nrf2* nuclear factor erythroid 2–related factor 2, *PRKCSH* protein kinase C substrate 80 K-H

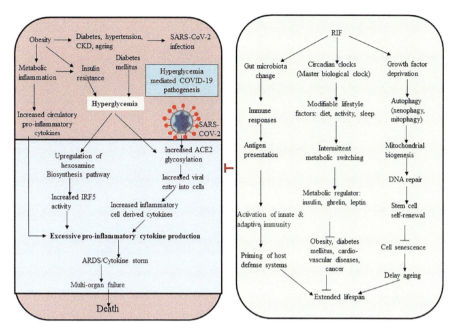

Fig. 5.2 Cellular and molecular mechanisms of RIF as an intervention tool

Ramadan intermittent fasting (RIF) is a potential intervention tool for combating several diseases, including SARS-CoV-2 infection. RIF can prime the immune system by activating several physiological processes, including immune responses and autophagy. In the context of hyperglycemia-mediated coronavirus disease 2019 (COVID-19) pathogenesis, hyperglycemia and poor glycemic control, characterized by insulin resistance, are independently associated with the severity of COVID-19 and increase the risk of mortality. Hyperglycemia is associated with increased severe acute respiratory syndrome coronavirus 2 (SARS-CoV-2) replication in obese diabetic patients, leading to sustained viral proliferation and the induction of a cytokine storm. Furthermore, hyperglycemia may potentiate the glycosylation of the SARS-CoV-2 receptor angiotensin-converting enzyme 2 (ACE2). *Abbreviations: IRF5* interferon regulatory factor-5, a marker of metabolic inflammation of obese individuals, *ARDS* acute respiratory distress syndrome, *BHB* 3-beta-hydroxybutyrate, *AcAc* acetoacetate, *SOD2* superoxide dismutase 2, *HO-1* heme oxygenase 1, *NQO1* NAD(P)H quinone dehydrogenase 1, *LDL* low-density lipoprotein, *CRP-C* C-reactive protein-C, *PKA* protein kinase A, *NGN3* neurogenin-3, *PDX1* insulin promoter factor 1

disrupt circadian metabolic regulation and induce various shift-work-associated diseases. The molecular mechanisms of the circadian rhythmicity, known as the "molecular clock," consist of a series of interlocked transcriptional–translational feedback loops involving clock genes, such as *brain and muscle Arnt-like protein 1 (BMAL1), CLOCK, PER1/2,* and *CRY1/2,* which, in turn, cause oscillations in a myriad of downstream targets. Furthermore, sirtuin 1 (SIRT1) and AMP-activated protein kinase (AMPK) interact with these circadian factors and modulate their activity via inducing autophagy [44, 45]. Table 5.2 displays the impact of RIF on key hormones of the circadian rhythm. The link of RIF to the circadian rhythm alteration is discussed elsewhere in this book.

Table 5.2 Ramadan fasting can affect the circadian rhythms of selected hormones

Hormone	Non-Ramadan	Ramadan
Hormones with a dominant circadian function		
Melatonin	Controls sleep–wake cycle	Reduced level during Ramadan
	Highest from midnight to 8 a.m.	
Cortisol	Stress hormone	Morning to evening ratio reduced to around 1.22
	Peaks in the morning	
	Low at night	
	Morning-to-evening ratio is typically 2.5	
Growth hormone	Pulsatile secretion with higher levels in the morning	Lower levels in the morning and evening
Hormones with a dominant function in controlling food intake		
Leptin	Satiety hormone	Much higher level in the morning
	Higher after meals (BF, L, and din)	Evening levels are similar or reduced compared to non-Ramadan
	Dependent on fat mass and higher in obese individuals	
	Peaks from 10 p.m. to 3 a.m.	
Ghrelin	Hunger hormone	No significant effect on normal-weight individuals
	High before meals (BF, L, and din)	Marked reduction in overweight and obese individuals during the last week of Ramadan
GLP-1	Rises with meals	No studies
	Increases insulin secretion	
	Reduces gastric motility	
	Reduces appetite	

Modified from Ali et al. [17]
BF breakfast, *L* lunch, *Din* dinner

5.3 Ramadan-Induced Autophagy in Human Health and Diseases

Autophagy (Greek for "self-eating")/macro-autophagy is a lysosome-dependent catabolic pathway in which cellular constituents are engulfed by autophagosomes and degraded upon autophagosome fusion with lysosomes. As a major cytoprotective process, autophagy maintains cellular, tissue, and organismal homeostasis and recycles cytoplasmic content for energy production [46] (Table 5.3). Autophagy can be either nonselective ("bulk"), which indiscriminately sequesters and degrades parts of the cytoplasmic content, or "selective" autophagy, which targets specific, often potentially harmful, cargos for degradation. Autophagy-related gene (ATG) products are the key components of autophagy, and more than 40 ATGs in brewer's yeast by genetic screening, and approximately one-half of these genes show clear homology to ATGs in mammals [48]. These *ATG* genes have diverse physiologically important roles in membrane trafficking and signaling pathways [48]. There

Table 5.3 The major actions of autophagy in cellular homeostasis in mammals

Organs	Role(s) of autophagy	
Brain	Regulates food intake, energy balance, and whole-body energy metabolism Controls axonal integrity and neuroprotective effect on neurological diseases	
Immune system	Regulates cytokine production and the development of T and B cells	
Myeloid cells	Modulates inflammasome and cytokine secretion	
Bone	Regulates bone mass and osteoclast and osteocyte function Maintains osteocyte homeostasis	
Heart	Regulates cardiac mitochondrial homeostasis and preserves cardiac structure Controls angiogenesis and prevents age-related dysfunction	
Kidney	Maintains podocyte integrity Maintains proximal tubule cell homeostasis Protects against ischemic injury	
Lung	Regulates the airway's responsiveness	
Adipose tissue	Adipogenesis/adipocyte differentiation	
BAT	Regulates BAT generation and adaptive thermogenesis	
WAT	Regulates insulin sensitivity, inflammation, lipolysis, and differentiation	
Skeletal muscle	Maintains muscle mass and myofiber integritypreserves skeletal muscle function during aging	
Muscles	Regulates the maintenance of muscle mass, positive metabolic effects of exercise, and release of myokines	
Digestive system	Stomach	Regulates gastric mucosal cells
	Intestine	Maintains barrier integrity and preserves intestinal homeostasis Regulates the function of Paneth cells Prevents invasion of pathogens and maintains mucosal immune response
	Liver	Regulates lipolysis, β-oxidation, glycogenolysis, gluconeogenesis, and hepatokine secretion Regulates homeostasis of hepatocytes and prevents hepatocellular degeneration Degrades lipid droplets and suppresses hepatic tumors
	Pancreas	Regulates β-cell mass, insulin content, secretion, and response to cellular stress
Reproductive system	Male	Spermiogenesis and spermiation Testosterone synthesis and acrosome biogenesis Flagella biogenesis and sperm motility Modulates ectoplasmic specialization assembly Maintains normal cytoskeletal organization
	Female	Follicular cell growth and differentiation and the promotion of progesterone synthesis Placentation, oogenesis, and embryogenesis

Modified from Kirat et al. [47]
Abbreviations: *BAT* brown adipose tissue, *WAT* white adipose tissue

are conclusive etiological links existing between mutations in genes that control autophagy (dysregulation of autophagy) and human disease, especially metabolic disorders such as diabetes, atherosclerosis and NAFLD, neurodegeneration, cancer, and aging [49–52], (Table 5.4). For example, autophagy is subjected to a complex regulatory network that involves AMPK and mechanistic target of rapamycin (mTOR) signaling to regulate its initiation, mediated through cellular responses to

Table 5.4 Key autophagy-related gene mutations and human diseases

Gene	Disease
Mutations in genes required for autophagy and lysosomal function	
ATG16L1	Crohn's disease (CD)
ATG16L2	Systemic lupus erythematosus (SLE)
ATG5	Ataxia with developmental delay, systemic sclerosis, SLE
ATG7	Mild-to-severe intellectual disability, ataxia, and tremor
ATP6AP2	X-linked parkinsonism with spasticity and multisystem disorder
Beclin 1 (*BECN1*)	Breast and ovarian cancers
CLEC16A	Diabetes Multiple sclerosis
CTNS	Cystinosis
EPG5	Vici syndrome
GBA	Gaucher's disease and Parkinson's disease (PD)
GRN	Frontotemporal dementia (heterozygous) or neuronal ceroid lipofuscinosis (homozygous)
LAMP2	Danon's cardiomyopathy
PIK3R4 (VPS15)	Cortical atrophy and epilepsy
SNX14	Autosomal recessive spinocerebellar ataxia
SPG11, SPG15 (ZFYVE26), and *SPG49 (TECPR)*	Hereditary spastic paraplegia
WDR45 (WIPI4)	Beta-propeller protein-associated neurodegeneration
Mutations in genes that regulate autophagy and lysosomal function	
APP	Alzheimer's disease
AT-1 (SLC33A1)	Spastic paraplegia Developmental delay Autism spectrum disorders (ASD)
C9orf72	Amyotrophic lateral sclerosis (ALS)frontotemporal dementia (FTD)
ERBB2	Breast cancer
GBA1	Gaucher's disease Parkinson's disease
GPR65	Inflammatory bowel disease (IBD)
Huntingtin (*HTT*)	Huntington's disease
IRGM	Nonalcoholic fatty liver disease (NAFLD)Crohn's disease Tuberculosis
LRRK2	Crohn's disease (CD)Parkinson's disease (PD)
MeCP2	Rett syndrome (X-linked neurodevelopmental disorder)

(continued)

Table 5.4 (continued)

Gene	Disease
MTMR3	Inflammatory bowel disease (IBD)
PLEKHM1	Osteopetrosis
RAB7A	Charcot–Marie–tooth type 2B disease
PS1	Alzheimer's disease
PTPN2	IBD Type 1 diabetes Juvenile arthritis
SMS	Snyder–Robinson syndrome (SRS)
TMEM230	Parkinson's disease
v-ATPase	Autosomal recessive osteoporosis
WASP	Wiskott–Aldrich syndrome
Mutations in genes required for cargo delivery in selective autophagy	
ALFY	Primary microcephaly ASD, schizophrenia, and microcephaly
CALC0C02 (NDP52)	Crohn's disease and AD
FAM134B	Hereditary sensory and autonomic neuropathy type II
FANC	Fanconi anemia (FA) congenital syndrome Hereditary breast and ovarian cancers Sporadic cancers
OPTN1	Amyotrophic lateral sclerosis (ALS) Primary open-angle glaucoma (POAG) Paget's disease of the bone (PGD)
PARK2/Parkin	Autosomal recessive and sporadic early-onset Parkinson's disease Colon, lung, and brain cancers
PARK6/PINK1	Autosomal recessive and sporadic early-onset Parkinson's disease
PEX13	Zellweger spectrum disorders
SQSTM1 (p62)	ALS FTD Paget's disease Distal myopathy
SMURF1	Ulcerative colitis
TBK1	ALS Frontotemporal dementia Other neurodegenerative phenotypes POAG
TRIM20	Familial Mediterranean fever
VPS13D	Ataxia with spasticity

stress conditions, including nutrient deprivation (Fig. 5.1). Fasting hormones, glucagon, and ghrelin enhance autophagy by activating AMPK in different target organs [53, 54]. The satiety hormone, leptin, which plays a cardinal role in the pathophysiology of obesity and diabetes, stimulates autophagy of long-lived proteins in adipocytes by activating AMPK [55]. Figure 5.3 illustrates the effect of RIF on regulating the autophagy pathways.

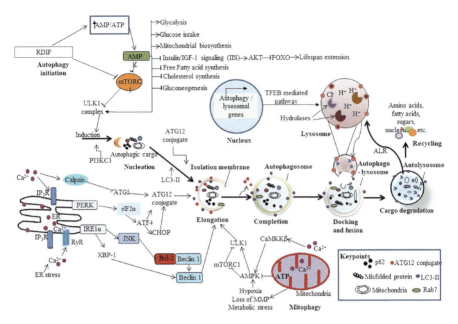

Fig. 5.3 Ramadan intermittent fasting (RIF) mediates the autophagy pathway and its regulation Autophagy receives RIF signals through two metabolic sensors, namely AMPK and mTOR. Under conditions of nutrient deprivation, AMPK is activated, which, in turn, negatively regulates mTOR, as well as directly activates the ULK1 complex, thereby acting as a positive regulator of autophagy. RIF suppresses mTOR and detaches from the ULK1 complex, leading to the activation of autophagy. Beclin 1 complex is another autophagy activator that mTOR negatively regulates. Once autophagy is initiated, the cytoplasmic cargo to be degraded is engulfed into double-membrane vesicles, called autophagosomes, which then fuse with lysosomes to form autolysosomes, where the cargo is degraded. *mTOR* mechanistic target of rapamycin, *AMPK* AMP-activated protein kinase, *RDIF* Ramadan diurnal intermittent fasting. (Modified from Al-Bari et al. [72])

The health benefits of fasting (at least 12 h) result from "flipping the metabolic switch" [56]. During fasting, most tissues utilize fatty acids as their primary source of energy. In contrast, the brain relies on glucose and ketone bodies (KBs), including β-hydroxybutyrate (BHB) and acetoacetate (AcAc), which are produced by hepatocytes from glucose. Thus, ketone bodies serve as crucial alternative energy sources for extrahepatic tissues under various physiological conditions, such as glucose deficiency and fasting, as well as a low-carbohydrate, high-fat ketogenic diet (KD). Ketone bodies (KBs) and KD demonstrate neuroprotective effects by orchestrating various cellular processes through metabolic and signaling functions. Additionally, KBs and KD contribute to reducing neuroinflammation and modulating autophagy, neurotransmission systems, and the gut microbiome [57]. BHB and KD have been shown to stimulate autophagic flux in glucose-starved cultured neurons and hypoglycemic brains.

BHB has been shown to increase NAD^+ levels, stimulating autophagy by activating the SIRT1–AMPK pathway. KBs and KD enhance autophagy through the transcription factor EB (TFEB), a key regulator of lysosomal biogenesis. Autophagy is upregulated in cerebral cortical and cerebellar neurons in response to fasting, and autophagy alters synaptic plasticity and neurogenesis in ways consistent with its involvement in neuronal network adaptations to intermittent metabolic switching [58]. Intriguingly, an 8–12-h IF with a modified diet may be exploited as a protective strategy against SARS-CoV-2 infection [38]. The gut microbiota can directly or indirectly influence host metabolism, cognition, and neuroinflammation by producing microbe-derived metabolites, including short-chain fatty acids (SCFAs), such as acetate, butyrate, and propionate [57]. As a regulator of the gut microbiota, ketone bodies modulate the microbiota and play a crucial role in brain function through the gut–brain axis [57].

Recently, one study investigated the effects of RIF on autophagy gene expression in overweight and obese individuals. The researchers found that 4 weeks of RIF led to significant upregulation of the autophagy genes *LAMP2, LC3B*, and *ATG5*, but not *ATG4D*, compared to pre-fasting levels. These changes were accompanied by reductions in body weight, BMI, and fat mass, as well as several inflammatory markers, along with increases in beneficial markers, such as high-density lipoprotein (HDL) and Interleukin (IL)-10. Interestingly, no significant association was found between high-energy intake, waist circumference, or obesity and the expression of these four autophagy genes. The study suggests that RIF may positively influence metabolic health and aging-related markers, at least partially, through the upregulation of autophagy [59].

Senescence is a hallmark of aging. Cellular senescence is an irreversible arrest of the cell cycle, accompanied by numerous characteristic changes and phenotypes. Accumulation of senescent cells can reduce cellular, tissue, and organ functions, thus leading to age-related morbidities or diseases [60]. Intermittent fasting prolongs lifespan and rejuvenates aged cells [61, 62]. Fasting has been suggested to reduce senescence via its induction of autophagy [63].

5.4   Effect of Gene Variation on Response to RIF

Only a few studies have investigated the changes in metabolic response to RIF based on genetic variation. A previous report showed that individuals who were overweight or obese and had the UCP2 gene with the GG genotype showed greater weight reduction with IF, compared to a low-calorie diet. However, there were no differences in weight loss between the two regimens for those with the AA or GA genotypes [64]. Furthermore, RIF data showed that in overweight and obese people, the Hp phenotype may have an independent impact on how IF affects lipid profiles, serum Hp, CD163, and inflammatory cytokines.

In humans, the acute-phase protein, haptoglobin, gene has two genotypes, Hp1 and Hp2, which give three phenotypes: Hp1-1, Hp2-1, and Hp2-2. Homozygous subjects have type 1 alleles encoding Hp and are characterized by high expression of Hp1-1. The Hp2-2 phenotype is encoded by the homozygous genotype, which only has type 2 alleles. A heterozygous genotype has type 1 and type 2 alleles associated with high expression of Hp2-1. Its structural phenotype determines the properties and functions of haptoglobin [65]. A previous study revealed that obese individuals with the Hp1-1 phenotype experienced a significant reduction in BMI and body weight (BW) in response to RIF, compared to those with the Hp2-2 or Hp2-1 phenotypes. Moreover, there were notable variations in the body weight (BW) change among the Hp phenotypes. The waist circumference reduction in obese individuals with the HP1-1 genotype after RIF was noteworthy, as it differed considerably from that of the Hp2-1 and Hp2-2 groups. The study also revealed that low-density lipoprotein (LDL) and TG significantly decreased in Hp2-2 and Hp2-1 patients in response to RIF. Furthermore, the IF advantages of Hp2-2 persons with overweight/obesity are presumably maximized, whereas participants carrying Hp1-1 and Hp2-1 responded less strongly to RIF with respect to anti-inflammatory effects. Additionally, the mean difference values of serum anti-inflammatory CD163 among Hp phenotypes showed a tendency to increase via Hp1-1, Hp2-1, and Hp2-2 in response to RIF. In contrast to Hp1-1, serum HP had substantially less expression in the Hp2-1 and Hp2-2 phenotypes. Hp2-2 displayed a greater anti-inflammatory response to RIF than Hp1-1 because of the beneficial effects of IF on the development and enhancement of adipocytokine pathways in patients with obesity [66]. According to Harney et al., intermittent fasting, the every-other-day fasting model, improves metabolic profile in mice without causing weight loss.

Paoli et al. (2020) studied a cohort of 107 male Caucasians. It demonstrated that candidate gene polymorphisms could be associated with interindividual variations in response to the sport-fasting protocol (three-phase protocol with gradual caloric restriction with a minimum of 189 kcal/d.) There was an association between the A-allele of the insulin-like growth factor 1 (IGF 1) rs35767 single-nucleotide polymorphism (SNP) with an 8% smaller change in total body mass [67].

At the proteomic level, there were depot-specific alterations in the extracellular matrix composition, inhibition of lipolysis, increased mitochondrial activity, and enhanced fatty acid production. They are also carried out by significantly reducing the catecholamine receptor's abundance (ADRB3). These changes are crucial in maintaining visceral lipid storage during fasting. Furthermore, the downregulation of inflammatory collagen IV in white adipose tissue (vWAT) is highlighted by enrichment analysis, which permits increased insulin sensitivity [68]. Proteomic analysis is conducted in another RIF study, employing tandem mass spectrometry and nano-ultrahigh-performance liquid chromatography. The levels of various tumor suppressor and DNA repair gene protein products (GPPs) were significantly higher than before RIF during the last week of RIF (KIT, CROCC, CALU, PIGR, and INTS6) and a week after RIF (CALU, SEMA4B,

IGFBP4, and CALR). Additionally, RIF upregulates H2B histone proteins as part of an antiaging proteome response during the last week of RIF, as well as a proteome response associated with anti-diabetes, by upregulating key regulatory proteins of insulin signaling at the end of RIF (IGFBP-5, POLRMT, and VPS8) and a week after RIF (PRKCSH). Furthermore, compared to the levels before RIF, they discovered a significant decrease in the levels of tumor promoter GPs during the last week of RIF (CD109, POLK, NIFK, SRGN, and CAMP) and 1 week after RIF (PLAC1 and CAMP) [32]. In the same direction, another study showed that the anticancer serum proteomic signature is associated with RIF by increasing the levels of LATS1, CFHR1, and COLEC10 GPs, which have anti-cancer properties. Conversely, there was a significant reduction of specific proteins that are overexpressed in several cancers, like B4GALT1, ASAP1, FMO5, RRBP1, TNKS2, HUWE1, ARHGEF28, PALB2, SMOC1, IRAK3, and MUC20 GPs. Also, RIF proteomic analysis upregulated key regulatory proteins of glucose and lipid metabolism by increasing the PLIN4, CFL1, and PKM expression, cytoskeleton remodeling, immune system, and cognitive function, metabolic syndrome by enhancing the PM3, TPM4, PLIN4, CFL1, and PKM GP expression, Alzheimer's disease which is associated with upregulation of HOMER1 expression and downregulation of APP and ARPP-21, and SYNE1, circadian clock by increment expression of NR1D1, DNA repair by upregulating expression of CEP164 levels, inflammation, and several neuropsychiatric disorders [69].

Moreover, alterations in the host plasma proteome are observed after 4 weeks of alternating fasting in mice. A significant anti-inflammatory impact of this dietary plan is confirmed by the decreased plasma concentration of acute-phase proteins, HPT, A1AT, SPA, and APO-E [70]. Another study obtained similar findings, investigating the peripheral blood mononuclear cell (PMBC) proteome in participants with metabolic syndrome in response to RIF, which induced an anti-inflammatory and anti-tumorigenic effect, as shown by the upregulation of tumor suppressor effect–associated proteins (TUBB4B, LSP1, and ACTR3B). In contrast, tumor promoter effect–associated proteins (CD36, CALM1, CALM2, CALM3, FLOT2, and PPIF) were downregulated, and differentially expressed lipid and atherosclerosis pathways revealed the anti-atherosclerotic effect was like APOB, HSPA8, CALM1, CALM2, CALM3, and CD36 [71].

5.5   Conclusion and Future Perspectives

Although several meta-analyses have reported weight loss following RIF, a complete weight regain is often observed within a month after Ramadan. Regaining weight after successful weight loss achieved by lifestyle interventions is a major challenge in managing overweight and obesity. Many Muslims engage in unhygienic post-Ramadan feasting. Like fasting, the post-fasting transition enables the body to gradually adjust its circadian rhythm, or body clock, thereby promoting the homeostasis of various bodily organs. Investigating the underlying mechanisms of weight regain can help researchers and clinicians develop effective strategies to address weight regain and mitigate obesity-associated metabolic and cardiovascular complications.

Fasting has long been associated with healthy sleep, as it helps regulate the circadian rhythm, making it easier to fall asleep at night. However, Ramadan-fasting Muslims may develop severe disturbances in sleep and feeding patterns. This can be attributed to the disruption of cortisol's circadian rhythm. This hormone regulates the expression of many other hormones and cytokines, including adipokines, which may simultaneously contribute to insulin resistance.

RIF has also been associated with disrupted circadian rhythms, changes in sleep–wake cycles, and alterations in hormones such as leptin, ghrelin, cortisol, and melatonin. The chrono-hormonal changes, including circadian-related hormones such as cortisol, melatonin, adipokines, resistin, and ghrelin, may significantly influence metabolic homeostasis and promote health. For example, melatonin regulates energy flow by controlling the intensity and circadian distribution of metabolic processes, including the proper synthesis, secretion, and action of insulin and, consequently, glucose homeostasis. These changes are associated with sudden changes in meal timings, diet composition, and sleep continuity during Ramadan, which may interfere with the metabolic impacts of RIF. Thus, increasing the intake of fruits, vegetables, and plant-based proteins is an important factor that could help improve healthy sleep for those observing RIF.

Table 5.5 Clinical trials of observing Ramadan fasting

Identifier	Study type	Study status	Duration (month)	Conditions	Interventions	Sponsor/location
NCT06043843	Intl	R	1	DM	Incidence rate of hypoglycemia	Sengkang General Hospital
NCT04923503	Intl	C	1	DM	Change acylated ghrelin, insulin	Universitas Diponegoro
NCT05331443	Ob	EI	1	Endothelial dysfunction	Reactive hyperemia-peripheral arterial tonometry index (RHI) tonometry	University of Monastir
NCT04862390	Ob	C	1	DM in pregnancy	Hypoglycemia incidence	King Abdullah International Medical Research Center
NCT00429390	Intl	C	1	Metabolic syndrome	Insulin sensitivity in metabolic syndrome	Free Islamic University of Medical Sciences
NCT01148303	Intl	C	1	Headache	Headache diary	Hartford Hospital
NCT01340768	Intl	C	1	Type 2 DM	Symptomatic hypoglycemic event	Merck Sharp & Dohme LLC
NCT03970772	Intl	C	1	Type 1 DM	Hypoglycemic events	Qassim University
NCT06033872	Intl	C	1	DM	Incidence rate of hypoglycemia	Sengkang General Hospital
NCT06105372	Ob	EI	1	Microbiota	Lipid profiles	Okan University
NCT02941367	Intl	C	1	Type 2 DM	Symptomatic hypoglycemia event	Sanofi
NCT05071950	Intl	C	1	DM	Postprandial glucose	University Putra Malaysia
NCT03079050	Intl	C	1	Heartburn	Heartburn relief	American University of Beirut Medical Center
NCT01758380	Intl	C	1	Type 2 DM	Hypoglycemic event	Novartis Pharmaceuticals
NCT01131182	Intl	C	1	Type 2 DM	Symptomatic hypoglycemic event	Merck Sharp & Dohme LLC

(continued)

Table 5.5 (continued)

Identifier	Study type	Study status	Duration (month)	Conditions	Interventions	Sponsor/location
NCT00433082	Intl	C	1	Metabolic syndrome	Measuring inflammatory markers	Free Islamic University of Medical Sciences
NCT05792982	Ob	C	1		FGF-21 levels	Hacettepe University
NCT05827965	Intl	ANR	1	Adrenal insufficiency	Prevalence of complications	Hopital La Rabta
NCT05359302	Ob	R	1	Sleep disorder	Change in sleep quality	University of Monastir
NCT01941238	Ob	C	1	Type 1 DM	Incidence of hypoglycemia	Reem Mohammad Alamoudi
NCT02292290	Intl	C	1	Type 2 DM	Composite	University of Leicester
NCT04804995	Ob	C	1	Headache, migraine	Headache frequency and phenotype	Danish Headache Center
NCT03098381	Ob	C	1		Alteration in body composition	Chulalongkorn University
NCT03314246	Intl	C	1	Type 2 DM	Change in HbA1c	Joyce Lee
NCT04772924	Intl	C	1	Coronary artery disease	Major adverse cardiovascular event	Shiraz University of Medical Sciences
NCT05592524	Ob	C	1	Liver transplantation	Effect of fasting on allograft function	Ain Shams University
NCT02720133	Ob	C	5	Cardiovascular risk factors	Clinical complications	University of Monastir
NCT01354925	Intl	C	1	Type 2 DM	Difference in mean four-point self-monitoring of blood glucose (SMBG)	Meir Medical Center
NCT04135248	Ob	U	1	Type 1 DM	Rate of self-reported hypoglycemia	Dasman Diabetes Institute
NCT02737657	Ob	C	1	Type 2 DM	Episode of hypoglycemia	Janssen-Cilag International NV
NCT00766441	Intl	T	1	DM, hypoglycemia	Occurrence of hypoglycemia	University of Manchester
NCT03988517	Intl	C	1	Hypothyroidism	Change in thyroid stimulating hormone (TSH) level	Hamad Medical Corporation

NCT number	Study type	Status	No.	Condition	Outcome	Institution
NCT05716724	Ob	C	1	Type 2 DM	Change in HbA1c	Novo Nordisk A/S
NCT03585829	Intl	C	1	Corticotropin deficiency	Occurrence of complications	University of Tunis El Manar
NCT05421468	Intl	R	2	Hypothyroidism	Thyroid function, change in TSH level	King Abdullah International Medical Research Center
NCT02499289	Ob	U	1	PCOS	Ovulation monitoring	Ain Shams University
NCT05571891	Ob	C	1	Health	Anthropometric measurements	University of Bari
NCT00757094	Ob	C	2	Chemotherapy, cancer	Safety of chemotherapy	King Fahad Medical City
NCT00263094	Intl	C	1	Headache	Incidence of headache	Sheba Medical Center
NCT04392570	Ob	C	1	Type 2 DM	Serum osmolarities	Istanbul Medeniyet University
NCT01624116	Intl	C	1	Type 2 DM	Change in fructosamine levels	Services Hospital, Lahore
NCT05747352	Ob	C	1	Type 1 DM	Glucose time	Centre Hospitalier Sud Francilien
NCT04237493	Intl	C	1	Type 2 DM	Hypoglycemia	University of Jordan
NCT03501511	Intl	C	1	Type 1 DM	Health education	Ain Shams University
NCT03246711	Ob	C	1	Fetal growth retardation	Fetal growth	Ain Shams Maternity Hospital
NCT04846075	Ob	U	1	Quality of life	Change in serotonin, BDNF, and NGF concentrations	Bastyr University
NCT04864483	Intl	C	1	Type 1 DM	Incidence of early-day hypoglycemia	King Abdullah International Medical Research Center
NCT05918497	Ob	ANR	1	Hypothyroidism	Variability regimen of L-thyroxine	Sohag University
NCT04356898	Ob	C	1	DM	Change in mean glucose level	Imperial College London Diabetes Centre
NCT05287633	Intl	R	1	Dyspepsia	Relief of dyspepsia symptoms	University of Monastir

C completed, *R* recruiting, *EI* enrolling by invitation, *ANR* active not recruiting, *U* unknown, *T* terminated, *Ob* observational, *Intl* interventional, *BDNF* brain-derived neurotrophic factor, *NGF* nerve growth factor, *DM* diabetes mellitus, *PCOS* polycystic ovary syndrome, *HbA1c* glycated hemoglobin

Intriguingly, RIF's recognized and potential health benefits have led to several clinical trials, which are expected to reveal further insights into the clinical and molecular aspects linking fasting to different biological processes (Table 5.5).

References

1. Pinches IJL, Pinches YL, Johnson JO, Haddad NC, Boueri MG, Oke LM, et al. Could "cellular exercise" be the missing ingredient in a healthy life? Diets, caloric restriction, and exercise-induced hormesis. Nutrition. 2022;99–100:111629.
2. Sarker G, Peleg-Raibstein D. Maternal overnutrition induces long-term cognitive deficits across several generations. Nutrients. 2018;11(1):7.
3. Wolfrum C, Peleg-Raibstein D. Maternal overnutrition leads to cognitive and neurochemical abnormalities in C57BL/6 mice. Nutr Neurosci. 2019;22(10):688–99.
4. Panebianco C, Potenza A, Pazienza V. Fasting and engineered diets as a powerful tool in the medical practice: an old approach in the new era. Ann Transl Med. 2017;5(21):429.
5. Tang D, Tang Q, Huang W, Zhang Y, Tian Y, Fu X. Fasting: from physiology to pathology. Adv Sci (Weinh). 2023;10(9):e2204487.
6. Khan MAB, BaHammam AS, Amanatullah A, Obaideen K, Arora T, Ali H, et al. Examination of sleep in relation to dietary and lifestyle behaviors during Ramadan: a multi-national study using structural equation modeling among 24,500 adults amid COVID-19. Front Nutr. 2023;10:1040355.
7. Mendelsohn AR, Larrick JW. Prolonged fasting and refeeding promote hematopoietic stem cell regeneration and rejuvenation. Rejuvenation Res. 2014;17(4):385–9.
8. Tagliafico L, Nencioni A, Monacelli F. Fasting and cognitive impairment. Nutrients. 2023;15:24.
9. Wang X, Yang Q, Liao Q, Li M, Zhang P, Santos HO, et al. Effects of intermittent fasting diets on plasma concentrations of inflammatory biomarkers: a systematic review and meta-analysis of randomized controlled trials. Nutrition. 2020;79–80:110974.
10. Faris ME, Laher I, Khaled MB, Mindikoglu AL, Zouhal H. Editorial: the model of Ramadan diurnal intermittent fasting: unraveling the health implications – Volume I. Front Nutr. 2022;9:971610.
11. Madkour MI, Malhab LJB, Abdel-Rahman WM, Abdelrahim DN, Saber-Ayad M, Faris ME. Ramadan diurnal intermittent fasting is associated with attenuated FTO gene expression in subjects with overweight and obesity: a prospective cohort study. Front Nutr. 2021;8:741811.
12. Jahrami HA, Faris ME, Janahi AI, Janahi MI, Abdelrahim DN, Madkour MI, et al. Does four-week consecutive, dawn-to-sunset intermittent fasting during Ramadan affect cardiometabolic risk factors in healthy adults? A systematic review, meta-analysis, and meta-regression. Nutr Metab Cardiovasc Dis. 2021;31(8):2273–301.
13. Jahrami HA, Alsibai J, Clark CCT, Faris MAE. A systematic review, meta-analysis, and meta-regression of the impact of diurnal intermittent fasting during Ramadan on body weight in healthy subjects aged 16 years and above. Eur J Nutr. 2020;59(6):2291–316.
14. Faris M, Jahrami H, Abdelrahim D, Bragazzi N, BaHammam A. The effects of Ramadan inter-mittent fasting on liver function in healthy adults: a systematic review, meta-analysis, and meta-regression. Diabetes Res Clin Pract. 2021;178:108951.
15. Faris MA-IE, Jahrami HA, Obaideen AA, Madkour MI. Impact of diurnal intermittent fasting during Ramadan on inflammatory and oxidative stress markers in healthy people: systematic review and meta-analysis. J Nutr Intermed Metab. 2019;15:18–26.
16. Faris MA-IE, Madkour MI, Obaideen AK, Dalah EZ, Hasan HA, Radwan H, et al. Effect of Ramadan diurnal fasting on visceral adiposity and serum adipokines in overweight and obese individuals. Diabetes Res Clin Pract. 2019;153:166–75.

17. Ali T, Lessan N. Chrononutrition in the context of Ramadan: potential implications. Diabetes Metab Res Rev. 2024;40(2):e3728.
18. Al-Rawi N, Madkour M, Jahrami H, Salahat D, Alhasan F, BaHammam A, et al. Effect of diurnal intermittent fasting during Ramadan on ghrelin, leptin, melatonin, and cortisol levels among overweight and obese subjects: a prospective observational study. PLoS One. 2020;15(8):e0237922.
19. Gudden J, Arias Vasquez A, Bloemendaal M. The effects of intermittent fasting on brain and cognitive function. Nutrients. 2021;13(9):3166.
20. Fekih S, Zguira MS, Koubaa A, Bettaieb A, Hajji J, Bragazzi NL, et al. Effects of mental training through imagery on the competitive anxiety of adolescent tennis players fasting during Ramadan: a randomized, controlled experimental study. Front Nutr. 2021;8:713296.
21. Wang Y, Wu R. The effect of fasting on human metabolism and psychological health. Dis Markers. 2022;2022:5653739.
22. Madkour MI, El-Serafi AT, Jahrami HA, Sherif NM, Hassan RE, Awadallah S, et al. Ramadan diurnal intermittent fasting modulates SOD2, TFAM, Nrf2, and sirtuins (SIRT1, SIRT3) gene expressions in subjects with overweight and obesity. Diabetes Res Clin Pract. 2019;155:107801.
23. Faris MA, Kacimi S, Al-Kurd RA, Fararjeh MA, Bustanji YK, Mohammad MK, et al. Intermittent fasting during Ramadan attenuates proinflammatory cytokines and immune cells in healthy subjects. Nutr Res (New York, NY). 2012;32(12):947–55.
24. Almeneessier AS, BaHammam AA, Alzoghaibi M, Olaish AH, Nashwan SZ, BaHammam AS. The effects of diurnal intermittent fasting on proinflammatory cytokine levels while controlling for sleep/wake pattern, meal composition, and energy expenditure. PLoS One. 2019;14(12):e0226034.
25. Rahbar AR, Safavi E, Rooholamini M, Jaafari F, Darvishi S, Rahbar A. Effects of intermittent fasting during Ramadan on insulin-like growth Factor-1, interleukin 2, and lipid profile in healthy Muslims. Int J Prev Med. 2019;10:7.
26. Aliasghari F, Izadi A, Gargari BP, Ebrahimi S. The effects of Ramadan fasting on body composition, blood pressure, glucose metabolism, and markers of inflammation in NAFLD patients: an observational trial. J Am Coll Nutr. 2017;36(8):640–5.
27. Akrami Mohajeri F, Ahmadi Z, Hassanshahi G, Akrami Mohajeri E, Ravari A, Ghalebi SR. Dose Ramadan fasting affects inflammatory responses: evidences for modulatory roles of this unique nutritional status via chemokine network. Iran J Basic Med Sci. 2013;16(12):1217–22.
28. Mari A, Khoury T, Baker M, Baker A, Mahamid M. The impact of Ramadan fasting on fatty liver disease severity: a retrospective case-control study from Israel. Isr Med Assoc J. 2021;23(2):94–8.
29. Zouhal H, Bagheri R, Ashtary-Larky D, Wong A, Triki R, Hackney AC, et al. Effects of Ramadan intermittent fasting on inflammatory and biochemical biomarkers in males with obesity. Physiol Behav. 2020;225:113090.
30. Mindikoglu AL, Abdulsada MM, Jain A, Choi JM, Jalal PK, Devaraj S, et al. Intermittent fasting from dawn to sunset for 30 consecutive days is associated with anticancer proteomic signature and upregulates key regulatory proteins of glucose and lipid metabolism, circadian clock, DNA repair, cytoskeleton remodeling, immune system, and cognitive function in healthy subjects. J Proteome. 2020;217:103645.
31. Al-Shafei AI. Ramadan fasting ameliorates arterial pulse pressure and lipid profile and alleviates oxidative stress in hypertensive patients. Blood Press. 2014;23(3):160–7.
32. Mindikoglu AL, Abdulsada MM, Jain A, Jalal PK, Devaraj S, Wilhelm ZR, et al. Intermittent fasting from dawn to sunset for four consecutive weeks induces anticancer serum proteome response and improves metabolic syndrome. Sci Rep. 2020;10(1):18341.
33. Tahapary DL, Astrella C, Kristanti M, Harbuwono DS, Soewondo P. The impact of Ramadan fasting on metabolic profile among type 2 diabetes mellitus patients: a meta-analysis. Diabetes Metab Syndr. 2020;14(5):1559–70.

34. Nematy M, Alinezhad-Namaghi M, Rashed MM, Mozhdehifard M, Sajjadi SS, Akhlaghi S, et al. Effects of Ramadan fasting on cardiovascular risk factors: a prospective observational study. Nutr J. 2012;11:69.
35. Su J, Wang Y, Zhang X, Ma M, Xie Z, Pan Q, et al. Remodeling of the gut microbiome during Ramadan-associated intermittent fasting. Am J Clin Nutr. 2021;113(5):1332–42.
36. Ozkul C, Yalinay M, Karakan T. Structural changes in gut microbiome after Ramadan fasting: a pilot study. Benefic Microbes. 2020;11(3):227–33.
37. Ali I, Liu K, Long D, Faisal S, Hilal MG, Ali I, et al. Ramadan fasting leads to shifts in human gut microbiota structured by dietary composition. Front Microbiol. 2021;12:642999.
38. Soliman S, Faris ME, Ratemi Z, Halwani R. Switching host metabolism as an approach to dampen SARS-CoV-2 infection. Ann Nutr Metab. 2020;76(5):297–303.
39. Bastani A, Rajabi S, Kianimarkani F. The effects of fasting during Ramadan on the concentration of serotonin, dopamine, brain-derived neurotrophic factor and nerve growth factor. Neurol Int. 2017;9(2):7043.
40. Elias A, Padinjakara N, Lautenschlager NT. Effects of intermittent fasting on cognitive health and Alzheimer's disease. Nutr Rev. 2023;81(9):1225–33.
41. Alkurd R, Mahrous L, Zeb F, Khan MA, Alhaj H, Khraiwesh HM, et al. Effect of calorie restriction and intermittent fasting regimens on brain-derived neurotrophic factor levels and cognitive function in humans: a systematic review. Medicina (Kaunas). 2024;60(1):191.
42. Riat A, Suwandi A, Ghashang SK, Buettner M, Eljurnazi L, Grassl GA, et al. Ramadan fasting in Germany (17–18 h/day): effect on cortisol and brain-derived neurotrophic factor in association with mood and body composition parameters. Front Nutr. 2021;8:697920.
43. Faris MA, Jahrami H, BaHammam A, Kalaji Z, Madkour M, Hassanein M. A systematic review, meta-analysis, and meta-regression of the impact of diurnal intermittent fasting during Ramadan on glucometabolic markers in healthy subjects. Diabetes Res Clin Pract. 2020;165:108226.
44. Ajabnoor GM, Bahijri S, Shaik NA, Borai A, Alamoudi AA, Al-Aama JY, et al. Ramadan fasting in Saudi Arabia is associated with altered expression of CLOCK, DUSP, and IL-1alpha genes, as well as changes in cardiometabolic risk factors. PLoS One. 2017;12(4):e0174342.
45. Wu Q, Gao ZJ, Yu X, Wang P. Dietary regulation in health and disease. Signal Transduct Target Ther. 2022;7(1):252.
46. Vargas JNS, Hamasaki M, Kawabata T, Youle RJ, Yoshimori T. The mechanisms and roles of selective autophagy in mammals. Nat Rev Mol Cell Biol. 2023;24(3):167–85.
47. Kirat D, Alahwany AM, Arisha AH, Abdelkhalek A, Miyasho T. Role of macroautophagy in mammalian male reproductive physiology. Cells. 2023;12(9):1322.
48. Liu S, Yao S, Yang H, Liu S, Wang Y. Autophagy: regulator of cell death. Cell Death Dis. 2023;14(10):648.
49. Levine B, Kroemer G. Biological functions of autophagy genes: a disease perspective. Cell. 2019;176(1–2):11–42.
50. Dikic I, Elazar Z. Mechanism and medical implications of mammalian autophagy. Nat Rev Mol Cell Biol. 2018;19(6):349–64.
51. Griffey CJ, Yamamoto A. Macroautophagy in CNS health and disease. Nat Rev Neurosci. 2022;23(7):411–27.
52. Yamamoto H, Zhang S, Mizushima N. Autophagy genes in biology and disease. Nat Rev Genet. 2023;24(6):382–400.
53. Ezquerro S, Frühbeck G, Rodríguez A. Ghrelin and autophagy. Curr Opin Clin Nutr Metab Care. 2017;20(5):402–8.
54. Yanagi S, Sato T, Kangawa K, Nakazato M. The homeostatic force of ghrelin. Cell Metab. 2018;27(4):786–804.
55. Goldstein N, Haim Y, Mattar P, Hadadi-Bechor S, Maixner N, Kovacs P, et al. Leptin stimulates autophagy/lysosome-related degradation of long-lived proteins in adipocytes. Adipocytes. 2019;8(1):51–60.

56. Anton SD, Moehl K, Donahoo WT, Marosi K, Lee SA, Mainous AG 3rd, et al. Flipping the metabolic switch: understanding and applying the health benefits of fasting. Obesity (Silver Spring). 2018;26(2):254–68.
57. Jang J, Kim SR, Lee JE, Lee S, Son HJ, Choe W, et al. Molecular mechanisms of neuroprotection by ketone bodies and ketogenic diet in cerebral ischemia and neurodegenerative diseases. Int J Mol Sci. 2023;25(1):124.
58. Mattson MP, Moehl K, Ghena N, Schmaedick M, Cheng A. Intermittent metabolic switching, neuroplasticity and brain health. Nat Rev Neurosci. 2018;19(2):63–80.
59. Bou Malhab LJ, Madkour MI, Abdelrahim DN, Eldohaji L, Saber-Ayad M, Eid N, et al. Dawn-to-dusk intermittent fasting is associated with overexpression of autophagy genes: a prospective study on overweight and obese cohort. Clin Nutr ESPEN. 2025;65:209–17.
60. Gasek NS, Kuchel GA, Kirkland JL, Xu M. Strategies for targeting senescent cells in human disease. Nat Aging. 2021;1(10):870–9.
61. Mahmoudi S, Xu L, Brunet A. Turning back time with emerging rejuvenation strategies. Nat Cell Biol. 2019;21(1):32–43.
62. Saad R. Effects of intermittent fasting on health, aging, and disease. N Engl J Med. 2020;382(18):1773.
63. Shetty AK, Kodali M, Upadhya R, Madhu LN. Emerging anti-aging strategies – scientific basis and efficacy. Aging Dis. 2018;9(6):1165–84.
64. Mo'ez Al-Islam EF, Jahrami HA, Obaideen AA, Madkour MI. Impact of diurnal intermittent fasting during Ramadan on inflammatory and oxidative stress markers in healthy people: systematic review and meta-analysis. J Nutr Intermed Metab. 2019;15:18–26.
65. Filipek A. Hp1-1 as a genetic marker in diabetes: measures, applications, and correlations. In: Patel VB, Preedy VR, editors. Biomarkers in diabetes. Cham: Springer; 2023. p. 681–701.
66. Madkour MI, Hassan RE, Sherif NM, Awadallah S, Abdelrahim DN, Jahrami HA, et al. Haptoglobin polymorphism modulates cardiometabolic impacts of four consecutive weeks, dawn to sunset Ramadan intermittent fasting among subjects with overweight/obesity. Diabetes Res Clin Pract. 2022;190:110024.
67. Delli Paoli G, van de Laarschot D, Friesema EC, Verkaik R, Giacco A, Senese R, et al. Short-term, combined fasting and exercise improves body composition in healthy males. Int J Sport Nutr Exerc Metab. 2020;30(6):386–95.
68. Harney DJ, Cielesh M, Chu R, Cooke KC, James DE, Stöckli J, et al. Proteomics analysis of adipose depots after intermittent fasting reveals visceral fat preservation mechanisms. Cell Rep. 2021;34(9):108804.
69. Mindikoglu AL, Abdulsada MM, Jain A, Choi JM, Jalal PK, Devaraj S, et al. Intermittent fasting from dawn to sunset for 30 consecutive days is associated with anticancer proteomic signature. It upregulates key regulatory proteins involved in glucose and lipid metabolism, the circadian clock, DNA repair, cytoskeleton remodeling, the immune system, and cognitive function in healthy subjects. J Proteome. 2020;217:103645.
70. Mascaro A, D'Antona G. Proteomic analysis of plasma after 4 weeks of intermittent fasting in mice. Mediterr J Nutr Metab. 2013;6(3):227–32.
71. Mindikoglu AL, Park J, Opekun AR, Abdulsada MM, Wilhelm ZR, Jalal PK, et al. Dawn-to-dusk dry fasting induces anti-atherosclerotic, anti-inflammatory, and anti-tumorigenic proteome in peripheral blood mononuclear cells in subjects with metabolic syndrome. Metabol Open. 2022;16:100214.
72. Al-Bari MAA, Ito Y, Ahmed S, Radwan N, Ahmed HS, Eid N. Targeting autophagy with natural products as a potential therapeutic approach for cancer. Int J Mol Sci. 2021;22(18):9807.

Chapter 6
Ramadan Fasting: Influences on Sleep, Circadian Rhythms, Mealtime, and Metabolic Health

Ahmed S. BaHammam and Shaden O. Qasrawi

Abstract This chapter examines the effects of Ramadan fasting on sleep and metabolic health, focusing on how changes in daily routines during the fasting period influence sleep patterns, sleepiness, circadian rhythms, and metabolism. It discusses the role of altered eating schedules and lifestyle during Ramadan in affecting sleep quality and architecture, noting that these factors, rather than the act of fasting, are likely to cause changes in sleep patterns. The chapter also addresses the importance of maintaining regular routines, such as consistent mealtimes and light exposure, to support the synchronization of the internal clocks of the body and prevent metabolic issues. The text presents findings that suggest that controlled lifestyle factors during Ramadan help preserve the circadian system's integrity. It emphasizes the critical role of meal timing in metabolic health, proposing that adhering to the religious practice of eating around dawn and dusk during Ramadan can enhance metabolic health and stabilize circadian rhythms. The chapter highlights the importance of consistent daily practices during Ramadan to safeguard against sleep disturbances and circadian disruptions and improve the health benefits of the fasting practice. It concludes that well-regulated fasting and lifestyle adjustments during Ramadan can positively impact sleep and metabolic health.

Keywords Intermittent fasting · Dietary patterns · Sleep quality · Lifestyle changes · Biological clocks · Sleepiness

A. S. BaHammam (✉)
Department of Medicine, College of Medicine, University Sleep Disorders Center,
King Saud University, Riyadh, Saudi Arabia

The Strategic Technologies Program of the National Plan for Sciences and Technology and
Innovation in the Kingdom of Saudi Arabia (08-MED511-02), Riyadh, Saudi Arabia
e-mail: ashammam@ksu.edu.sa

S. O. Qasrawi
Sleep Disorders Unit, Kingdom Hospital, Riyadh, Saudi Arabia

M. E. Faris et al. (eds.), *Health and Medical Aspects of Ramadan Intermittent Fasting*, https://doi.org/10.1007/978-981-96-6783-3_6

83

6.1 Introduction

During the month of Ramadan, around 1.5 billion Muslims observe Ramadan globally by engaging in diurnal intermittent fasting from dawn to dusk, which significantly alters their usual dietary patterns and daily schedules [1, 2]. Although Ramadan fasting does not mandate calorie restriction, it significantly changes meal timing and frequency, with most eating happening at night and less often [3]. This behavioral change has prompted scientific inquiry into its potential health effects, providing researchers with a unique opportunity to explore how this mass practice of fasting during Ramadan can physically and behaviorally influence individuals, affecting aspects such as sleep patterns, circadian rhythms, and metabolic processes [1, 2].

It is important to realize that the health effects of Ramadan fasting are not solely due to the act of fasting itself but are also significantly influenced by the lifestyle changes that accompany Ramadan (Fig. 6.1). These include shifts in sleep patterns, meal timings, physical activity levels, and social interactions, all of which

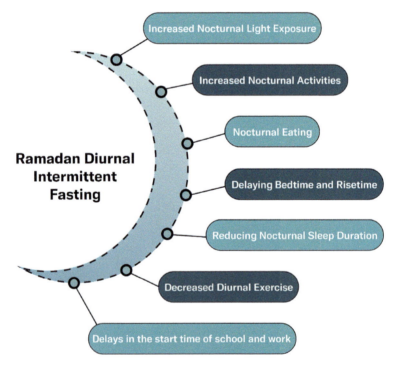

Fig. 6.1 Adjustments in daily routines during Ramadan affecting cardiometabolic risk. This diagram illustrates various daily habit changes that occur during the month of Ramadan, which could potentially impact cardiometabolic health. The month-long observance significantly transforms nocturnal behaviors and routines, such as heightened nocturnal exposure to artificial light, increased after-dark activities, and a shift in eating patterns that now include frequent nighttime meals. These changes may lead to a delay in the typical bedtime, contributing to a reduction in nocturnal sleep duration. Concurrently, daytime physical activity levels often reduce, and often, there is a postponement in the commencement times for schools and workplaces. Together, these shifts in daily life during the observance of Ramadan could influence the cardiometabolic health of individuals

contribute to the overall impact on health outcomes. Despite its significance, this multifaceted aspect may sometimes be overlooked by researchers, leading to a narrow interpretation of the effects of the fasting practice.

In this chapter, we provide a comprehensive overview of the latest and most relevant research exploring the complex relationship between Ramadan fasting and various physiological processes, offering valuable insights into the holistic impact of this practice. We also address the interplay between fasting and the lifestyle changes associated with Ramadan, aiming to provide a comprehensive understanding of their combined influence on health.

6.2   The Effects of Ramadan Intermittent Fasting on Sleep

Studies that investigated the influence of Ramadan fasting on sleep duration, quality, and architecture have yielded heterogeneous outcomes. Some studies report negligible differences in sleep parameters during Ramadan in comparison to control periods, while others document variations such as delayed onset of sleep and wake times.

6.2.1   Sleep Pattern

In certain Islamic nations, the work schedule is adjusted during the month of Ramadan to accommodate the needs of those fasting. Working hours tend to be shorter, and work commencement is postponed [4]. Research conducted across many Islamic countries demonstrated a significant shift in bedtime and wake-up times [5]. Surprisingly, this alteration in bedtime is evident even among non-Muslim residents in Saudi Arabia, even though there are no changes in work timings for non-Muslims, suggesting that lifestyle changes, not fasting, influence the sleeping pattern during Ramadan [6]. While the delayed start of work during Ramadan may contribute to delayed bedtime and rise time during Ramadan, other factors, such as adjusted operating hours for stores, malls, TV programs, and restaurants, as well as late socializing, may also influence this [2, 7].

A recent systematic review included 24 studies involving 646 participants to analyze sleep quality measures, specifically total sleep time (TST) in the free-living environment with no interventions [1]. The meta-analysis revealed that during Ramadan, participants experienced a reduction in TST by approximately 1 h, from an average of 7.2 h per night before Ramadan to 6.4 h. A decrease in sleep duration of 1 h has been reported to be associated with increased metabolic and vascular risks [8, 9]. Subsequently, subgroup analyses were conducted to assess the effects of age, sex, and physical activity levels. The results indicated that TST decreased across all subgroups, with athletes showing a higher overall pooled estimate of TST compared to nonathletes [1]. The effect of Ramadan fasting on TST was moderate, with a Hedges' g value of -0.43, suggesting a medium effect size [1]. The analysis also highlighted that the observed changes in sleep patterns during Ramadan are not solely due to fasting but also due to lifestyle changes associated with the holy month, such as altered mealtimes, social activities, and work schedules. The authors suggest that these lifestyle changes, along with fasting, collectively influence sleep duration and daytime alertness [1].

Another recent systematic review and meta-analysis specifically focused on athletes and physically active individuals during Ramadan, which showed a reduction in sleep duration and quality and an increase in daily nap duration. However, daytime sleepiness levels remained unchanged [10].

The impact of cultural and social activities, such as staying up late because of the nighttime eating schedule or socializing, as well as getting up early for the predawn meal and prayer, can affect both the amount and quality of sleep during Ramadan [10]. This is supported by research in Saudi Arabia [11], which highlighted poor sleep quality and sleep habits during Ramadan, noting that factors like marital status, student status, financial status, and family size have an influence on sleep during this month [11].

A recent Joint Consensus Statement by the Saudi Public Health Authority provided a conditional recommendation for optimal health during Ramadan, suggesting that adults should aim for sufficient nocturnal sleep of 4–6 h, supplemented by a daytime nap of 1.5–2 h [12].

In summary, during Ramadan, adjustments in work and social schedules across Islamic nations lead to notable shifts in sleep patterns for both fasting individuals and non-Muslims, with a decrease in total sleep time and a slight increase in daytime sleepiness. This suggests that lifestyle changes during Ramadan, rather than fasting alone, play a significant role in altering sleep habits, underlining the broader impact of the holy month on daily routines and health.

6.2.2 Daytime Sleepiness

Numerous investigations have explored the impact of Ramadan fasting on daytime drowsiness, employing both subjective measures, like the Epworth Sleepiness Scale (ESS) [6, 13–19], and objective tools, such as the Multiple Sleep Latency Test (MSLT) [16–18]. The findings from these studies present a mixed picture, potentially due to methodological variances, the absence of objective evaluations, or the failure to account for external factors that might influence alertness and cognitive performance during the day. A recent systematic review analyzed 24 studies involving 646 participants to evaluate excessive daytime sleepiness (EDS) during Ramadan [1]. Using the Epworth Sleepiness Scale (ESS) in an unrestricted environment, the review found a slight increase in the ESS score from 6.1 before Ramadan to 7.0 during the holy month, indicating a minor rise in daytime sleepiness.

Subjective evaluations based on the ESS have yielded inconsistent outcomes. While some studies indicate a noticeable rise in daytime drowsiness during Ramadan [13, 15], other studies have not identified any significant changes [6, 14, 16].

Regarding objective assessments, three studies have utilized the MSLT under controlled conditions to measure sleepiness [16–18]. One particular study observed an increase in sleepiness during the 10:00 and 12:00 MSLT naps as Ramadan progressed [18]. It is crucial to acknowledge that this study employed a portable polysomnography device, which necessitated the operator to terminate the test 20 min after it started, irrespective of when sleep commenced. To circumvent this issue, another investigation conducted a standard MSLT in a sleep laboratory [16]. This research found no significant differences in sleep latency, the time it takes to fall asleep, and sleep efficiency between the initial and final weeks of Ramadan, compared to baseline data [16]. Additionally, an analysis of EEG activity during nap times did not show any variance between the baseline and during Ramadan [16].

A third study aimed to objectively determine the effects of Ramadan fasting on daytime sleepiness in eight healthy participants. This was achieved by maintaining a consistent sleep–wake cycle, ensuring a stable caloric intake, and controlling light exposure. The study assessed both MSLT and ESS at four different times: 3 weeks before Ramadan, following a week of Islamic fasting (baseline fasting); 1 week before Ramadan (non-fasting baseline); 2 weeks into Ramadan; and 2 weeks post-Ramadan (recovery phase) [17]. The findings indicated no significant changes in ESS scores across the four periods. Similarly, the MSLT results showed no significant variation in sleep latency across the "non-fasting baseline," "baseline fasting," "Ramadan," and "recovery" phases.

A case-crossover study indicated that under controlled conditions, Islamic intermittent fasting does not impact drowsiness, vigilance, or psychomotor performance, as measured by the Johns Drowsiness Scale; blink total duration; and mean reaction time [20]. The study controlled for factors such as light/dark exposure, caloric intake, sleep/wake schedule, and sleep quality and found no significant changes in these measures during the fasting period, compared to non-fasting times. Another study investigated the impact of diurnal intermittent fasting (DIF) on plasma orexin-A levels, a neurotransmitter associated with wakefulness, and reported that orexin-A levels increased during the daytime fasting hours and decreased at night compared to non-fasting baseline levels, with significant differences observed at several time points throughout the day and night [21]. These results suggest that DIF can enhance alertness during fasting hours, supporting previous findings from animal studies.

In summary, the examination of diurnal intermittent fasting and its influence on daytime sleepiness yields conflicting outcomes attributed to differences in study methods and external lifestyle influences. Controlled studies, meticulously accounting for factors like sleep patterns and duration, caloric intake, and light exposure, generally find no significant increase in sleepiness during fasting periods. This suggests that the impact of fasting on alertness may be minimal when lifestyle factors are consistently maintained, highlighting the complexity of isolating fasting effects from other variables affecting daytime drowsiness.

6.2.3 Sleep Architecture

Four investigations have examined the effects of Ramadan on sleep architecture utilizing polysomnography, with two of them employing unattended polysomnography in participants' homes [22, 23] and the other two conducting attended polysomnography within laboratory settings [16, 17]. When sleep/wake cycles, light exposure, and meal timings were controlled and accounted for, these studies observed no significant alterations in non-rapid eye movement sleep (NREM) sleep stages, arousal index, stage transitions, or cardiorespiratory metrics during Ramadan [16, 17]. However, one study focusing on young athletes found that while sleep duration remained unchanged, the frequency of awakenings experienced a significant increase during Ramadan [22]. This particular study also noted a drastic shift in the primary sleep period from night to daytime, without controlling for daytime napping. This sudden change in sleep schedule and pattern is believed to be responsible for the observed modifications in sleep architecture in this context [24, 25].

A study that accounted for various lifestyle adjustments associated with Ramadan found a decrease in rapid eye movement sleep (REM) sleep during the night compared to baseline levels; however, REM sleep levels normalized post-Ramadan [17]. This reduction in REM sleep during Ramadan has also been documented in three other studies [16, 22, 23]. These results are supported by an animal study that investigated the impact of experimental fasting on sleep architecture, revealing an absence of REM sleep in piglets after 18 hours of fasting, which improved following feeding [26]. Multiple hypotheses have been suggested to account for the reduction in REM sleep observed during fasting periods; however, the exact reasons behind this decrease and the potential clinical consequences remain unclear.

The results have been mixed regarding the impact of fasting during Ramadan on sleep latency. A previous study found a marked rise in the time it takes to fall asleep and a considerable decrease in overall sleep duration [23]. However, the main meal timing in this research, at 11:30 PM, could have affected the onset of sleep. On the other hand, subsequent research, which offered meals earlier in the evening (3–3.5 hours before sleep) and prohibited naps during the day, observed no notable alteration in the time it takes to fall asleep [16, 17]. These insights suggest that when meals are scheduled for early evening and daytime naps are avoided, intermittent fasting has minimal impact on sleep architecture, aside from reducing REM sleep. However, in environments where meal timings and daytime napping are not regulated, as is often the case during Ramadan, sleep latency and overall sleep architecture may be adversely affected.

In summary, studies on the effects of Ramadan fasting on sleep architecture reveal no significant changes in various sleep metrics when lifestyle factors are controlled. However, variations were noted in REM sleep reduction and sleep latency, influenced by meal timings and napping habits. These findings suggest that while fasting itself has minimal impact on sleep architecture, except for a decrease in REM sleep, unregulated mealtimes, increased nocturnal light exposure, and daytime napping during Ramadan can lead to alterations in sleep patterns.

6.3 Biological Clocks and Circadian Rhythm

6.3.1 Biological Clocks

Every organ, tissue, and cell within our bodies operates on a circadian rhythm, guided not only by the central biological clock located in the suprachiasmatic nucleus (SCN) in the hypothalamus but also by peripheral biological clocks inherent to each cell. These peripheral clocks ensure that our entire body works in a coordinated manner, adapting physiological functions and gene expression to the near-24-h cycle that defines our internal timekeeping system [27, 28]. Essential for our health and well-being, these rhythms rely on external cues—such as light, which directly influences the SCN central clock, and factors including meal timings and hormones—to synchronize the activities of the peripheral clocks [29–33].

Optimal metabolic function necessitates that the central clock is in sync with the external environment, with light exposure playing a pivotal role in signaling the day-to-night transitions essential for regulating processes like glucose metabolism [30]. Simultaneously, the harmony between the central clock and the cell-specific peripheral clocks, which is significantly influenced by the timing of meals, is critical for managing metabolic functions and insulin secretion, crucial for maintaining energy balance [34–41].

Disruptions in the alignment between these internal clocks and external factors—due to irregular patterns of light exposure or inconsistent eating schedules—can lead to a cascade of health issues, including metabolic dysfunctions, heightened risk for diseases such as nonalcoholic fatty liver disease, obesity, and a spectrum of cardiometabolic diseases [42–48]. This misalignment emphasizes the critical importance of consistent daily routines involving regular light exposure and meal timings to ensure that the internal biological clocks are synchronized with the natural environment.

This intricate relationship between light exposure, meal timing, hormonal signals, and the synchronization between central and peripheral clocks underlines the necessity of a harmonized circadian system for optimal metabolic function. Maintaining synchronized daily routines is vital for minimizing health risks associated with circadian rhythm misalignments. Further research is essential to deepen our understanding of the long-term effects of circadian disruptions and find effective strategies for mitigating their adverse impacts on health [49, 50].

6.3.2 The Impact of Ramadan Intermittent Fasting on Circadian Rhythm

During Ramadan, fasting individuals typically adjust their mealtimes to after sunset, consuming breakfast at sunset and a predawn meal, potentially affecting their circadian rhythms and biological clocks. Evidence suggests that consuming high-calorie meals at unusual times may disrupt the alignment between the body's central and peripheral clocks, impacting metabolism and possibly leading to weight gain [25, 51, 52]. However, the effect of Ramadan fasting on circadian rhythms varies across studies, which fall into two categories: [1] those conducted in a free-living environment without control for lifestyle variables [3, 6, 53] and [2] those that account for changes in sleep patterns, diet, and light exposure during Ramadan [16, 54–56].

Research in the free-living setting indicates shifts in circadian rhythms during Ramadan, with alterations in body temperature and melatonin levels showing a delayed pattern [57, 58]. For instance, body temperature rhythms were observed to reverse, with notable temperature drops during the day and increases at night [58]. Similarly, melatonin levels exhibited a delayed peak and a flattened slope [57]. These findings suggest that factors beyond meal timing shifts contribute to changes in circadian rhythms during Ramadan [53].

Contrastingly, studies that controlled for lifestyle modifications during Ramadan revealed no significant shifts in circadian rhythms, suggesting that the previously observed changes might primarily reflect lifestyle adjustments associated with the fasting month [59]. For example, a study adjusting for sleep and meal timings found no significant impact of diurnal intermittent fasting on the melatonin circadian pattern [54]. This indicates that the synchronization between central and peripheral clocks, crucial for metabolic function, remains intact when lifestyle factors are consistent.

Furthermore, the circadian patterns of leptin and ghrelin, hormones influenced by fasting, meal timings, and sleep, were examined. While one study reported a significant delay in leptin levels in a free-living setting [60], controlled studies found no changes in the circadian rhythms of leptin or ghrelin, highlighting the importance of controlling for external factors to assess the impact of Ramadan fasting on these hormones accurately [55].

In summary, while Ramadan fasting introduces changes in meal patterns that could impact circadian rhythms, controlled studies reveal that these rhythms remain stable when lifestyle factors are consistently managed. This suggests that under controlled conditions, Ramadan fasting does not adversely affect the circadian system, emphasizing the importance of maintaining synchronized daily routines to safeguard health against circadian misalignments.

6.4   Mealtime and Metabolism

Growing research underscores the crucial role of meal timing in regulating metabolism and its significant interaction with the body's circadian rhythm [61]. Chrononutrition, an emerging field, explores the relationship between meal timing, circadian rhythms, and metabolic control [62] (Fig. 6.2). Recent studies suggest that the timing of meals affects the circadian rhythm, metabolic processes, and body weight management [30]. Eating at inappropriate times can cause a mismatch between the body's peripheral clocks and

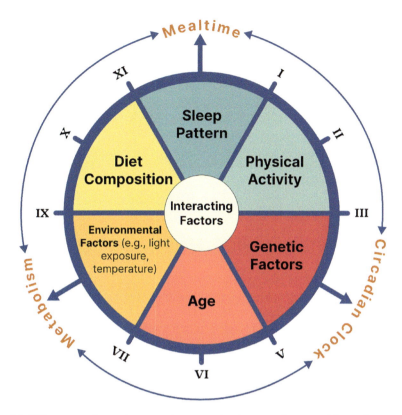

Fig. 6.2 This presentation underscores the connection between chrononutrition and a range of influencing factors. Chrononutrition, an advancing field of investigation, explores the detailed association between the timing of meals, circadian rhythms, and metabolic functions. However, determining the impact of chrononutrition becomes complex due to the multitude of interacting variables. These variables cover an individual's chronotype, lifestyle factors including shift work, disturbances in sleep patterns, the makeup and size of meals, the degree of physical activity, environmental influences such as light exposure at night, and age and genetic determinants

the central biological clock in the SCN, raising the risk of cardiometabolic diseases [29, 61]. In nocturnal animals like mice, which consume the majority of their food at night (70–80% during the dark phase), shifting food intake to their inactive daylight hours leads to weight gain and disrupts the alignment between their internal clocks [63, 64]. Studies have found that limiting food intake to the active phase can protect against weight gain and metabolic syndrome, highlighting the importance of meal timing beyond just calorie restriction [65, 66].

Human studies mirror these findings, with late-night eating linked to a higher risk of cardiometabolic issues [29]. A large Swedish study found a significant association between late-night eating and increased obesity risk [67], and a systematic review confirmed the adverse effects of late meal timing on weight and metabolism [68]. Late meal timing has also been associated with increased blood sugar levels and diabetes risk [68].

In shift workers, night eating correlates with metabolic problems. Research on female nurses showed that meals consumed at night led to higher blood sugar and insulin levels, compared to those eaten during the day [69]. A study on nonobese males demonstrated similar increases in blood sugar and fats after nighttime meals [70].

Experiments on restricted eating periods—limiting food intake to daytime—have shown benefits, such as weight loss and improved metabolic markers, compared to unrestricted eating [71]. Early time-restricted eating (TRE), aligning mealtimes with human circadian rhythms, has improved blood pressure, reduced oxidative stress, and enhanced insulin sensitivity, illustrating the potential health benefits of synchronizing meal timing with our natural biological rhythms [72–74].

6.4.1   Ramadan Fasting, Mealtime, and Metabolism

Given this context, could it be hypothesized that altering eating schedules to nighttime during Ramadan might have detrimental effects? Such a hypothesis contradicts the current body of data and systematic reviews, which highlight the beneficial impacts of diurnal intermittent fasting during Ramadan on metabolic health [5, 48, 50, 75–79]. Current evidence indicates that people who fast from dawn to sunset display two high points (acrophases) in cortisol levels at both dawn and dusk, in contrast to those who do not fast and experience just one high point [57].

Glucocorticoids are pivotal in synchronizing both the peripheral body clocks and the central SCN clock with the day–night cycle, serving as vital timing markers. They ensure that the peripheral oscillators are correctly aligned with the light–dark (LD) cycle, a mechanism especially critical in mitigating desynchronization risks that arise from alternating fasting and refeeding patterns [30, 80]. Their role extends to preventing sudden shifts in the timing of these peripheral clocks within the circadian rhythm, particularly important through sequences of fasting and subsequent refeeding that could otherwise disrupt clock harmony [81]. Therefore, having two peaks of cortisol during Ramadan fasting at dawn and dusk may help synchronize the peripheral clocks with the central clock, which is proposed as one of the mechanisms to explain the beneficial effects of Ramadan fasting on metabolic health [30, 82, 83].

Current evidence indicates that eating meals just before dawn and right after dusk helps the biphasic cortisol circadian rhythm synchronize the peripheral clocks with the central clock [30]. This ensures that they work together, preventing any timing differences between the central and peripheral clocks. The link between meal timing and daily cortisol changes has been documented, pointing to both adrenal and non-adrenal influences [84]. By aligning meals with dawn and dusk, the fasting-induced dual-phase cortisol rhythm aids in coordinating the timing between the peripheral and central clocks, thus maintaining harmony and avoiding misalignments and, hence, metabolic derangements [83]. However, to explore the impact of this meal timing on people with chronic metabolic diseases and metabolic syndrome more deeply, randomized controlled trials are needed. These trials should use a comprehensive multi-omics approach, including studies on circadian gene expression, metabolomics, and proteomics.

Therefore, changing Ramadan nights to an open buffet or random eating and drinking patterns, along with not scheduling meals in sync with dawn and dusk, can disrupt the synchrony between peripheral clocks in the body and the central clock within the SCN. However, eating main meals at dawn and dusk is likely to regulate the circadian oscillators that are specifically responsive to the light at dawn and dusk. Adopting a fasting regimen from dawn to dusk, where meals are consumed shortly before starting the fast (predawn) and immediately after it ends (dusk) over several consecutive days, could effectively serve as a strong cue for realigning meal timings with the natural cycles of dawn and dusk [83]. Such alignment of eating schedules with dawn and dusk is likely to resynchronize the rhythm of peripheral clocks with the central clock in the SCN (leading to a uniform circadian timing after the fasting period), thus normalizing the circadian phase and enhancing the regularity and intensity of mRNA oscillations (and therefore, protein synthesis) [30].

Recently, we cautioned against the disruptions to circadian rhythms caused by delaying school and office timings during Ramadan, drawing parallels to the well-documented negative health impacts of Daylight Saving Time (DST) [4, 85, 86]. The argument is that such practices could undermine the health benefits of fasting during Ramadan by disturbing the body's internal clock, echoing widespread scientific consensus against DST due to its adverse effects on cardiometabolic and immune functions [4]. Advocating for a fixed year-round schedule aligned with human circadian biology underscores the necessity of further research to fully grasp the health and safety implications of timing adjustments during Ramadan. This stance is reinforced by the growing movement to abolish DST in favor of promoting public health and safety.

A recent Joint Consensus Statement by the Saudi Public Health Authority provided a conditional recommendation for optimal health during Ramadan: To maintain circadian rhythm and sleep quality, it is recommended to limit food intake to two main meals at night, one at sunset and another before dawn, with an optional snack in between, if needed [12].

In summary, the evidence suggests that timing meals just before and after fasting from dawn to dusk during Ramadan generates a dual-peak cortisol pattern, crucial for syncing the peripheral clocks with its central clock. This synchronization ensures consistent timing across the circadian system, avoiding misalignments between the peripheral clocks and the central brain clock. Essentially, this practice underscores the value of traditional Ramadan fasting rituals in maintaining circadian harmony, highlighting the risks of deviating toward nocturnal eating or irregular meal timings. By aligning mealtimes with natural light cycles, leveraging glucocorticoids for synchronization, such fasting practices affirm the role of dietary timing in enhancing overall metabolic health and circadian rhythm stability.

6.5 Conclusion

During Ramadan, changes are not limited to when and how much people eat but also affect their entire daily routine, including sleep schedules and social behaviors. This widespread alteration in lifestyle during Ramadan provides a unique opportunity to study the effects of fasting and lifestyle changes on human health. Research has shown varied effects on sleep quality and duration during Ramadan, with some people experiencing a shift delay in their sleep patterns and others seeing little to no change. These discrepancies emphasize the role of individual differences and the influence of lifestyle adjustments beyond fasting itself. Furthermore, the relationship between meal timings during Ramadan and metabolic health underscores the importance of aligning eating schedules with natural circadian rhythms. Properly timed meals can help synchronize the central and peripheral clocks of the body, contributing to better metabolic outcomes and overall health.

In conclusion, Ramadan fasting presents a complex interplay between fasting, sleep, and metabolism, significantly influenced by lifestyle changes during the holy month. The findings underscore the necessity of maintaining regular routines and meal timings to minimize health risks and enhance the benefits of Ramadan fasting on the body's circadian rhythm and metabolic health. This holistic approach to understanding the impact of Ramadan offers valuable insights into the benefits of fasting and lifestyle regulation for health and well-being.

Acknowledgments We extend our gratitude to Abdulrahman A. Bahammam for his artistic contributions to Figs. 6.1 and 6.2.

References

1. Faris MAE, Jahrami HA, Alhayki FA, Alkhawaja NA, Ali AM, Aljeeb SH, et al. Effect of diurnal fasting on sleep during Ramadan: a systematic review and meta-analysis. Sleep Breath. 2020;24(2):771–82.
2. Qasrawi SO, Pandi-Perumal SR, BaHammam AS. The effect of intermittent fasting during Ramadan on sleep, sleepiness, cognitive function, and circadian rhythm. Sleep Breath. 2017;21(3):577–86.
3. Alzhrani A, Alhussain MH, BaHammam AS. Changes in dietary intake, chronotype and sleep pattern upon Ramadan among healthy adults in Jeddah, Saudi Arabia: a prospective study. Front Nutr. 2022;9:966861.
4. Bahammam AS, Pirzada AR. Delaying school and office timings during Ramadhan: boon or bane? Ann Thorac Med. 2021;16(1):1–3.
5. Almeneessier AS, Pandi-Perumal SR, BaHammam AS. Intermittent fasting, insufficient sleep, and circadian rhythm: interaction and effects on the cardiometabolic system. Curr Sleep Med Rep. 2018;4:179–95.
6. BaHammam A. Assessment of sleep patterns, daytime sleepiness, and chronotype during Ramadan in fasting and nonfasting individuals. Saudi Med J. 2005;26(4):616–22.
7. Bahammam A. Does Ramadan fasting affect sleep? Int J Clin Pract. 2006;60(12):1631–7.

8. Li W, Wang D, Cao S, Yin X, Gong Y, Gan Y, et al. Sleep duration and risk of stroke events and stroke mortality: a systematic review and meta-analysis of prospective cohort studies. Int J Cardiol. 2016;223:870–6.
9. Wang X, Sparks JR, Bowyer KP, Youngstedt SD. Influence of sleep restriction on weight loss outcomes associated with caloric restriction. Sleep. 2018;41(5)
10. Trabelsi K, Ammar A, Glenn JM, Boukhris O, Khacharem A, Bouaziz B, et al. Does observance of Ramadan affect sleep in athletes and physically active individuals? A systematic review and meta-analysis. J Sleep Res. 2022;31(3):e13503.
11. Al Harbi KM, Alsaleem LS, Alsaidan AI, Almalki BS, Qutub R, Alammari Y. Quality of sleep in the Saudi population during the holy month of Ramadan. Cureus. 2023;15(12):e50897.
12. Alfawaz RA, Aljuraiban GS, AlMarzooqi MA, Alghannam AF, BaHammam AS, Dobia AM, et al. The recommended amount of physical activity, sedentary behavior, and sleep duration for healthy Saudis: a joint consensus statement of the Saudi public health authority. Ann Thorac Med. 2021;16(3):239–44.
13. Taoudi Benchekroun M, Roky R, Toufiq J, Benaji B, Hakkou F. Epidemiological study: chronotype and daytime sleepiness before and during Ramadan. Therapie. 1999;54(5):567–72.
14. Margolis SA, Reed RL. Effect of religious practices of Ramadan on sleep and perceived sleepiness of medical students. Teach Learn Med. 2004;16(2):145–9.
15. Bahammam. Sleep pattern, daytime sleepiness, and eating habits during the month of Ramadan. Sleep Hypnosis. 2003;5:165–74.
16. Bahammam. Effect of fasting during Ramadan on sleep architecture, daytime sleepiness and sleep pattern. Sleep Biol Rhythm. 2004;2:2.
17. Bahammam AS, Almushailhi K, Pandi-Perumal SR, Sharif MM. Intermittent fasting during Ramadan: does it affect sleep? J Sleep Res. 2014;23(1):35–43.
18. Roky R, Chapotot F, Benchekroun MT, Benaji B, Hakkou F, Elkhalifi H, et al. Daytime sleepiness during Ramadan intermittent fasting: polysomnographic and quantitative waking EEG study. J Sleep Res. 2003;12(2):95–101.
19. Bahammam AS, Alaseem AM, Alzakri AA, Sharif MM. The effects of Ramadan fasting on sleep patterns and daytime sleepiness: an objective assessment. J Res Med Sci. 2013;18(2):127–31.
20. Bahammam AS, Nashwan S, Hammad O, Sharif MM, Pandi-Perumal SR. Objective assessment of drowsiness and reaction time during intermittent Ramadan fasting in young men: a case-crossover study. Behav Brain Funct. 2013;9(1):32.
21. Almeneessier AS, Alzoghaibi M, BaHammam AA, Ibrahim MG, Olaish AH, Nashwan SZ, et al. The effects of diurnal intermittent fasting on the wake-promoting neurotransmitter orexin-a. Ann Thorac Med. 2018;13(1):48–54.
22. Chamari K, Briki W, Farooq A, Patrick T, Belfekih T, Herrera CP. Impact of Ramadan intermittent fasting on cognitive function in trained cyclists: a pilot study. Biol Sport. 2016;33(1):49–56.
23. Roky R, Chapotot F, Hakkou F, Benchekroun MT, Buguet A. Sleep during Ramadan intermittent fasting. J Sleep Res. 2001;10(4):319–27.
24. Fond G, Macgregor A, Leboyer M, Michalsen A. Fasting in mood disorders: neurobiology and effectiveness. A review of the literature. Psychiatry Res. 2013;209(3):253–8.
25. Oosterman JE, Kalsbeek A, la Fleur SE, Belsham DD. Impact of nutrients on circadian rhythmicity. Am J Physiol Regul Integr Comp Physiol. 2015;308(5):R337–50.
26. Oike H, Oishi K, Kobori M. Nutrients, clock genes, and Chrononutrition. Curr Nutr Rep. 2014;3(3):204–12.
27. Rumanova VS, Okuliarova M, Foppen E, Kalsbeek A, Zeman M. Exposure to dim light at night alters daily rhythms of glucose and lipid metabolism in rats. Front Physiol. 2022;13:973461.
28. Van Laake LW, Lüscher TF, Young ME. The circadian clock in cardiovascular regulation and disease: lessons from the Nobel prize in physiology or medicine 2017. Eur Heart J. 2018;39(24):2326–9.
29. St-Onge MP, Ard J, Baskin ML, Chiuve SE, Johnson HM, Kris-Etherton P, et al. Meal timing and frequency: implications for cardiovascular disease prevention: a scientific statement from

the American Heart Association. Circulation. 2017;135(9):e96–e121. https://doi.org/10.1161/CIR.0000000000000476.

30. BaHammam AS, Pirzada A. Timing matters: the interplay between early mealtime, circadian rhythms, gene expression, circadian hormones, and metabolism-a narrative review. Clocks Sleep. 2023;5(3):507–35.

31. Manella G, Bolshette N, Golik M, Asher G. Input integration by the circadian clock exhibits nonadditivity and fold-change detection. Proc Natl Acad Sci USA. 2022;119(44):e2209933119.

32. Ripperger JA, Schibler U. Rhythmic CLOCK-BMAL1 binding to multiple E-box motifs drives circadian Dbp transcription and chromatin transitions. Nat Genet. 2006;38(3):369–74.

33. Zelinski EL, Deibel SH, McDonald RJ. The trouble with circadian clock dysfunction: multiple deleterious effects on the brain and body. Neurosci Biobehav Rev. 2014;40:80–101.

34. Aschoff J, von Goetz C, Wildgruber C, Wever RA. Meal timing in humans during isolation without time cues. J Biol Rhythm. 1986;1(2):151–62.

35. Crespo M, Leiva M, Sabio G. Circadian clock and liver cancer. Cancers (Basel). 2021;13(14)

36. Daan S, Albrecht U, van der Horst GT, Illnerova H, Roenneberg T, Wehr TA, et al. Assembling a clock for all seasons: are there M and E oscillators in the genes? J Biol Rhythm. 2001;16(2):105–16.

37. Froy O, Garaulet M. The circadian clock in white and brown adipose tissue: mechanistic, endocrine, and clinical aspects. Endocr Rev. 2018;39(3):261–73.

38. Hira T, Trakooncharoenvit A, Taguchi H, Hara H. Improvement of glucose tolerance by food factors having glucagon-like Peptide-1 releasing activity. Int J Mol Sci. 2021;22(12)

39. Sinturel F, Gos P, Petrenko V, Hagedorn C, Kreppel F, Storch KF, et al. Circadian hepatocyte clocks keep synchrony in the absence of a master pacemaker in the suprachiasmatic nucleus or other extrahepatic clocks. Genes Dev. 2021;35(5–6):329–34.

40. Stenvers DJ, Jongejan A, Atiqi S, Vreijling JP, Limonard EJ, Endert E, et al. Diurnal rhythms in the white adipose tissue transcriptome are disturbed in obese individuals with type 2 diabetes compared with lean control individuals. Diabetologia. 2019;62(4):704–16.

41. Jakubowicz D, Rosenblum RC, Wainstein J, Twito O. Influence of fasting until noon (extended Postabsorptive state) on clock gene mRNA expression and regulation of body weight and glucose metabolism. Int J Mol Sci. 2023;24(8)

42. Lajoie P, Aronson KJ, Day A, Tranmer J. A cross-sectional study of shift work, sleep quality and cardiometabolic risk in female hospital employees. BMJ Open. 2015;5(3):e007327. https://doi.org/10.1136/bmjopen-2014-.

43. Nagata C, Tamura T, Wada K, Konishi K, Goto Y, Nagao Y, et al. Sleep duration, nightshift work, and the timing of meals and urinary levels of 8-isoprostane and 6-sulfatoxymelatonin in Japanese women. Chronobiol Int. 2017;34(9):1187–96.

44. Wang F, Zhang L, Zhang Y, Zhang B, He Y, Xie S, et al. Meta-analysis on night shift work and risk of metabolic syndrome. Obes Rev. 2014;15(9):709–20. https://doi.org/10.1111/obr.12194.

45. Perez-Diaz-Del-Campo N, Castelnuovo G, Caviglia GP, Armandi A, Rosso C, Bugianesi E. Role of circadian clock on the pathogenesis and lifestyle management in non-alcoholic fatty liver disease. Nutrients. 2022;14(23)

46. Reutrakul S, Knutson KL. Consequences of circadian disruption on cardiometabolic health. Sleep Med Clin. 2015;10(4):455–68. https://doi.org/10.1016/j.jsmc.2015.07.005.

47. Saran AR, Dave S, Zarrinpar A. Circadian rhythms in the pathogenesis and treatment of fatty liver disease. Gastroenterology. 2020;158(7):1948–66 e1.

48. Alasmari AA, Al-Khalifah AS, BaHammam AS, Alshiban NMS, Almnaizel AT, Alodah HS, et al. Ramadan fasting model exerts hepatoprotective, anti-obesity, and anti-hyperlipidemic effects in an experimentally-induced nonalcoholic fatty liver in rats. Saudi J Gastroenterol. 2024;30(1):53–62.

49. Arble DM, Bass J, Behn CD, Butler MP, Challet E, Czeisler C, et al. Impact of sleep and circadian disruption on energy balance and diabetes: a summary of workshop discussions. Sleep. 2015;38(12):1849–60. https://doi.org/10.5665/sleep.226.

50. BaHammam AS, Almeneessier AS. Recent evidence on the impact of Ramadan diurnal intermittent fasting, mealtime, and circadian rhythm on Cardiometabolic risk: a review. Front Nutr. 2020;7:28.
51. Garaulet M, Gomez-Abellan P. Timing of food intake and obesity: a novel association. Physiol Behav. 2014;134:44–50.
52. Bandin C, Scheer FA, Luque AJ, Avila-Gandia V, Zamora S, Madrid JA, et al. Meal timing affects glucose tolerance, substrate oxidation and circadian-related variables: a randomized, crossover trial. Int J Obes. 2015;39(5):828–33.
53. BaHammam A, Alrajeh M, Albabtain M, Bahammam S, Sharif M. Circadian pattern of sleep, energy expenditure, and body temperature of young healthy men during the intermittent fasting of Ramadan. Appetite. 2010;54(2):426–9.
54. Almeneessier AS, Bahammam AS, Sharif MM, Bahammam SA, Nashwan SZ, Pandi Perumal SR, et al. The influence of intermittent fasting on the circadian pattern of melatonin while controlling for caloric intake, energy expenditure, light exposure, and sleep schedules: a preliminary report. Ann Thorac Med. 2017;12(3):183–90.
55. Alzoghaibi MA, Pandi-Perumal SR, Sharif MM, BaHammam AS. Diurnal intermittent fasting during Ramadan: the effects on leptin and ghrelin levels. PLoS One. 2014;9(3):e92214.
56. Bahammam A. Intermittent fasting does not influence the circadian pattern of melatonin when controlling for meals, light exposure and sleep schedules. Sleep Med. 2013;14:e68.
57. Bogdan A, Bouchareb B, Touitou Y. Ramadan fasting alters endocrine and neuroendocrine circadian patterns. Meal-time as a synchronizer in humans? Life Sci. 2001;68(14):1607–15.
58. Roky R, Iraki L, HajKhlifa R, Lakhdar Ghazal N, Hakkou F. Daytime alertness, mood, psychomotor performances, and oral temperature during Ramadan intermittent fasting. Ann Nutr Metab. 2000;44(3):101–7.
59. Almeneessier AS, BaHammam AS. How does diurnal intermittent fasting impact sleep, daytime sleepiness, and markers of the biological clock? Curr Insights Nat Sci Sleep. 2018;10:439–52.
60. Kotrbacek V, Schweigel M, Honig Z. The effect of short-term fasting on sleep in pigs. Vet Med (Praha). 1990;35(9):547–52.
61. Kessler K, Pivovarova-Ramich O. Meal timing, aging, and metabolic health. Int J Mol Sci. 2019;20(8):1911. https://doi.org/10.3390/ijms20081911.
62. Pot GK. Chrono-nutrition – an emerging, modifiable risk factor for chronic disease? Nutr Bull. 2021;46(2):114–9. https://doi.org/10.1111/nbu.12498.
63. Damiola F, Le Minh N, Preitner N, Kornmann B, Fleury-Olela F, Schibler U. Restricted feeding uncouples circadian oscillators in peripheral tissues from the central pacemaker in the suprachiasmatic nucleus. Genes Dev. 2000;14(23):2950–61.
64. Yasumoto Y, Hashimoto C, Nakao R, Yamazaki H, Hiroyama H, Nemoto T, et al. Short-term feeding at the wrong time is sufficient to desynchronize peripheral clocks and induce obesity with hyperphagia, physical inactivity and metabolic disorders in mice. Metabolism. 2016;65(5):714–27.
65. Chaix A, Zarrinpar A, Miu P, Panda S. Time-restricted feeding is a preventative and therapeutic intervention against diverse nutritional challenges. Cell Metab. 2014;20(6):991–1005.
66. Hatori M, Vollmers C, Zarrinpar A, DiTacchio L, Bushong EA, Gill S, et al. Time-restricted feeding without reducing caloric intake prevents metabolic diseases in mice fed a high-fat diet. Cell Metab. 2012;15(6):848–60.
67. Berg C, Lappas G, Wolk A, Strandhagen E, Toren K, Rosengren A, et al. Eating patterns and portion size associated with obesity in a Swedish population. Appetite. 2009;52(1):21–6. https://doi.org/10.1016/j.appet.2008.07.008.
68. Beccuti G, Monagheddu C, Evangelista A, Ciccone G, Broglio F, Soldati L, et al. Timing of food intake: sounding the alarm about metabolic impairments? A Syst Rev Pharmacol Res. 2017;125(Pt B):132–41. https://doi.org/10.1016/j.phrs.2017.09.005.
69. Knutsson A, Karlsson B, Ornkloo K, Landstrom U, Lennernas M, Eriksson K. Postprandial responses of glucose, insulin and triglycerides: influence of the timing of meal intake during night work. Nutr Health. 2002;16(2):133–41.

70. Al-Naimi S, Hampton SM, Richard P, Tzung C, Morgan LM. Postprandial metabolic profiles following meals and snacks eaten during simulated night and day shift work. Chronobiol Int. 2004;21(6):937–47.
71. Gill S, Panda S. A smartphone app reveals erratic diurnal eating patterns in humans that can be modulated for health benefits. Cell Metab. 2015;22(5):789–98.
72. Jamshed H, Beyl RA, Della Manna DL, Yang ES, Ravussin E, Peterson CM. Early time-restricted feeding improves 24-hour glucose levels and affects markers of the circadian clock, aging, and autophagy in humans. Nutrients. 2019;11(6)
73. Sutton EF, Beyl R, Early KS, Cefalu WT, Ravussin E, Peterson CM. Early time-restricted feeding improves insulin sensitivity, blood pressure, and oxidative stress even without weight loss in men with prediabetes. Cell Metab. 2018;27(6):1212–21 e3.
74. Ravussin E, Beyl RA, Poggiogalle E, Hsia DS, Peterson CM. Early time-restricted feeding reduces appetite and increases fat oxidation but does not affect energy expenditure in humans. Obesity (Silver Spring). 2019;27(8):1244–54.
75. Faris AE, Jahrami HA, Alsibai J, Obaideen AA. Impact of Ramadan diurnal intermittent fasting on the metabolic syndrome components in healthy, non-athletic Muslim people aged over 15 years: a systematic review and meta-analysis. Br J Nutr. 2020;123(1):1–22.
76. Pieczynska-Zajac JM, Malinowska A, Lagowska K, Leciejewska N, Bajerska J. The effects of time-restricted eating and Ramadan fasting on gut microbiota composition: a systematic review of human and animal studies. Nutr Rev. 2023;82:777.
77. Yan S, Wang C, Zhao H, Pan Y, Wang H, Guo Y, et al. Effects of fasting intervention regulating anthropometric and metabolic parameters in subjects with overweight or obesity: a systematic review and meta-analysis. Food Funct. 2020;11(5):3781–99.
78. Al-Jafar R, Wahyuni NS, Belhaj K, Ersi MH, Boroghani Z, Alreshidi A, et al. The impact of Ramadan intermittent fasting on anthropometric measurements and body composition: evidence from LORANS study and a meta-analysis. Front Nutr. 2023;10:1082217.
79. Faris MAE, Madkour MI, Obaideen AK, Dalah EZ, Hasan HA, Radwan H, et al. Effect of Ramadan diurnal fasting on visceral adiposity and serum adipokines in overweight and obese individuals. Diabetes Res Clin Pract. 2019;153:166–75.
80. Pezuk P, Mohawk JA, Wang LA, Menaker M. Glucocorticoids as entraining signals for peripheral circadian oscillators. Endocrinology. 2012;153(10):4775–83.
81. Le Minh N, Damiola F, Tronche F, Schutz G, Schibler U. Glucocorticoid hormones inhibit food-induced phase-shifting of peripheral circadian oscillators. EMBO J. 2001;20(24):7128–36.
82. Mindikoglu AL, Opekun AR, Gagan SK, Devaraj S. Impact of time-restricted feeding and Dawn-to-sunset fasting on circadian rhythm, obesity, metabolic syndrome, and nonalcoholic fatty liver disease. Gastroenterol Res Pract. 2017;2017:3932491.
83. Mindikoglu AL, Park J, Opekun AR, Abdulsada MM, Wilhelm ZR, Jalal PK, et al. Dawn-to-dusk dry fasting induces anti-atherosclerotic, anti-inflammatory, and anti-tumorigenic proteome in peripheral blood mononuclear cells in subjects with metabolic syndrome. Metabol Open. 2022;16:100214.
84. Stimson RH, Mohd-Shukri NA, Bolton JL, Andrew R, Reynolds RM, Walker BR. The postprandial rise in plasma cortisol in men is mediated by macronutrient-specific stimulation of adrenal and extra-adrenal cortisol production. J Clin Endocrinol Metab. 2014;99(1):160–8.
85. Rishi MA, Ahmed O, Barrantes Perez JH, Berneking M, Dombrowsky J, Flynn-Evans EE, et al. Daylight saving time: an American Academy of sleep medicine position statement. J Clin Sleep Med. 2020;16(10):1781–4.
86. Roenneberg T, Wirz-Justice A, Skene DJ, Ancoli-Israel S, Wright KP, Dijk DJ, et al. Why should we abolish daylight saving time? J Biol Rhythm. 2019;34(3):227–30.

Part III
Organ Systems and Disease

·

Chapter 7
Impact of Ramadan Intermittent Fasting on Cardiovascular Health and Disease

Huma Naqeeb, Iftikhar Alam, Sharifa AlBlooshi, MoezAlIslam E. Faris, and Falak Zeb

Abstract Intermittent fasting (IF) is a dietary approach involving alternating periods of fasting and eating, which has garnered attention for its potential health benefits and flexibility. This chapter examines the efficacy of various IF protocols, such as alternate-day fasting (ADF) and time-restricted feeding/eating (TRF/E), in improving health markers among different populations, including those at increased risk of cardiovascular diseases (CVD). While the practice of fasting can enhance longevity and reduce chronic illness indicators, like oxidative stress and inflammation, individual responses may vary depending on specific protocols and demographic factors. The chapter emphasizes the significance of Ramadan fasting, a form of IF practiced by millions globally, showcasing its impact on lipid profile, blood pressure, and overall cardiovascular health. Challenges associated with fasting during Ramadan, particularly for individuals

H. Naqeeb
Department of Human Nutrition and Dietetics, Women's University Mardan, Mardan, Pakistan
e-mail: huma.naqeeb@wumardan.edu.pk

I. Alam (✉)
Department of Human Nutrition and Dietetics, Faculty of Sciences, Bacha Khan University, Charsadda, Khyber Pakhtunkhwa (KPK), Pakistan
e-mail: iftikharalam@aup.edu.pk

S. AlBlooshi
College of Natural and Health Sciences, Zayed University, Dubai, United Arab Emirates
e-mail: Sharifa.Alblooshi@zu.ac.ae

M. E. Faris
Department of Clinical Nutrition and Dietetics, Faculty of Allied Medical Sciences, Applied Science Private University, Amman, Jordan

F. Zeb (✉)
Research Institute of Medical and Health Sciences (RIMHS), University of Sharjah, Sharjah, United Arab Emirates

© The Author(s), under exclusive license to Springer Nature Singapore Pte Ltd. 2025
M. E. Faris et al. (eds.), *Health and Medical Aspects of Ramadan Intermittent Fasting*, https://doi.org/10.1007/978-981-96-6783-3_7

predisposed to CVD, are discussed alongside recommended health assessments. Additionally, the chapter highlights potential metabolic and circadian rhythm disturbances induced by altered eating patterns. Overall, IF, including Ramadan fasting, appears to facilitate better health outcomes, particularly in weight management and cardiovascular risk reduction, warranting further investigation to substantiate these findings across diverse populations.

Keywords Intermittent fasting · Cardiovascular diseases · Ramadan fasting · Health markers · Metabolism

7.1   Introduction

Intermittent fasting (IF) is a dietary approach characterized by alternating periods of fasting and eating, offering flexibility in timing and duration [1–3]. It has gained popularity for both health improvement and religious reasons, making it a relatively straightforward intervention to study [4]. Various protocols exist, including alternate-day fasting (ADF) and time-restricted feeding/eating (TRF/E), with fasting periods ranging from 12 to 20 h [2–4]. A commonly accepted practice involves fasting for 16 h, followed by an 8-h eating window. Research indicates that IF can significantly improve health indicators in healthy individuals and those with chronic illnesses, potentially increasing longevity and reducing oxidative stress and inflammation [2, 3, 6]. However, the outcomes may vary depending on the fasting protocol and the population studied. Overall, incorporating fasting into dietary strategies may significantly improve health indicators.

Ramadan fasting (RF) has been linked to notable enhancements in multiple variables involved in cardiovascular etiology. Studies have demonstrated that RF leads to reductions in visceral adiposity and body weight among overweight and obese individuals. For instance, Madkour et al. [7] observed a significant decrease in body mass and fat mass after 29–30 days of RIF, independent of caloric intake changes. In addition to anthropometric benefits, RIF positively influences adipocytokine profiles and inflammatory markers. Madkour et al. [7] reported that RIF is associated with significant reductions in pro-inflammatory cytokines, such as interleukin-6 (IL-6) and tumor necrosis factor-alpha (TNF-α), along with an increase in the anti-inflammatory biomarker interleukin-10 (IL-10). These alterations indicate an improvement in systemic inflammation, a significant factor in cardiovascular diseases. Furthermore, RIF has been linked to favorable modifications in lipid metabolism. The same study by Madkour et al. [7] also found that RIF resulted in decreased plasma levels of sphingosine and sphinganine, as well as their phosphorylated derivatives, sphingosine-1-phosphate and sphinganine-1-phosphate. Additionally, reductions in specific sphingomyelin species were observed. These lipidomic changes are significant, as sphingolipids play a crucial role in the development of insulin resistance and atherosclerosis. These changes indicate an improvement in systemic inflammation. Collectively, these findings suggest that RIF may confer protective effects against cardiovascular diseases by modulating body fat distribution, improving adipocytokine profiles, reducing systemic inflammation, and altering lipidomic pathways.

7.2 Cardiovascular Diseases and Risk Factors

Cardiovascular diseases (CVD), including coronary artery disease, heart failure, stroke, and peripheral vascular disease, present significant global health challenges [8, 9]. In regions like Asia, such as Pakistan, CVD burdens are disproportionately high, contributing to 19% of total mortality [10, 11]. The development of CVD is influenced by multifactorial elements, including genetic predisposition, environmental factors, and lifestyle choices, such as hypertension, high cholesterol, smoking, diabetes, obesity, physical inactivity, and poor dietary habits [12]. Addressing CVD necessitates prioritizing cost-effective policies aligned with Sustainable Development Goal 3, aiming to reduce premature mortality from noncommunicable diseases [10, 11]. Special considerations are essential for fasting during Ramadan due to potential challenges, particularly for those at higher cardiovascular risk. Pre-Ramadan health assessments and monitoring during fasting periods are recommended to manage deviations in health parameters [13].

7.3 Intermittent Fasting

Intermittent fasting (IF) has gained attention as a dietary strategy to promote health, particularly in addressing the challenges posed by the obesogenic environment. IF involves alternating periods of fasting and eating, using various protocols such as ADF and TRF. Studies have shown that IF can reduce weight and improve body mass index (BMI), waist circumference (WC), and lipid profile. It also decreases inflammatory responses, as evidenced by changes in serum levels of adipocytokines and inflammatory cytokines. These findings suggest that IF may offer a viable and accessible strategy for some individuals seeking to manage overweight and obesity [14] (Table 7.1).

Table 7.1 Some selected studies showing the health benefits of IF

Title	Author(s)	Study type	Results/discussion
The effect of intermittent energy and carbohydrate restriction vs. daily energy restriction on weight loss and metabolic disease risk markers in overweight women	Harvie et al. [15]	Randomized trial	Intermittent energy restriction showed better insulin sensitivity and weight control results than daily energy restriction
A low-fat over high-fat diet benefits vascular health during alternate-day fasting	Klempel et al. [16]	Randomized study	Alternate-day fasting (ADF) with a low-fat (LF) diet improves brachial artery flow-mediated dilation (FMD). Whether these beneficial effects can be reproduced with a high-fat (HF) diet is unclear
Restricting night-time eating reduces daily energy intake in healthy young men: a short-term cross-over study	Lecheminant et al. [17]	Cross-sectional	Few experimental data support the notion that reducing night-time eating (NER) alters healthy adults' total daily energy intake (EI) or body weight. During the NER condition, participants consumed less total energy per day than during the control condition. There was a significant difference in weight change between the NER and control conditions ($F = 22.68$; $P < 0.001$)
Practicality of intermittent fasting in humans and its effect on oxidative stress and genes related to aging and metabolism	Wegman et al. [18]	Double-blinded randomized clinical trial	Participants found the diet tolerable, with no adverse clinical findings or changes in body weight. It was also found that IF decreased plasma insulin levels (1.01 μU / mL)
A randomized pilot study comparing zero-calorie alternate-day fasting to daily caloric restriction in adults with obesity	Catenacci et al. [19]	Randomized clinical trial	Alternate-day fasting (ADF) is a safe and tolerable weight loss approach. Alternate-day fasting (ADF) produced similar changes in weight, body composition, lipids, and insulin sensitivity index (IS Si) at 8 weeks and did not appear to increase the risk of recovery from weight 24 weeks after completion of the intervention

(continued)

Table 7.1 (continued)

Title	Author(s)	Study type	Results/discussion
Comparison of high-protein, intermittent fasting low-calorie diet and heart healthy diet for vascular health of the obese	Zuo et al. [19]	Longitudinal study	The results suggest that a high-protein diet and a low-calorie intermittent fasting diet are associated with similar reductions in BMI and blood lipids in obese men and women. This diet has also demonstrated an advantage in minimizing weight gain and increasing arterial compliance compared to a heart-healthy diet after one year
Effects of intermittent fasting on health markers in those with type 2 diabetes: a pilot study	Arnason, Bowen [20]	Observational study	The data demonstrated noticeable trends during intermittent fasting (IF) toward lower energy, carbohydrate, and fat intake. The results indicate that short-term intermittent fasting may be a safe and tolerable nutritional intervention in patients with type 2 diabetes (T2D) by improving their weight, fasting glucose, and postprandial variability
Potential benefits and harms of intermittent energy restriction and intermittent fasting amongst obese, overweight and Normal weight subjects-a narrative review of human and animal evidence	Harvie; Howell [21]	Review	The review's studies highlight the potential beneficial and adverse effects of intermittent energy restriction compared to continuous energy restriction on ectopic and visceral fat stores, size of adipocytes, insulin resistance, and metabolic flexibility
Metabolic effects of intermittent fasting	Patterson; Sears [23]	Review	Modified fasts appear to promote weight loss and may improve metabolic health. Intermittent fasting is hypothesized to influence metabolic regulation through its effects on circadian biology, the gut microbiome, and modifiable lifestyle behaviors such as sleep
Is 2 days of intermittent energy restriction per week a feasible weight loss approach in obese males? A randomised pilot study	Conley et al. [24]	Randomized pilot study (n = 24)	After 6 months, participants in both groups significantly reduced body weight, waist circumference (WC), and systolic blood pressure. There was no significant change in diastolic blood pressure, fasting blood glucose, or lipids

(continued)

Table 7.1 (continued)

Title	Author(s)	Study type	Results/discussion
Energy metabolism and intermittent fasting: The Ramadan perspective	Lessan, Ali [25]	Review	Observing Ramadan fasting is accompanied by changes in sleep and activity patterns and circadian rhythm hormones, including cortisol, insulin, leptin, ghrelin, growth hormone, prolactin, sex hormones, and adiponectin
Effects of time-restricted feeding in weight loss, metabolic syndrome and cardiovascular risk in obese women	Schroder et al. [26]	Non-randomized controlled trial	A time-restricted feeding regimen lowers body weight without altering metabolic syndrome–related biomarkers
Feasibility of time-restricted eating and impacts on cardiometabolic health in 24-h shift workers	Manoogian et al. [27]	Randomized controlled trial	No notable variations were found in metabolic syndrome indicators between the groups that underwent intermittent and continuous calorie restriction
Time-restricted eating without calorie counting for weight loss in a racially diverse population: A randomized controlled trial	Lin et al. [28]	Randomized controlled trial	Time-restricted eating is more effective in achieving weight loss when compared with control but not more effective than claoric restriction (CR) in a racially diverse population
The effect of fasting on cardiovascular diseases: a systematic review	Hailu et al. [29]	Systematic review	Fasting is beneficial in lowering a population's cardiovascular risk. This result holds for all types of fasting used as an intervention in the clinical trials we reviewed. The result is pronounced when fasting regimens are combined with a regular exercise routine

7.4   Intermitting Fasting: Not a Compelling Option Because of Food Availability

Food is a fundamental requirement for life, and throughout history, humans have experienced periods of food scarcity, leading to adaptive physiological and behavioral responses for survival [21]. Intermittent fasting involves partial or total energy restriction for 1–3 days per week or specific hours of the day, either as a dietary habit or for religious reasons [25]. Intermittent fasting impacts metabolic regulation by influencing the circadian rhythm, gut microbiome, and lifestyle behaviors [23]. Different IF protocols include ADF, full-day fasting, and time-restricted eating (TRE). ADF alternates between fasting and non-fasting days, while full-day fasting involves complete fasting for 1 or 2 days per week, with limited caloric intake on other days [30]. TRE involves eating within a specific time window each day, with the remaining hours designated for fasting [31]. Intermittent fasting can benefit individuals with average weight by improving health markers, such as cardioprotection, fasting glucose reduction, cancer prevention, and body composition improvement, regardless of weight loss [22].

7.5 Intermittent Fasting and Corrections of Metabolic Abnormalities

The World Health Organization [9] identifies overweight and obesity as significant contributors to chronic noncommunicable diseases (NCDs). Recent evidence challenges the traditional belief that increasing meal frequency aids in weight loss, suggesting that reducing meal frequency may be more beneficial [32]. Intermittent fasting (IF) has emerged as a promising weight loss strategy. A study by Klempel et al. [16] has shown significant weight loss, reduced BMI, favorable body composition, and lipid profile changes following IF interventions. Although Hoddy et al. [33] did not evaluate all parameters, they observed weight reduction with IF. Overall, IF presents a viable option for weight management, demonstrating comparable efficacy to daily calorie restriction in promoting weight loss and improving body composition.

Experimental studies have demonstrated that fasting effectively corrects metabolic abnormalities, such as obesity, diabetes, cardiovascular diseases, cancer, and neurodegenerative diseases [34]. Fasting involves abstaining from food, leading to weight loss, cellular repair, and rejuvenation. Intermittent fasting (IF) has shown comparable weight loss and improved body composition compared to daily energy restriction in both healthy individuals and obese populations [22, 24]. Intervention with IF has significantly reduced weight and waist circumference and improved lipid profile [22]. Studies also suggest that IF may increase life expectancy and improve various health markers, including insulin resistance and arterial compliance [35]. Intermittent fasting induces weight loss by reducing caloric intake while preserving lean body mass. IF offers potential benefits similar to calorie restriction, but prolonged fasting periods should be conducted under medical supervision.

7.6 Effect of Fasting on Glucose and Lipid Metabolism

The human body maintains internal stability and homeostasis by regulating temperature, blood glucose levels (BGL), and pH [36]. Fasting disrupts dietary glucose intake, causing BGL to drop and triggering responses to restore normal levels [37]. Glucagon, released by the pancreas, stimulates glycogenolysis and lipolysis in liver and muscle cells, releasing stored glucose and converting fat stores into glucose. Adrenaline also stimulates glycogenolysis and lipolysis to restore BGL [38]. During fasting, the liver's glycogen stores provide glucose at about 4 grams per hour. Short-term fasting minimally affects metabolism, with oxidative metabolism meeting energy needs [39]. Hence, even toward the end of a fasting cycle, glycogen stores are likely not fully depleted, and muscle glycogen could further sustain glucose supply [40]. Practical limitations led to fitness tests assessing glycogen depletion effects, such as reduced strength and power, instead of direct BGL assessment [41]. Grip strength and standing broad jump tests were employed in this study.

7.7   Effect of Fasting on Circadian Rhythm

Eating at different times, particularly during fasting, can impact the body's circadian rhythm, affecting organ cycles concerning the sleep–wake cycle. The human body possesses internal clocks in all cells, classified as central clocks in the suprachiasmatic nucleus (SCN) and peripheral clocks in various organs and tissues. These clocks regulate tissue-specific gene expression to maintain the circadian rhythm. Shifting mealtimes, especially during fasting, can disrupt the normal circadian pattern of food intake, potentially disrupting the circadian rhythm and biological clock of individuals practicing intermittent fasting. During Ramadan, studies have shown a reduction in nocturnal sleep time among 16-year-old Muslims compared to pre-Ramadan baselines. The circadian rhythm adapts to individuals' sleep–wake cycles, controlling core body temperature, hormone secretions, and other physiological processes. The disrupted sleep cycle during Ramadan, due to waking before sunrise for the predawn meal (*Suhoor*), is associated with reduced neuromuscular coordination, impaired reaction time, increased fatigue, and perceived exhaustion early in the day. These disturbances may impact overall performance and well-being during fasting periods.

7.8   Intermittent Fasting and Melatonin

The circadian rhythm, closely tied to melatonin secretion, reflects the body's internal clock and is influenced by environmental cues. Measuring melatonin levels provides a precise marker for investigating circadian rhythm, with studies during Ramadan fasting revealing delayed night-time peaks and flattened slopes in melatonin secretion. While IF can subtly impact melatonin, sleep, and body temperature following circadian rhythm fluctuations, the body quickly adapts to eating patterns and environmental changes. Short-term adjustments are unlikely to disrupt balance, but long-term changes prompt recalibrated adaptations. Intermittent fasting elicits various physiological and biochemical changes, notably weight loss, reduced BMI, and waist circumference, along with correcting metabolic abnormalities, like obesity, diabetes, cardiovascular diseases, cancer, and neurodegenerative diseases. Moreover, it improves cellular biomarkers, reduces disease risks, promotes health, and enhances longevity. However, more long-term human studies are needed to establish clear benefits and potential adverse effects of IF, ensuring robust scientific evidence of its therapeutic efficacy on human health.

A recent study explored the effects of Ramadan fasting (RF) on melatonin levels. Its findings align with those of previous research, indicating that RF significantly decreases serum melatonin concentrations. For instance, Al-Rawi et al. [42] observed a notable reduction in melatonin levels among overweight and obese individuals during Ramadan fasting. Similarly, Roky et al. [43] reported that the circadian distribution of melatonin was affected during Ramadan, with a decrease in amplitude and a shift in acrophase. These studies suggest that altered meal timings and sleep patterns during RF may disrupt the circadian rhythm of melatonin secretion.

According to their findings, this research contributes to this body of knowledge by demonstrating that RF leads to a significant decrease in nocturnal melatonin peaks, potentially delaying its secretion. This alteration in melatonin rhythm could have implications for sleep quality and overall circadian biology during fasting periods. Understanding these changes is crucial for developing strategies to mitigate potential adverse effects on health associated with disrupted melatonin cycles during intermittent fasting practices.

7.9 Ramadan Fasting: An Effective Form of Intermittent Fasting

Ramadan is the holiest and most awaited month for the Muslim community worldwide. Each year, around 1.8 billion believers perform this ritual for 30 days, during which they undertake to deprive themselves of water and food from the time of *Salat Al-Fajr* (dawn prayer) to *Salat Al-Maghrib* (evening prayer). Eating for approximately 40 min is allowed before sunrise (*Suhur*). Feeding can resume only after the evening (iftar), after which a vast quantity of food is consumed in the community (Al-Quran, 2:182). This ritual, however, has been attracting attention due to its benefits, not only spiritually but also for the health of the individual, from improvement in lipid profile, blood pressure, anthropometric measurements to the regulation of hunger and satiety [44, 46, 48]. This summary aims to present a bibliographical review of studies and previous studies on the topic, in which the benefits of body weight and profile biochemistry of IF throughout Ramadan, carried out by this great community, are discussed and clarified (Fig. 7.1).

Azizi [44] observes a temporary increase in serum uric acid levels during fasting due to decreased glomerular filtration and uric acid clearance, with prolonged fasting leading to a drastic rise in uric acid levels. Conversely, al Hourani et al. [45] note minimal to no increase in uric acid levels during fasting, attributing weight loss to increased fatty acid oxidation and fat loss rather than lean mass loss.

Regarding lipid profile changes during fasting, Temizhan et al. [46] report reductions in total cholesterol, low density lipoprotein (LDL), very low density

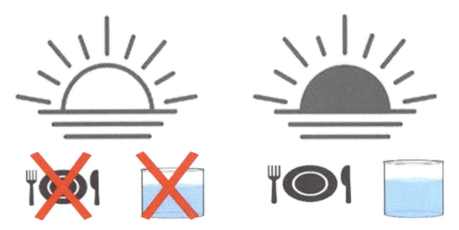

Fig. 7.1 Ramadan fasting as a form of intermittent fasting starts at dawn and finishes at sunset in the evening. The complete restriction of food and drinks characterizes Ramadan fasting

lipoprotein (VLDL), and triglycerides post-fasting, with no significant change in high density lipoprotein (HDL) levels. This improvement, particularly in females, may be linked to dietary fat intake changes and metabolic alterations during fasting, as suggested by Asgary et al. [47]. Additionally, al Hourani et al. [48] observe a gradual but nonsignificant increase in HDL cholesterol, potentially associated with weight loss during fasting. Al Zunaidy et al. [49] found significant reductions in triglycerides, total cholesterol, HDL, and LDL post–Ramadan fasting. Research by Bouhlel et al. [50] indicates that fasting during Ramadan is associated with decreased body mass and fat during Ramadan. Trabelsi et al. [51] observed reductions in body weight and body fat percentage among physically active men during and after Ramadan fasting, concluding that Ramadan fasting leads to decreases in both parameters. Temizhan [46] investigated patients with coronary disease during Ramadan fasting and found a significantly lower number of coronary heart disease events compared to other times of the year, suggesting that fasting during Ramadan does not increase the risk of such events. Shehab et al. [52] studied the effect of Ramadan fasting on blood pressure in healthy individuals, noting changes in systolic blood pressure by the end of Ramadan. They observed similar incidences of acute coronary syndrome, fibrillation, decompensated heart failure, and stroke during Ramadan compared to other months. Cansel [53] examined heart rate variability during Ramadan fasting, concluding that heartbeats become more pronounced, stimulating parasympathetic activity associated with calm, rest, and digestion control.

Fasting during Ramadan has significantly impacted various health aspects, including lipid profile, inflammatory markers, cancer risk, coronary heart disease, blood pressure, and overall well-being. However, conflicting findings among studies underscore the importance of considering regional dietary habits and participant demographics, such as health status and socioeconomic factors. Future research should adopt a multiethnic and geographically diverse approach to address these discrepancies, considering variables like gender, race, physical activity, dietary patterns, and sleep habits.

Alam et al. (2019) highlighted the benefits of recurrent circadian fasting, particularly for individuals at risk of cardiometabolic and inflammatory disorders. Adherence to recommended dietary behaviors regulating carbohydrate and caloric intake was crucial for maximizing these benefits, especially among older adults with abnormal cardiovascular, metabolic, and inflammatory profiles. Studies by Gul et al. [3] and Alam et al. [2] demonstrated reductions in body weight and improvements in blood chemistry and cytokine profiles among individuals observing Ramadan fasting. Chronic inflammation, a key contributor to atherosclerosis, insulin resistance, and cardiovascular diseases, involves pro-inflammatory cytokines such as interleukins (ILs) and tumor necrosis factor-alpha (TNF-α). Fasting has shown the potential to mitigate inflammation and lower inflammatory markers, benefiting healthy individuals and those with underlying health conditions. Ramadan fasting (RF) has been shown to induce metabolic and physiological adaptations that contribute to reductions in body weight and improvements in blood chemistry. A study by Faris et al. [54] observed significant weight loss and favorable changes in lipid profiles during RF, which can be attributed to enhanced lipolysis and decreased insulin levels, promoting fat utilization as an energy source. Similarly, Adawi et al. [55] reported decreased body mass index (BMI) and improved glycemic control, likely due to the prolonged fasting state enhancing insulin sensitivity and reducing glucose fluctuations. Chronic inflammation, a key driver of atherosclerosis, insulin resistance, and cardiovascular diseases, involves pro-inflammatory cytokines such as interleukins (ILs) and tumor necrosis factor-alpha (TNF-α). Fasting modulates inflammatory responses by reducing oxidative stress and regulating immune cell activity. Faris et al. [54] demonstrated that RF significantly decreases IL-6 and TNF-α levels, potentially through the activation of autophagy and the suppression of pro-inflammatory signaling pathways. These mechanisms contribute to improved immune homeostasis, benefiting both healthy individuals and those with metabolic disorders.

RF has been associated with a significant decrease in nocturnal melatonin peaks, potentially delaying its secretion. This alteration in melatonin rhythm may have implications for sleep quality and overall circadian biology during fasting periods. Understanding these changes is crucial for developing strategies to mitigate potential adverse effects on health associated with disrupted melatonin cycles during intermittent fasting practices. Pro-inflammatory cytokines play critical roles in the pathogenesis of various diseases, with fasting potentially modulating their levels and promoting anti-inflammatory responses. These findings suggest fasting could be an alternative strategy for managing inflammation and enhancing cardiovascular health, emphasizing its potential as a therapeutic intervention, as depicted in Fig. 7.2.

Heat shock protein-27 (Hsp27), a member of the small Hsp family, functions as a chaperone and influences cellular processes like apoptosis, cell movement, and embryogenesis. Autophagy, a vital cellular recycling process, maintains cell survival by degrading organelles, proteins, and macromolecules. adenosine

Fig. 7.2 The putative mechanism for the beneficial effects of fasting involves increased or reduced levels of specific cytokines/chemokines

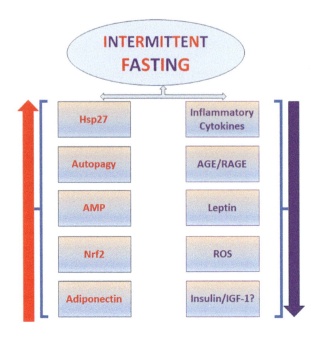

monophosphate (AMP)-activated protein kinase (AMPK) regulates metabolism in response to nutrient deficits, promoting glucose uptake and lipid oxidation while inhibiting energy-consuming processes. Nuclear factor erythroid 2-related factor 2 (NRF2) controls genes involved in metabolic pathways like glycolysis and lipid metabolism. Adiponectin, secreted by adipocytes, regulates glucose and lipid metabolism and insulin sensitivity through anti-inflammatory and antioxidant effects. Pro-inflammatory cytokines contribute to metabolic diseases, such as obesity and atherosclerosis. The Advanced Glycation Endproducts- Receptor for Advanced Glycation Endproducts (AGE–RAGE) interaction induces cellular damage through inflammation and oxidative stress. Leptin regulates lipid metabolism independently of food intake by inhibiting lipogenesis and stimulating lipolysis. Reactive oxygen species (ROS) generated during metabolism regulate cellular functions via redox signaling. Insulin-like growth factor-I (IGF-I) promotes cell survival, protein synthesis, hypertrophy, and cell division based on nutrient availability. These mechanisms underscore the intricate regulation of metabolism and its role in physiological processes and diseases.

7.10   Conclusion

Intermittent fasting in its various forms, including Ramadan fasting, has generally demonstrated a significant improvement in coronary heart disease risk score and other cardiovascular risk factors, such as weight, BMI, and waist circumference. This suggests that IF and Ramadan fasting may help improve CVD risk factors.

7.11   Future Directions

More multicenter studies with larger sample sizes and other habitual changes controlled with a matched control group are warranted. We also suggest establishing special research groups and centers to undertake more robust research on IF in different parts of the world.

Acknowledgments   We acknowledge the Nutrition, Education, Awareness, and Training (NEAT) organization, Cooperative Society Charsadda KP, Pakistan, for its technical support in compiling this chapter.

Conflict of Interest   Nil

References

1. Mentzelou M, Papadopoulou SK, Psara E, Voulgaridou G, Pavlidou E, Androutsos O, Giaginis C. Chrononutrition in the prevention and management of metabolic disorders: a literature review. Nutrients. 2024;16(5):722.
2. Gul R, Khan I, Alam I, Almajwal A, Hussain I, Sohail N, Hussain M, Cena H, Shafiq S, Aftab A. Ramadan-specific nutrition education improves cardio-metabolic health and inflammation—a prospective nutrition intervention study from Pakistan. Front Nutr. 2023;10:1204883.
3. Alam I, Gul R, Chong J, Tan CT, Chin HX, Wong G, Doggui R, Larbi A. Recurrent circadian fasting (RCF) improves blood pressure, biomarkers of cardiometabolic risk and regulates inflammation in men. J Transl Med. 2019;17:1–29.
4. Moro T, Tinsley G, Longo G, Grigoletto D, Bianco A, Ferraris C, Guglielmetti M, Veneto A, Tagliabue A, Marcolin G, Paoli A. Time-restricted eating effects on performance, immune function, and body composition in elite cyclists: a randomized controlled trial. J Int Soc Sports Nutr. 2020;17:1–1.
5. Jahrami HA, Alsibai J, Obaideen AA. Impact of Ramadan diurnal intermittent fasting on the metabolic syndrome components in healthy, non-athletic Muslim people aged over 15 years: a systematic review and meta-analysis. Br J Nutr. 2020;123(1) 1st ed. Cambridge University Press.
6. Madkour MI, Islam MT, Tippetts TS, Chowdhury KH, Lesniewski LA, Summers SA, Zeb F, Abdelrahim DN, AlKurd R, Khraiwesh HM, AbuShihab KH. Ramadan intermittent fasting is associated with ameliorated inflammatory markers and improved plasma sphingolipids/ceramides in subjects with obesity: lipidomics analysis. Sci Rep. 2023;13(1):17322. Persynaki A, Karras S, Pichard C. Unraveling the metabolic health benefits of fasting related to religious beliefs: a narrative review. Nutrition. 2017;35:14–20.
7. Roth GA, Mensah GA, Johnson CO, Addolorato G, Ammirati E, Baddour LM, et al. Global burden of cardiovascular diseases and risk factors, 1990–2019: update from the GBD 2019 study. J Am Coll Cardiol. 2020;76(25):2982–3021.
8. World Health Organization. Obesity and overweight 2016. Available from: https://www.who.int/news-room/fact-sheets/detail/obesity-and-overweight
9. Hussain SM, Oldenburg B, Wang Y, Zoungas S, Tonkin AM. Assessment of cardiovascular disease risk in South Asian populations. Int J Vasc Med. 2013;123(1) 1st ed. Hindawi.
10. Liaquat A, Javed Q. Current trends of cardiovascular risk determinants in Pakistan. Cureus. 2018;123(1) 1st ed. Cureus Inc. 10 (10)
11. Mensah GA, Roth GA, Fuster V. The global burden of cardiovascular diseases and risk factors: 2020 and beyond. J Am Coll Cardiol. 2019;74(20):2529–32.

12. Beshyah S, Badi A, El-Ghul A, Gabroun A, Dougman K, Eledrisi M. The year in "Ramadan fasting and health" (2018): a narrative review. Ibnosina J Med Biomed Sci. 2019;11(4):151–70.
13. Wilson RA, Deasy W, Stathis CG, Hayes A, Cooke MB. Intermittent fasting with or without exercise prevents weight gain and improves lipids in diet-induced obese mice. Nutrients. 2018;10(3):346.
14. Harvie M, Wright C, Pegington M, McMullan D, Mitchell E, Martin B, Cutler RG, Evans G, Whiteside S, Maudsley S, Camandola S. The effect of intermittent energy and carbohydrate restriction v. daily energy restriction on weight loss and metabolic disease risk markers in overweight women. Br J Nutr. 2013 Oct;110(8):1534–47.
15. Klempel MC, Kroeger CM, Norkeviciute E, Goslawski M, Phillips SA, Varady KA. Benefit of a low-fat over high-fat diet on vascular health during alternate day fasting. Nutr Diabetes. 2013;3(5):e71.
16. LeCheminant JD, Christenson ED, Bailey BW, Tucker LA. Restricting night-time eating reduces daily energy intake in healthy young men: a short-term cross-over study. Br J Nutr. 2013;110(11):2108–13.
17. Wegman MP, Guo MH, Bennion DM, Shankar MN, Chrzanowski SM, Goldberg LA, Xu J, Williams TA, Lu X, Hsu SI, Anton SD. Practicality of intermittent fasting in humans and its effect on oxidative stress and genes related to aging and metabolism. Rejuvenation Res. 2015;18(2):162–72.
18. Catenacci VA, Pan Z, Ostendorf D, Brannon S, Gozansky WS, Mattson MP, Martin B, MacLean PS, Melanson EL, Troy DW. A randomized pilot study comparing zero-calorie alternate-day fasting to daily caloric restriction in adults with obesity. Obesity. 2016;24(9):1874–83.
19. Zuo L, He F, Tinsley GM, Pannell BK, Ward E, Arciero PJ. Comparison of high-protein, intermittent fasting low-calorie diet, and heart-healthy diet for vascular health of the obese. Front Physiol. 2016;29(7):209013.
20. Arnason TG, Bowen MW, Mansell KD. Effects of intermittent fasting on health markers in those with type 2 diabetes: a pilot study. World J Diabetes. 2017;8(4):154.
21. Harvie M, Howell A. Potential benefits and harms of intermittent energy restriction and intermittent fasting amongst obese, overweight and normal weight subjects—a narrative review of human and animal evidence. Behav Sci. 2017;7(1):4.
22. Patterson RE, Sears DD. Metabolic effects of intermittent fasting. Annu Rev Nutr. 2017;37(1):371–93.
23. Conley M, Le Fevre L, Haywood C, Proietto J. Is two days of intermittent energy restriction per week a feasible weight loss approach in obese males? A randomized pilot study. Nutr Diet. 2018;75(1):65–72.
24. Lessan N, Ali T. Energy metabolism and intermittent fasting: the Ramadan perspective. Nutrients. 2019;11(5):1192.
25. Schroder JD, Falqueto H, Mânica A, Zanini D, de Oliveira T, de Sá CA, Cardoso AM, Manfredi LH. Effects of time-restricted feeding in weight loss, metabolic syndrome and cardiovascular risk in obese women. J Transl Med. 2021;19:1–1.
26. Manoogian EN, Zadourian A, Lo HC, Gutierrez NR, Shoghi A, Rosander A, Pazargadi A, Ormiston CK, Wang X, Sui J, Hou Z. Feasibility of time-restricted eating and impacts on cardiometabolic health in 24-h shift workers: the healthy heroes randomized control trial. Cell Metab. 2022;34(10):1442–56.
27. Lin S, Cienfuegos S, Ezpeleta M, Gabel K, Pavlou V, Mulas A, Chakos K, McStay M, Wu J, Tussing-Humphreys L, Alexandria SJ. Time-restricted eating without calorie counting for weight loss in a racially diverse population: a randomized controlled trial. Ann Intern Med. 2023;176(7):885–95.
28. Hailu KT, Salib K, Nandeesha SS, Kasagga A, Hawrami C, Ricci E, Hamid P. The effect of fasting on cardiovascular diseases: a systematic review. Cureus. 2024;16(1):e53221.
29. Pettit MJ. Effects of fasting on autophagy, immune and inflammatory response. University of Bridgeport; 2023.

30. Rothschild JA, Kilding AE, Broome SC, Stewart T, Cronin JB, Plews DJ. Pre-exercise carbohydrate or protein ingestion influences substrate oxidation but not performance or hunger compared with cycling in the fasted state. Nutrients. 2021;13(4):1291.
31. Hutchison AT, Heilbronn LK. Metabolic impacts of altering meal frequency and timing–does when we eat matter? Biochimie. 2016;124:187–97.
32. Hoddy KK, Bhutani S, Phillips SA, Varady KA. Effects of different degrees of insulin resistance on endothelial function in obese adults undergoing alternate day fasting. Nutrition and Healthy Aging. 2016;4(1):63–71.
33. Mattson MP, Longo VD, Harvie M. Impact of intermittent fasting on health and disease processes. Aging Res Rev. 2017;39:46–58.
34. Zuo L, He F, Tinsley GM, Pannell BK, Ward E, Arciero PJ. Comparison of high-protein, intermittent fasting, low-calorie diet, and heart-healthy diet for vascular health of the obese. Front Physiol. 2016;7:209013.
35. Odeh A. Effect of Ramadan intermittent fasting on swimming performance. Intersect. 2023;16(3):1–23.
36. Allott EH, Howard LE, Cooperberg MR, Kane CJ, Aronson WJ, Terris MK, Amling CL, Freedland SJ. Serum lipid profile and risk of prostate cancer recurrence: results from the SEARCH database. Cancer Epidemiol Biomarkers Prev. 2014;23(11):2349–56.
37. Pedersen C, Kraft G, Edgerton DS, Scott M, Farmer B, Smith M, Laneve DC, Williams PE, Moore LM, Cherrington AD. The kinetics of glucagon action on the liver during insulin-induced hypoglycemia. Am J Physiol Endocrinol Metab. 2020;318(5):E779–90.
38. Murray B, Rosenbloom C. Fundamentals of glycogen metabolism for coaches and athletes. Nutr Rev. 2018;76(4):243–59.
39. Jensen MV, Joseph JW, Ronnebaum SM, Burgess SC, Sherry AD, Newgard CB. Metabolic cycling in control of glucose-stimulated insulin secretion. Am J Physiol Endocrinol Metab. 2008 Dec;295(6):E1287–97.
40. Ørtenblad N, Westerblad H, Nielsen J. Muscle glycogen stores and fatigue. J Physiol. 2013 Sep;591(18):4405–13.
41. Al-Rawi N, Madkour M, Jahrami H, Salahat D, Alhasan F, BaHammam A, Al-Islam Faris ME. Effect of diurnal intermittent fasting during Ramadan on ghrelin, leptin, melatonin, and cortisol levels among overweight and obese subjects: a prospective observational study. PLoS One. 2020;15(8):e0237922.
42. Roky R, Houti I, Moussamih S, Qotbi S, Aadil N. Physiological and chronobiological changes during Ramadan intermittent fasting. Ann Nutr Metab. 2004;48(4):296–303.
43. Azizi F. Research in Islamic fasting and health. Ann Saudi Med. 2002;22(3–4):186–91.
44. Mirsane SA, Shafagh S, Oraei N. Effects of fasting in the holy month of Ramadan on the uric acid, urea, and creatinine levels: a narrative review. J Fasting Health. 2016;4(4):130.
45. Temizhan A, Tandogan I, Dönderici Ö, Demirbas B. The effects of Ramadan fasting on blood lipid levels. Am J Med. 2000;109(4):341.
46. Asgary S, Aghaei F, Naderi GA, Kelishadi R, Gharipour M, Azali S. Effects of Ramadan fasting on lipid peroxidation, serum lipoproteins, and fasting blood sugar. Med J Islam World Acad Sci. 2000;13(1):35–8.
47. Al Hourani HM, Atoum MF, Akel S, Hijjawi N, Awawdeh S. Effects of Ramadan fasting on some hematological and biochemical parameters. Jordan J Biol Sci. 2009;2(3):103–8.
48. AlZunaidy NA, Al-Khalifa AS, Hussain MH, Mohammed MA, Alfheeaid HA, Althwab SA, Faris ME. The effect of Ramadan intermittent fasting on food intake, anthropometric indices, and metabolic markers among premenopausal and postmenopausal women: a cross-sectional study. Medicina. 2023;59(7):1191.
49. Bouhlel E, Denguezli M, Zaouali M, Tabka Z, Shephard RJ. Ramadan fasting's effect on plasma leptin, adiponectin concentrations, and body composition in trained young men. Int J Sport Nutr Exerc Metab. 2008;18(6):617–27.

50. Trabelsi K, El Abed K, Stannard SR, Jammoussi K, Zeghal KM, Hakim A. Effects of fed-versus fasted-state aerobic training during Ramadan on body composition and some metabolic parameters in physically active men. Int J Sport Nutr Exerc Metab. 2012;22(1):11–8.
51. Shehab A, Abdulle A, El Issa A, Al Suwaidi J, Nagelkerke N. Favorable changes in lipid profile: the effects of fasting after Ramadan. PLoS One. 2012;7(10):e47615.
52. Cansel M, Taşolar H, Yağmur J, Ermiş N, Açıkgöz N, Eyyüpkoca F, Pekdemir H, Özdemir R. The effects of Ramadan fasting on heart rate variability in healthy individuals: a prospective study. Anatol J Cardiol. 2014;14(5):413.
53. Faris ME, Kacimi S, Ref'at A, Fararjeh MA, Bustanji YK, Mohammad MK, Salem ML. Intermittent fasting during Ramadan attenuates proinflammatory cytokines and immune cells in healthy subjects. Nutr Res. 2012;32(12):947–55.
54. Adawi M, Watad A, Brown S, Aazza K, Aazza H, Zouhir M, Sharif K, Ghanayem K, Farah R, Mahagna H, Fiordoro S. Ramadan fasting exerts immunomodulatory effects: insights from a systematic review. Front Immunol. 2017;8:1144.

Chapter 8
The Effect of Ramadan Fasting on Liver Diseases

Mohamed H. Emara, Hanan H. Soliman, Ebada Mohamed Said,
Hassan E. Elbatae, Tarik I. Zaher, Ahmed Abdel-Razik,
and Mohamed Elnadry

Abstract Ramadan intermittent fasting (RIF) offers several health benefits, particularly for individuals in good health and those diagnosed with metabolic dysfunction–associated fatty liver disease (MAFLD). By realigning circadian rhythms in tissues involved in metabolic processes linked to MAFLD, RIF could reduce the likelihood of developing MAFLD in healthy individuals and help manage the progression of the condition to metabolic dysfunction–associated steatohepatitis (MASH) in those already affected. Positive outcomes include enhanced body composition, better blood pressure control, improved lipid levels, normalized liver enzyme activity, and reduced liver fat accumulation.

M. H. Emara (✉) · H. E. Elbatae
Faculty of Medicine, Department of Hepatology, Gastroenterology and Infectious Diseases,
Kafrelsheikh University, Kafr El-Sheik, Egypt
e-mail: mohamed_emara@med.kfs.edu.eg; hassanelbatae_68@med.kfs.edu.eg

H. H. Soliman
Faculty of Medicine, Tropical Medicine and Infectious Diseases Department,
Tanta University, Tanta, Egypt
e-mail: Hanan.soliman@med.tanta.edu.eg

E. M. Said
Faculty of Medicine, Hepatology, Gastroenterology and Infectious Diseases Department,
Benha University, Benha, Egypt
e-mail: ebada.abdelhamid@fmed.bu.edu.eg

T. I. Zaher
Faculty of Medicine, Department of Hepatology, Gastroenterology and Infectious Diseases,
Zagazig University, Zagazig, Egypt
e-mail: ajied@medicine.zu.edu.eg

A. Abdel-Razik
Faculty of Medicine, Department of Tropical Medicine, Mansoura University, Mansoura, Egypt
e-mail: ahmedabdelrazik76@mans.edu.eg

M. Elnadry
Faculty of Medicine, Hepato-gastroenterology and Infectious Diseases Department,
Al-Azhar University, Cairo, Egypt
e-mail: prof_nadry@azhar.edu.eg

© The Author(s), under exclusive license to Springer Nature Singapore Pte
Ltd. 2025
M. E. Faris et al. (eds.), *Health and Medical Aspects of Ramadan Intermittent
Fasting*, https://doi.org/10.1007/978-981-96-6783-3_8

117

However, individuals with advanced cirrhosis, particularly those classified as Child–Pugh B or C, may experience worsening symptoms such as fluid retention (ascites), elevated bilirubin leading to jaundice, cognitive impairment (encephalopathy), and even life-threatening outcomes. Therefore, fasting is strongly discouraged for this high-risk group. Patients with cirrhosis face heightened risks of gastrointestinal (GI) bleeding, both from enlarged veins (varices) and ulcers, exacerbated by fasting-induced stress on the portal system.

Emerging research explores intermittent fasting (IF), including RIF, for its possible protective effects against certain cancers, such as liver cancer (hepatocellular carcinoma). Individuals who have undergone liver transplantation require close monitoring during RIF due to risks like dehydration, inconsistent use of immunosuppressive medications, and missed medical appointments. Regular checks of liver function, electrolyte balance, and drug levels (e.g., tacrolimus and cyclosporine) are essential. Fasting should be halted if health declines. Individuals with Gilbert syndrome may initially experience an increase in bilirubin levels during fasting, but these typically stabilize without any serious consequences.

To summarize, while RIF could improve metabolic markers and reduce steatosis in MAFLD, clinical deterioration and bleeding risks were observed in cirrhotic patients. Gilbert syndrome patients generally tolerate RIF safely, but close monitoring for transplant recipients is recommended.

Keywords Ramadan fasting · Intermittent fasting · Metabolic dysfunction–associated fatty liver disease (MAFLD) · Nonalcoholic fatty liver disease (NAFLD) · Cirrhosis · Calorie restriction

8.1 Introduction

During fasting, the liver becomes the central hub for glucose production through glycogenolysis, the breakdown of stored glycogen into glucose. In this process, glucose-6-phosphate (G6P) is transported to the endoplasmic reticulum, where the enzyme glucose-6-phosphatase removes its phosphate group, releasing free glucose into the bloodstream. Concurrently, lipolysis in adipose tissue liberates free fatty acids, which are then converted into ketone bodies by hepatocytes via ketogenesis in their mitochondria. These glucose and ketone molecules act as vital energy substrates for peripheral tissues during fasting or intense physical activity. The shift between the liver's fed and fasting metabolic states is precisely controlled by hormonal and neural signaling pathways [1].

As fasting progresses and glycogen reserves are depleted, the liver transitions to gluconeogenesis, synthesizing glucose from noncarbohydrate sources, including amino acids, lactate, pyruvate, and glycerol. While the liver produces some of these precursors internally, others are supplied via circulation from muscle and adipose tissue [1]. Notably, glycogenolysis and gluconeogenesis overlap temporally: Glycogenolysis maintains glucose levels for 12–24 h in response to declining blood sugar, while gluconeogenesis begins within 8 h and becomes the dominant glucose source after the first day of fasting [1].

Chronic liver disease (CLD), particularly alcoholic liver disease and severe cirrhosis, significantly affects glucose homeostasis [2]. Glucose intolerance and frank diabetes are frequently observed in those patients. They exhibit distorted diurnal patterns of gluconeogenic precursors, with elevated fasting blood lactate levels and exaggerated sustained elevation postprandially. Hyperlactatemia in cirrhosis correlates with the Child–Pugh score, which represents the degree of hepatic compensation, and impaired hepatic lactate clearance contributes to lactic acidosis in severe liver disease [3].

CLD was linked to hyperinsulinemia, hyperglucagonemia, insulin resistance, downregulation of insulin receptors, and impaired glucose tolerance or even frank diabetes. Fasting blood glucose levels may be lower in patients with cirrhosis than in controls [4].

8.2   Ramadan Fasting

Various intermittent fasting (IF) protocols have gained traction as non-pharmacological strategies to enhance health by promoting weight management and modifying dietary behaviors. Popular methods include time-restricted eating (TRE), alternate-day fasting, the 5:2 approach (where two fasting days are observed per week), and extended 24-h fasts. TRE involves confining caloric intake to a defined daily window, typically spanning 4–10 h, with or without caloric reduction [5].

Ramadan intermittent fasting (RIF), the focus of this discussion, represents a unique form of dry fasting combined with TRE, requiring abstention from all food and liquids from sunrise to sunset. Observers consume their entire caloric intake during nighttime hours.

The suprachiasmatic nucleus (SCN) in the brain acts as the central regulator of circadian rhythms, coordinating metabolic processes with peripheral tissue clocks and the natural light–dark cycle. However, the precise mechanisms governing this synchronization remain unclear [6]. Dietary patterns misaligned with the body's intrinsic rhythms can disrupt metabolic homeostasis. Meal timing serves as a potent external signal, recalibrating hepatic energy metabolism to align with feeding periods, irrespective of daylight cycles. Consuming over one-third of daily calories in the evening significantly increases the risk of obesity [2, 7].

Notably, Ramadan's nighttime fasting regimen alters hormonal profiles, particularly leptin—a hormone that regulates satiety. This shift suppresses leptin's typical nocturnal rise and delays its peak levels following evening meals [8, 9]. Additionally, RIF independently modulates skeletal muscle amino acid transport, bypassing the body's innate clock mechanisms [10]. It also activates genes associated with fat cell formation, adipose tissue browning, and lipid synthesis pathways, thereby enhancing insulin sensitivity [11]. The interplay between meal timing, hepatic function, and circadian regulation underscores their intricate connection [12].

A recent meta-analysis of 20 studies demonstrated the beneficial effects of RIF on liver function markers (e.g., bilirubin, aspartate aminotransferase (AST), alkaline phosphatase (ALP), and gamma-glutamyl transpeptidase (GGT) in healthy populations [13]. However, RIF may still have pros and cons for different hepatic diseases, which we will highlight next.

8.2.1 Acute Hepatitis

Patients with acute hepatitis of any etiology (viral, autoimmune, drug-induced, etc.) need supportive parameters, including eating frequent small meals [14]. So RIF was not studied in those patients because fasting is potentially unsafe and medically prohibited [15].

8.2.2 Chronic Hepatitis

In contrast to acute hepatitis, chronic hepatitis typically follows a fluctuating course with milder, nonspecific symptoms. Maintaining regular food intake is essential for preserving adequate hepatic blood flow. Previous studies have noted that RIF may exacerbate the severity of otherwise stable chronic liver diseases [16]. Additionally, adherence to antiviral therapy has been found to decline during fasting periods [14]. While baseline liver function tests (LFTs) in patients with chronic hepatitis B and C generally show minimal variation before, during, and after RIF, regular monitoring is still recommended for those who choose to fast [17].

8.2.3 Metabolic Dysfunction–Associated Fatty Liver Disease (MAFLD)

In 2020, the terms *metabolic dysfunction–associated fatty liver disease (MAFLD)* and *metabolic dysfunction–associated steatohepatitis (MASH)* were introduced, replacing the older nomenclature *nonalcoholic fatty liver disease (NAFLD)* and *nonalcoholic steatohepatitis (NASH),* to more accurately reflect the metabolic underpinnings of the condition. Subsequently, in July 2023, the terminology evolved further to *metabolic dysfunction–associated steatotic liver disease (MASLD)* and *metabolic-associated steatohepatitis (MASH)* to avoid the stigma associated with the word "fatty."

MAFLD is defined as hepatic steatosis involving more than 5% of the liver, confirmed via imaging or biopsy, in the presence of at least one cardiometabolic risk factor (overweight/obesity, visceral adiposity, dysglycemia, hypertension, or dyslipidemia) [18]. By contrast, NAFLD was characterized by >5% macrovesicular steatosis in individuals with minimal or no alcohol intake and only after excluding other identifiable causes of liver fat accumulation, which makes it a negative diagnosis made by exclusion [19]. Importantly, the MAFLD/MASLD framework shifts the paradigm from one of diagnosis by exclusion to one of inclusion, thereby broadening the scope of patients affected. For consistency, this article adopts the updated terminology.

According to current clinical guidelines issued by European [20, 21], American [19], Asian, and Korean [22] liver disease societies, the cornerstone of MAFLD management remains lifestyle modification—primarily weight reduction and regular physical activity. Although the 2018 guidelines from the American Association for the Study of Liver Diseases (AASLD) expressed uncertainty regarding the superiority of any specific dietary pattern for histologic improvement [23], more recent updates align with the European Society for Clinical Nutrition and Metabolism (ESPEN) recommendations in supporting the Mediterranean diet and regular exercise, with weight loss as the primary therapeutic target. Notably, weight reduction has demonstrated a dose-dependent improvement in hepatic steatosis, fibrosis, and MASH [19]. Significant histological improvement has been observed following weight loss in both lean and obese patients with MASH [24].

Both the American Gastroenterological Association (AGA) (2021) and AASLD (2022) clinical practice guidelines endorse intermittent fasting (IF), particularly time-restricted eating (TRE), for patients with MAFLD [19, 25]. RIF represents a time-restricted intermittent fasting regimen with exclusive nighttime food intake. This raises the question: Does RIF confer similar benefits?

Emerging evidence suggests that the timing of food intake, such as skipping breakfast, delayed meals, irregular eating patterns, or nocturnal eating, is associated with increased obesity rates [26], metabolic dysfunction [27], and a heightened risk or severity of MAFLD and MASH, especially in obese individuals [28–30]. Based on these associations, RIF might theoretically worsen MAFLD by concentrating food intake at night. Contrary to this expectation, multiple meta-analyses have demonstrated that RIF is associated with reductions in body weight, fat mass [31, 32], and improvements in cardiometabolic markers, including lipid profiles [33] and glycemic indices [34, 35].

In patients with MAFLD, RIF has been associated with reductions in fasting glucose and the homeostasis model assessment-estimated insulin resistance (HOMA-IR), paralleled by decreased levels of inflammatory cytokines and C-reactive protein [36]. Additionally, anthropometric improvements and favorable changes in serum vaspin and omentin-1 levels (adipokines linked to insulin resistance and hepatocyte ballooning, respectively) have been reported [37].

Notably, patients with MAFLD who observe RIF have experienced significant weight loss despite maintaining a consistent daily caloric intake [38]. The 2023 London Ramadan Study (LORANS) observed reductions in waist circumference, hip circumference, and BMI among 146 participants (70% of whom were diabetic or hypertensive) following Ramadan intensive follow-up. These improvements began in the second week of Ramadan and persisted for at least three weeks afterward [39]. The same study included a systematic review and meta-analysis of 66 studies, demonstrating that RIF led to reductions in anthropometric indices, including waist and hip circumferences, BMI, total body weight, and fat mass, without significantly affecting lean mass [39]. However, this meta-analysis was limited by population heterogeneity, as it included healthy individuals and those with cirrhosis, diabetes, hypertension, renal disease, NAFLD, and metabolic syndrome.

A recent Egyptian cohort study involving 40 MAFLD patients reported significant reductions in BMI and hepatic steatosis, assessed by FibroScan-controlled attenuation parameter (CAP), although dietary restrictions during the study were not specified [40]. In another study of seven patients with metabolic syndrome, reductions in ALT levels were observed post-Ramadan, accompanied by declines in pro-inflammatory cytokines, including IL-2, IL-8, and TNF-α [41]. Similarly, a cohort of 50 patients with MAFLD showed reduced ALT, serum insulin, and blood pressure, with increased high density lipoprotein (HDL-c) after approximately 27 days of RIF [42].

In contrast, a study involving 60 patients with MAFLD found that among the 36 who fasted, ALT levels increased significantly compared to their pre-Ramadan levels, and this rise was greater than that observed in the 24 non-fasting controls [43].

Other findings support the metabolic benefits of caloric restriction during RIF. In obese individuals, RIF has been associated with reductions in leptin levels and body weight [44]. Among patients with metabolic syndrome, RIF resulted in a decrease in fat mass and visceral adiposity while preserving lean body mass [45]. Even without deliberate caloric restriction, RIF has been shown to reduce visceral fat and adipokines (e.g., adiponectin, Interleukin 6 (IL-6), tumor necrosis factor alpha (TNF-α) and IGF-1) while maintaining glucose homeostasis in overweight and obese individuals [46].

Furthermore, a study comparing 83 fasting MAFLD patients with 40 non-fasting controls found significant improvements in cholesterol levels, atherogenic index, visceral fat, ultrasound steatosis grading, and liver enzymes despite no imposed dietary restrictions [47]. Most recently, a retrospective case-control study involving 155 patients with MAFLD/MASH (74 fasting and 81 non-fasting) reported RIF-associated improvements in inflammatory markers, HOMA-IR, and noninvasive indicators of MASH severity [48].

8.2.4   Liver Cirrhosis

Liver cirrhosis is a progressive, degenerative condition with diverse etiologies, including chronic viral hepatitis, alcohol-related liver disease, and metabolic dysfunction–associated fatty liver disease (MAFLD). It is characterized by hepatic functional impairment and the development of portal hypertension.

The liver plays a central role in maintaining glucose homeostasis during fasting states [1]. Consequently, patients with cirrhosis—particularly those with diabetes on pharmacological treatment—are at increased risk of hypoglycemia during fasting hours.

The impact of RIF on patients with cirrhosis has not been extensively studied. Limited observational data suggest that RIF may negatively affect decompensated cirrhotic patients, particularly those with Child–Pugh class B or C who choose to fast despite medical advice. Reported complications include the development of new ascites in 25–41% of patients and worsening ascites in 64% of those with pre-existing fluid accumulation. Additionally, 13–15% of patients experienced progression to Child–Pugh class C, accompanied by clinical jaundice and elevated serum bilirubin. Isolated cases of hepatic encephalopathy and gastrointestinal (GI) bleeding were also noted, along with a mortality rate of approximately 1% (three out of 300 patients). In contrast, patients with compensated cirrhosis generally showed no significant clinical or biochemical deterioration during RIF [16, 49, 50].

Given the variability in clinical presentation, individualized assessment of cirrhotic patients prior to fasting is essential. This should include a comprehensive clinical evaluation, laboratory tests, imaging, medication review, dietary planning, and endoscopic assessment in select cases. One recent review recommends that patients with Child–Pugh class B or C cirrhosis abstain from fasting, while patients with class A may be permitted to fast with caution [15].

The long-term impact of RIF on the natural course of cirrhosis remains poorly understood, as most available studies assess outcomes only during Ramadan and up to one month thereafter. It is plausible that the risk of decompensation may increase if fasting patients are followed over a longer duration. Moreover, several relevant variables—such as patient age, occupational demands, and the etiology of cirrhosis—have not been adequately addressed in existing studies. This highlights the need for a structured, individualized risk assessment tool to inform clinical decision-making regarding fasting in patients with cirrhosis [51].

8.2.5   Portal Hypertension, Variceal Bleeding, and Peptic Ulcer Risk

Portal hypertension and bleeding from gastroesophageal varices are major contributors to morbidity and mortality in patients with liver cirrhosis [52]. Under normal physiological conditions, postprandial hyperemia leads to increased portal and mesenteric blood flow [53]. In cirrhotic patients, this is accompanied by an increase in the hepatic venous pressure gradient (HVPG) and enhanced collateral circulation. While individuals with well-developed portosystemic collaterals may exhibit a smaller postprandial increase in HVPG, they often experience substantial surges in collateral blood flow, which can potentially predispose them to variceal dilation and rupture [54]. Moreover, the portal flow's congestive index significantly rises from fasting to postprandial states in Child–Pugh class A and B patients, further elevating the risk of variceal hemorrhage [50]. This physiologic mechanism may underlie the clinical observation of increased variceal bleeding episodes in cirrhotic patients with portal hypertension during nighttime, particularly after the iftar meal during Ramadan [15].

Peptic ulcers—whether symptomatic or silent—are also common in cirrhotic patients. Fasting significantly heightens the risk of gastrointestinal bleeding from peptic ulcers in both cirrhotic and non-cirrhotic individuals. Furthermore, the risk of ulcer perforation is notably increased during fasting, particularly among females and elderly patients. As a result, individuals with active peptic ulcer disease are strongly advised against observing Ramadan fasting. For patients with stable chronic liver disease, a screening upper gastrointestinal endoscopy is recommended at least one month before Ramadan. This allows for early identification and management of varices and ulcers, thereby minimizing the risk of bleeding during the fasting period [15].

8.2.6 Hepatocellular Carcinoma (HCC)

Emerging evidence suggests that pharmacological agents mimicking the metabolic effects of fasting can suppress hypoxia-induced metastasis, angiogenesis, and metabolic reprogramming in hepatocellular carcinoma (HCC). Similar outcomes have been observed with sodium-glucose cotransporter 2 (SGLT2) inhibitors, highlighting the potential anticarcinogenic benefits derived from fasting-like states [55].

Fasting activates multiple cellular pathways that enhance autophagy while inhibiting protein synthesis and cell proliferation, primarily through the downregulation of the mechanistic target of the rapamycin (mTOR) signaling pathway, which plays a central role in HCC pathogenesis. Furthermore, intermittent fasting—particularly during Ramadan—has been shown to help resynchronize the circadian rhythm and reset key metabolic pathways involved in cellular growth, repair, and defense mechanisms. These effects may help prevent the progression of CLD to HCC [56].

Obesity is a well-established risk factor for HCC, increasing both its incidence and associated mortality by approximately two- to fourfold [57]. Fasting, especially when combined with caloric restriction, promotes weight loss and may mitigate obesity-related cancer risks. Additionally, fasting induces a state of ketosis, during which ketone bodies, such as β-hydroxybutyrate, not only serve as alternative energy sources but also function as endogenous histone deacetylase inhibitors. This contributes to protection against oxidative stress and may delay tumor progression [56–58].

To date, no studies have directly investigated the impact of Ramadan intermittent fasting (RIF) on the development or progression of HCC. However, patients with advanced HCC typically exhibit significant hepatic decompensation and related complications, rendering any form of fasting, including RIF, inadvisable for this population [14, 15].

8.2.7 Liver Transplantation

Liver transplantation (LT) significantly enhances both survival and quality of life (QoL) in appropriately selected patients. In Islam, the obligation to perform religious rituals is contingent upon an individual's ability to do so, and Ramadan fasting is no exception. Islamic principles make fasting facultative for any diseased person. However, many Muslim transplant recipients consider the ability to participate in spiritual and religious practices—such as Ramadan fasting—to be a vital component of their overall QoL. Consequently, many individuals seek guidance from their healthcare providers regarding the safety of fasting after transplantation.

Indeed, RIF—a form of dry fasting that involves abstaining from both food and water for more than 12 h daily—may pose clinical risks for transplant recipients, including dehydration, accumulation of toxic metabolites, and potential impairment of renal function. These factors may increase the likelihood of graft rejection, particularly if medication timing is disrupted or adherence to immunosuppressive medication declines. Therefore, a comprehensive risk assessment is essential when evaluating a liver transplant recipient's suitability for fasting.

Patients are classified as high-risk if they meet any of the following criteria: transplantation within the previous 12 months, twice-daily immunosuppressive regimens, fluid restriction or susceptibility to dehydration, pregnancy, diabetes, unstable or reduced graft function, or the presence of multiple organ transplants. Those not meeting these criteria are generally considered to be at moderate or low risk of adverse outcomes during fasting [59].

One study assessing the safety of fasting in LT recipients found no significant differences in tacrolimus trough levels between fasting and non-fasting groups. The authors concluded that Ramadan fasting may be safe for patients with stable graft function and no evidence of cirrhosis [60]. Another study supported this conclusion, reporting that RIF did not adversely affect renal or hepatic parameters in LT recipients, provided that a structured protocol for adjusting immunosuppressive regimens and follow-up monitoring was followed. Ideally, any transition to a once-daily immunosuppression schedule should be initiated at least one month before Ramadan. For moderate- or low-risk patients, fasting decisions should be individualized based on baseline estimated glomerular filtration rate and the type of immunosuppressive therapy used. Continuous monitoring of graft function, serum electrolytes, and drug trough levels (e.g., tacrolimus or cyclosporine) is recommended throughout Ramadan. Patients should be advised to break the fast if any signs of clinical deterioration occur [61].

8.3 Gilbert Syndrome

Gilbert syndrome is a benign autosomal recessive disorder characterized by impaired bilirubin metabolism, leading to recurrent episodes of unconjugated hyperbilirubinemia. These episodes are typically harmless and do not impact life expectancy. Triggers include dehydration, fever, certain medications, and prolonged fasting that exceeds 12 h. Therefore, episodes of hyperbilirubinemia are justified to occur during Ramadan fasting, as observed in a case series. Nevertheless, patients maintained stable bilirubin levels without experiencing significant complications [62]. So we cannot recommend against fasting in those patients.

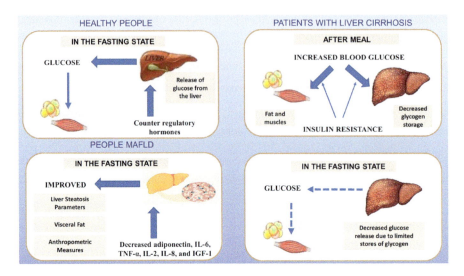

Fig. 8.1 Graphical abstract for the key findings of the current review

The key findings of this study are visually represented in the accompanying graphical abstract (Fig. 8.1).

8.4 Conclusion

RIF is a model of intermittent dry fasting with TRE, which involves no caloric restriction. The daytime fasting state and eating behavior during RIF hold potential for therapeutic intervention through modification of body energy and modulation of various hormonal and cytokine pathways. It has been investigated through observational and clinical trials as a potentially beneficial regimen for MAFLD. However, it was found harmful for patients with decompensated cirrhosis and patients with active GI bleeding, and it looks potentially detrimental for LT recipients who are not adopting modified immunosuppression regimens. Advising patients with liver diseases to observe fasting should be individualized on a case-by-case basis, depending on various parameters and risk stratification. Those with chronic liver disease (CLD) should be evaluated at least one month before undergoing a radiological intervention (RIF) to implement prophylactic interventions.

The abstract is attached in the following link:

https://drive.google.com/file/d/1BgD0ajXS8gWAdOh89Go8TM2w6FC7NcXJ/view?usp=sharing

References

1. Rui L. Energy metabolism in the liver. Compr Physiol. 2014;4(1):177–97.
2. García-Compeán D, Jáquez-Quintana JO, Lavalle-González FJ, Reyes-Cabello E, González-González JA, Muñoz-Espinosa LE, et al. The prevalence and clinical characteristics of glucose metabolism disorders in patients with liver cirrhosis. A prospective study. Ann Hepatol. 2012;11(2):240–8.
3. Zeng G, Penninkilampi R, Chaganti J, Montagnese S, Brew BJ, Danta M. Meta-analysis of magnetic resonance spectroscopy in the diagnosis of hepatic encephalopathy. Neurology. 2020;94(11):e1147–56.
4. Petrides AS, Vogt C, Schulze-Berge D, Matthews D, Strohmeyer G. Pathogenesis of glucose intolerance and diabetes mellitus in cirrhosis. Hepatology. 1994;20(5):1366–74.
5. Cleveland Clinic. Intermittent Fasting: 4 Different Types Explained [Internet] 2022. [Cited 2022 January 30]. Available from: https://health.clevelandclinic.org/intermittent-fasting-4-different-types-explained/. Accessed 20 Sept 2023.
6. Rijo-Ferreira F, Takahashi JS. Genomics of circadian rhythms in health and disease. Genome Med. 2019;11(1):82.
7. Han AL. Association between nonalcoholic fatty liver disease and dietary habits, stress, and health-related quality of life in Korean adults. Nutrients. 2020;12(6):1555.
8. Bogdan A, Bouchareb B, Touitou Y. Response of circulating leptin to Ramadan daytime fasting: a circadian study. Br J Nutr. 2005;93:515–8.
9. Gaeini Z, Mirmiran P, Bahadoran Z. Effects of Ramadan intermittent fasting on leptin and adiponectin: a systematic review and meta-analysis. Hormones (Athens). 2021;20:237–46.
10. Lundell LS, Parr EB, Devlin BL, Ingerslev LR, Altıntaş A, Sato S, Sassone-Corsi P, et al. Time-restricted feeding alters lipid and amino acid metabolite rhythmicity without perturbing clock gene expression. Nat Commun. 2020;11(1):4643.
11. Zhao L, Hutchison AT, Liu B, Wittert GA, Thompson CH, Nguyen L, et al. Time-restricted eating alters the 24-hour profile of adipose tissue transcriptome in men with obesity. Obesity (Silver Spring). 2023;31(Suppl 1):63–74.
12. Marjot T, Tomlinson JW, Hodson L, Ray DW. Timing of energy intake and the therapeutic potential of intermittent fasting and time-restricted eating in NAFLD. Gut. 2023;72(8):1607–19.
13. Faris ME, Jahrami H, Abdelrahim D, Bragazzi N, BaHammam A. The effects of Ramadan intermittent fasting on liver function in healthy adults: a systematic review, meta-analysis, and meta-regression. Diabetes Res Clin Pract. 2021;178:108951.
14. Staff Members of Tropical Medicine Department, Faculty of Medicine, Zagazig University, Egypt. Liver disease and fasting during the month of Ramadan. Afro-Egypt J Infect Endem Dis. 2014;4:112–3.
15. Emara MH, Soliman HH, Elnadry M, Mohamed Said E, Abd-Elsalam S, Elbatae HE, et al. Ramadan fasting and liver diseases: a review with practice advice and recommendations. Liver Int. 2021;41:436–48.
16. Elnadry MH, Nigm IA, Abdel Aziz IM, Elshafee AM, Elazhary SS, Abdel Hafeez MA, et al. Effect of Ramadan fasting on Muslim patients with chronic liver diseases. J Egypt Soc Parasitol. 2011;41:337–46.
17. Hickman IJ, Clouston AD, Macdonald GA, Purdie DM, Prins JB, Ash S, et al. Effect of weight reduction on liver histology and biochemistry in patients with chronic hepatitis C. Gut. 2002;51:89–94.
18. Rinella ME, Lazarus JV, Ratziu V, Francque SM, Sanyal AJ, Kanwal F, et al. A multisociety Delphi consensus statement on new fatty liver disease nomenclature. Ann Hepatol. 2023;29(1):101133.
19. Rinella ME, Neuschwander-Tetri BA, Siddiqui MS, Abdelmalek MF, Caldwell S, Barb D, et al. AASLD practice guidance on the clinical assessment and management of the nonalcoholic fatty liver disease. Hepatology. 2023;77(5):1797–835.

20. European Association for the Study of the Liver (EASL), European Association for the Study of Diabetes (EASD), European Association for the Study of Obesity (EASO) EASL-EASDEASO clinical practice guidelines for the management of the nonalcoholic fatty liver disease. J Hepatol. 2016;64:1388–402.
21. Plauth M, Bernal W, Dasarathy S, Merli M, Plank LD, Schütz T, et al. ESPEN guideline on clinical nutrition in liver disease. Clin Nutr. 2019;38:485–521.
22. Eslam M, Sarin SK, Wong VW, Fan JG, Kawaguchi T, Ahn SH, et al. The Asian Pacific Association for the Study of the Liver clinical practice guidelines for the diagnosis and management of metabolic-associated fatty liver disease. Hepatol Int. 2020;14:889–919.
23. The diagnosis and management of nonalcoholic fatty liver disease: practice guidance from the American Association for the Study of Liver Diseases. Clin Liver Dis (Hoboken). 2018;11(4):81.
24. Alam S, Hasan MJ, Khan AS, Alam M, Hasan N. Effect of weight reduction on histological activity and fibrosis of lean nonalcoholic steatohepatitis patient. J Transl Int Med. 2019;7:106–14.
25. Younossi ZM, Corey KE, Lim JK. AGA clinical practice update on lifestyle modification using diet and exercise to achieve weight loss in the management of nonalcoholic fatty liver disease: an expert review. Gastroenterology. 2021;160:912.
26. Maukonen M, Kanerva N, Partonen T, Männistö S. Chronotype and energy intake timing in relation to changes in anthropometrics: a 7-year follow-up study in adults. Chronobiol Int. 2019;36:27–41.
27. Yu JH, Yun C-H, Ahn JH, Suh S, Cho HJ, Lee SK, et al. The evening chronotype is associated with an increased risk of metabolic disorders and altered body composition in middle-aged adults. J Clin Endocrinol Metab. 2015;100(4):1494–502.
28. Xie J, Huang H, Chen Y, Xu L, Xu C. Skipping breakfast is associated with an increased long-term cardiovascular mortality in metabolic dysfunction-associated fatty liver disease (MAFLD) but not MAFLD-free individuals. Aliment Pharmacol Ther. 2022;55:212–24.
29. Vetrani C, Barrea L, Verde L, Sarno G, Docimo A, de Alteriis G, et al. The evening chronotype is associated with severe NAFLD in obesity. Int J Obes. 2022;46(9):1638–43.
30. Younes R, Rosso C, Petta S, Cucco M, Marietti M, Caviglia GP, et al. The usefulness of the index of NASH–ION for the diagnosis of Steatohepatitis in patients with nonalcoholic fatty liver: an external validation study. Liver Int. 2018;38:715–23.
31. Sadeghirad B, Motaghipisheh S, Kolahdooz F, Zahedi MJ, Haghdoost AA. Islamic fasting and weight loss: a systematic review and meta-analysis. Public Health Nutr. 2014;17:396–406.
32. Fernando HA, Zibellini J, Harris RA, Seimon RV, Sainsbury A. Effect of Ramadan fasting on weight and body composition in healthy non-athlete adults: a systematic review and meta-analysis. Nutrients. 2019;11:478.
33. Jahrami HA, Faris M, Abdulrahman IJ, Mohamed IJ, Abdelrahim DN, Madkour MI, et al. Does four-week consecutive, dawn-to-sunset intermittent fasting during Ramadan affect Cardiometabolic risk factors in healthy adults? A systematic review, meta-analysis, and meta-regression. Nutr Metab Cardiovasc Dis. 2021;31:2273–301.
34. Aydın N, Kul S, Karadağ G, Tabur S, Araz M. Effect of Ramadan fasting on Glycaemic parameters & body mass index in type II diabetic patients: a meta-analysis. Indian J Med Res. 2019;150:546.
35. Faris ME, Jahrami H, BaHammam A, Kalaji Z, Madkour M, Hassanein M. A systematic review, meta-analysis, and meta-regression of the impact of diurnal intermittent fasting during Ramadan on glucometabolic markers in healthy subjects. Diabetes Res Clin Pract. 2020;165:108226.
36. Aliasghari F, Izadi A, Gargari BP, Ebrahimi S. The effects of Ramadan fasting on body composition, blood pressure, glucose metabolism, and markers of inflammation in NAFLD patients: an observational trial. J Am Coll Nutr. 2017;36(8):640–5.

37. Ebrahimi S, Gaargari BP, Izadi A, Imani B, Asjodi F. The effects of Ramadan fasting on serum concentrations of vaspin and omentin-1 in patients with nonalcoholic fatty liver disease. Eur J Integr Med. 2018;19:110–4.
38. Mindikoglu AL, Opekun AR, Gagan SK, Devaraj S. Impact of time-restricted feeding and dawn-to-sunset fasting on circadian rhythm, obesity, metabolic syndrome, and nonalcoholic fatty liver disease. Gastroenterol Res Pract. 2017;2017:3932491.
39. Al-Jafar R, Wahyuni NS, Belhaj K, Ersi MH, Boroghani Z, Alreshidi A, et al. The impact of Ramadan intermittent fasting on anthropometric measurements and body composition: evidence from LORANS study and a meta-analysis. Front Nutr. 2023;10:1082217.
40. Gad AI, Abdel-Ghani HA, Barakat AAEA. Effect of Ramadan fasting on hepatic steatosis as quantified by controlled attenuation parameter (CAP): a prospective observational study. Egypt Liver J. 2022;12:22.
41. Unalacak M, Kara IH, Baltaci D, Erdem O, Bucaktepe PG. Effects of Ramadan fasting on biochemical and hematological parameters, as well as cytokines, in healthy and obese individuals. Metab Syndr Relat Disord. 2011;9(2):157–61.
42. Arabi SM, Hejri ZaRIFi S, Nematy M, Safarian M. The effect of Ramadan fasting on nonalcoholic fatty liver disease (NAFLD) patients. J Fasting Health. 2015;3(2):74–80.
43. Rahimi H, Habibi ME, Gharavinia A, Emami MH, Baghaei A, Tavakol N. Effect of Ramadan fasting on alanine aminotransferase (ALT) in nonalcoholic fatty liver disease (NAFLD). J Fasting Health. 2017;5(3):107–12.
44. Muhammad H, Latifah FN, Susilowati R. The yo-yo effect of Ramadan fasting on overweight/obese individuals in Indonesian: a prospective study. Mediterr J Nutr Metab. 2018;11:127–33.
45. Alinezhad-Namaghi M, Eslami S, Nematy M, Khoshnasab A, Rezvani R, Philippou E, et al. Intermittent fasting during Ramadan and its effects in individuals with metabolic syndrome. Nutr Today. 2019;54(4):159–64.
46. Faris MAE, Madkour MI, Obaideen AK, Dalah EZ, Hasan HA, Radwan H, et al. Effect of Ramadan diurnal fasting on visceral adiposity and serum adipokines in overweight and obese individuals. Diabetes Res Clin Pract. 2019;153:166–75.
47. Ebrahimi S, Gargari BP, Aliasghari F, Asjodi F, Izadi A. Ramadan fasting improves liver function and total cholesterol in patients with nonalcoholic fatty liver disease. Int J Vitam Nutr Res. 2020;90(1–2):95–102.
48. Mari A, Khoury T, Baker M, Said Ahmad H, Abu Baker F, Mahamid M. The impact of Ramadan fasting on fatty liver disease severity: a retrospective case-control study from Israel. Isr Med Assoc J. 2021;23(2):94–8.
49. Elfert AA, AbouSaif SA, Kader NA, AbdelAal E, Elfert AY, Moez AT, et al. A multicenter pilot study of the effects of Ramadan fasting on patients with liver cirrhosis. Tanta Med Sci J. 2011;6:25–33.
50. Mohamed SY, Emara MH, Hussien HI, Elsadek HM. Changes in portal blood flow and liver functions in cirrhotics during Ramadan in the summer: a pilot study. Gastroenterol Hepatol Bed Bench. 2016;9:180–8.
51. Emara MH, Abdelaty AI, Elbatae HE, Abdelrazik OM, Elgammal NE. The need for a risk-assessment tool among patients with chronic liver diseases interested in intermittent fasting: Ramadan model. Nutr Rev. 2024;82(2):240–3.
52. Gunarathne LS, Rajapaksha H, Shackel N, Angus PW, Herath CB. Cirrhotic portal hypertension: from pathophysiology to novel therapeutics. World J Gastroenterol. 2020;26(40):6111–40.
53. Chou CC. Splanchnic and overall cardiovascular hemodynamics during eating and digestion. Fed Proc. 1983;42(6):1658–61.
54. Albillos A, Bañares R, González M, Catalina MV, Pastor O, Gonzalez R, et al. The extent of the collateral circulation influences the postprandial increase in portal pressure in patients with cirrhosis. Gut. 2007;56(2):259–64.
55. Arvanitakis K, Koufakis T, Kotsa K, Germanidis G. The effects of sodium-glucose cotransporter 2 inhibitors on hepatocellular carcinoma: from molecular mechanisms to potential clinical implications. Pharmacol Res. 2022;181:106261.

56. Minciuna I, Kleef LAV, Stefanescu H, Procopet B. Is fasting good when one is at risk of liver cancer? Cancers (Basel). 2022;14(20):5084.
57. Gupta A, Das A, Majumder K, Arora N, Mayo HG, Singh PP, et al. Obesity is independently associated with increased risk of hepatocellular cancer-related mortality: a systematic review and meta-analysis. Am J Clin Oncol. 2018;41:874.
58. Longo VD, Di Tano M, Mattson MP, Guidi N. Intermittent and periodic fasting, longevity, and disease. Nat Aging. 2021;1:47–59.
59. Shafi Malik A, Rizwan Hamer B, Shabir S, Youssef S, Morsy M, Rashid R, et al. Effects of fasting on solid organ transplant recipients during Ramadan—a practical guide for healthcare professionals. Clin Med (Lond). 2021;21(5):e492–8.
60. Derbala M, Elbadri M, Amer A, Al Kaabi S, Mohiuddin S, Elsayd E. Safety and the deleterious effect of fasting Ramadan in liver transplant recipients. J Gastroenterol Metabol. 2018;1:301.
61. Montasser IF, Dabbous H, Sakr MM, Ebada H, Massoud YM, Salaheldin MM, et al. Effect of Ramadan fasting on Muslim recipients after living donor liver transplantation: a single center study. Arab J Gastroenterol. 2020;21(2):76–9.
62. Ashraf W, van Someren N, Quigley EM, Saboor SA, Farrow LJ. Gilbert's syndrome and Ramadan: exacerbation of unconjugated hyperbilirubinemia by religious fasting. J Clin Gastroenterol. 1994;19:122–4.

Chapter 9
Ramadan Intermittent Fasting, Gut Microbiota, and Gastrointestinal Health

Huma Naqeeb, Iftikhar Alam, Leila Cheikh Ismail, MoezAlIslam E. Faris, and Falak Zeb

Abstract Ramadan intermittent fasting (RIF) is a one-month religious practice observed by Muslims worldwide, characterized by abstinence from drinks and food from dawn to sunset. Beyond its spiritual significance, RIF has gained attention for its potential health benefits, including its impact on the gut microbiota and gastrointestinal (GI) health. RIF induces a shift in the gut microbial composition, promoting the production of gut metabolites and aligning the microbial rhythmicity. Additionally, RIF modulates the microbial metabolic pathways, leading to enhanced production of short-chain fatty acids (SCFAs) and other gut metabolites. These metabolites play a crucial role in maintaining gut integrity, regulating immune responses, and providing an energy source for colonocytes. RIF contributes to enhanced microbial diversity and SCFA produc-

H. Naqeeb
Department of Human Nutrition and Dietetics, Women University Mardan, Mardan, Pakistan
e-mail: huma.naqeeb@wumardan.edu.pk

I. Alam
Department of Human Nutrition and Dietetics, Faculty of Sciences, Bacha Khan University, Charsadda, Khyber Pakhtunkhwa (KPK), Pakistan
e-mail: iftikharalam@aup.edu.pk

L. C. Ismail
Department of Clinical Nutrition and Dietetics, College of Health Sciences, University of Sharjah, Sharjah, United Arab Emirates

Research Institute for Medical and Health Sciences (RIMHS), University of Sharjah, Sharjah, United Arab Emirates

Department of Women's and Reproductive Health, University of Oxford, Oxford, UK
e-mail: lcheikhismail@sharjah.ac.ae

M. E. Faris
Department of Clinical Nutrition and Dietetics, Faculty of Allied Medical Sciences, Applied Science Private University, Amman, Jordan

F. Zeb (✉)
Research Institute for Medical and Health Sciences (RIMHS), University of Sharjah, Sharjah, United Arab Emirates

M. E. Faris et al. (eds.), *Health and Medical Aspects of Ramadan Intermittent Fasting*, https://doi.org/10.1007/978-981-96-6783-3_9

131

tion, as well as improved gut hormones and other biomarkers, which have been associated with reduced inflammation, strengthened gut barrier function, and regulation of appetite and metabolism. Furthermore, RIF may mitigate the risk of gastrointestinal disorders, including peptic ulcer, inflammatory bowel disease (IBD), and colorectal cancer (CRC). Longitudinal studies assessing the long-term effects of RIF on microbial composition and its clinical implications are warranted. In conclusion, RIF appears to shape the gut microbiota in a manner conducive to gastrointestinal health. The modulation of microbial composition and metabolism during fasting holds promise for the prevention and management of GI disorders, highlighting the importance of integrating dietary practices with microbial therapeutics for promoting overall well-being.

Keywords Ramadan intermittent fasting · Gut microbiota · Gut health · Peptic ulcer · Microbial diversity

9.1 Introduction

Ramadan intermittent fasting (RIF), as observed by about 1.5 billion Muslims worldwide, involves refraining from eating food and drinking from dawn until sunset. The practice can have implications for individuals with gastrointestinal (GI) diseases and the gut microbiota. RIF has demonstrated several gut-related health benefits, such as improving gut microbiota composition and function [1], modifying gut hormone levels, enhancing migrating motor complex (MMC) autophagy, and decreasing the level of pro-inflammatory cytokines [2]. Patients suffering from inflammatory bowel disease (IBD) have a low chance of their illness worsening, according to the research currently available on the effects of RIF on gastrointestinal diseases. On the other hand, older men with ulcerative colitis (UC) were more likely to experience flare-ups when fasting. Similarly, following RIF, patients with duodenal ulcers were more likely to experience bleeding. In contrast, studies on liver disease patients have shown improvements in liver enzymes, cholesterol, and bilirubin after RIF, albeit with contradictory results [2].

Meal timings, dietary composition, and diet quality during Ramadan can enhance the therapeutic effect of RIF. For instance, these cues (meal timings and diet quality) of RIF may increase the abundance and diversity of gut microbiota upon the availability of nutrients [3]. Further, the increased microbial richness may stimulate the production of gut metabolites, such as SCFAs and amino acid derivatives, as well as enhance the bioavailability of polyphenols. Moreover, the time and caloric restriction, as well as gut metabolites, act as signaling molecules for oscillating the peripheral rhythmicity of the gut. This peripheral rhythmicity aligns the gut hormones with the gut biomarkers for normal gut function and homeostasis, thereby reducing the burden of gut-associated diseases like IBD, gastroesophageal reflux disease (GERD), colorectal cancer (CRC), and peptic ulcer (Fig. 9.1).

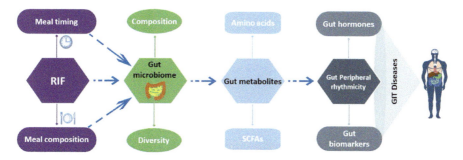

Fig. 9.1 RIF acts as a key for 3Ms (mediation, moderation, and modification) of 3Gs (increasing gut microbial diversity, enhancing gut metabolite production, and oscillating gut rhythmicity). Meal timing and composition are two clues that RIF (purple color) enhances microbial composition and diversity (green color) and the production of gut metabolites (sky blue color). It also targets gut rhythmicity, which improves gut hormones and other biomarkers (gray color)

9.2   RIF Shaping the Gut Microbiota

Several factors associated with fasting, including changes in dietary patterns, meal timing, and overall lifestyle during this period, may contribute to alterations in the gut microbiota [4], including colonic changes in the availability of fiber, polyphenols, prebiotics, proteins, and bile [5]. Further, Ramadan, with daily fasting from dawn to sunset, introduces a potential influence on the circadian rhythm of the gut microbiota. Disruptions to circadian rhythms, suggested by research, may contribute to alterations in the function and composition of the microbiota, thus affecting gut health. Fasting during Ramadan may also lead to changes in the production of crucial metabolites and short-chain fatty acids (SCFAs) produced during the fermentation of dietary fibers by gut bacteria. Given the essential role of SCFAs in maintaining gut health, alterations in their production could have implications for overall gastrointestinal well-being [6].

In addition to changing meal timing, RIF alters dietary habits and lifestyle, both of which play a significant role in shaping the gut microbiota. Proper hydration is identified as a key factor in supporting gut health by promoting the growth and activity of beneficial bacteria. Individuals who fast during Ramadan are advised to prioritize adequate hydration during non-fasting hours to maintain optimal conditions for the gut microbiota. It is crucial to recognize that responses to fasting, including its impact on the gut microbiota, exhibit considerable variability among individuals. Factors such as physical activity, diet quality, meal timing, and dietary habits are determinants of microbial composition and contribute to the diverse ways in which fasting affects the microbiota [7]. Some research indicates improved microbial diversity and changes in the abundance of beneficial bacteria [8], highlighting potential advantages linked to fasting practices for gastrointestinal well-being [5]. However, it is important to note that research on the specific effects of Ramadan fasting on the gut microbiota is still evolving, and individual responses can vary. The majority of human research shows that RIF has a beneficial impact on

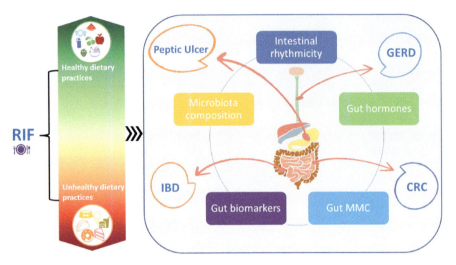

Fig. 9.2 RIF targeting gut biomarkers for gut health. Dietary practices during RIF may influence the overall environment of the gut microbiota, including gut hormone levels, gut rhythmicity, gut MMC, and other biomarkers that are associated with various gut diseases

the structure and composition of the gut microbiome by targeting the gut hormones, gut biomarkers, gut rhythmicity (peripheral), and migrating motor complex (MMC), thereby reducing the burden of gastrointestinal tract (GIT) diseases (Fig. 9.2) [2]. As previously reported, positive changes in the gut microbiota, such as the overexpression of bacteria that produce butyric acid, including *Lachnospiraceae, Prevotellaceae, Akkermansia muciniphila, and Bacteroides*, have been linked to better health markers and a reduction in the development of disease during RIF [5, 9]. In contrast, a study observed the increased microbial diversity following Ramadan and the decrease in SCFA and beneficial bacteria levels during fasting, raising the possibility that the daily diet during Ramadan may not supply enough nutrients to support a healthy gut microbiota [10].

RIF can influence the hormones associated with the gut that play a significant role in maintaining gut health. In a previous study on the effects of RIF on gut hormone levels in males with obesity, there was a decrease in Glucagon-Like Peptide-1 (GLP-1) concentrations and an increase in leptin concentrations, which may indicate a role in satiety. During Ramadan fasting, there is a decrease in body fat percentage and a corresponding reduction in GLP-1 levels, which further reduces the risk of obesity-associated GIT dysfunction. Furthermore, the study demonstrated that a decrease in food consumption during Ramadan led to a significant reduction in peptide YY (PYY) and cholecystokinin (CCK) concentrations [11].

The migrating motor complex (MMC) is another important component that improves gut health during RIF. MMC is a periodic, cyclic motility pattern that happens in the small intestine and stomach during fasting and is broken by food. The removal of any remaining undigested material from the gastrointestinal tract is the main function of the MMC during digestion. During MMC, extra bile secretions are also seen, which is important for preserving a favorable environment for cultures of beneficial bacteria. During the RIF, the MMC essentially serves as an intestinal house cleaner.

Furthermore, bile begins to destroy any leftover bacteria as it passes through the digestive system, preventing them from adhering to the gut wall [12]. In general, Ramadan fasting practices can enhance the MMC's gastrointestinal motility, facilitating the smooth passage of intestinal contents through the GI tract. Fasting enables the intestinal lining to be strengthened and cleansed. It can activate autophagy, a process that aids in the body's recycling, elimination of deteriorated cell components, and stimulation of cellular renewal. When the body experiences a modest form of nutritional stress, known as RIF, the cellular processes change from a growth phase to a repair phase [13]. Fasting enhances the removal process of toxins and causes the skin, kidneys, intestines, bladder, and sinuses to release more toxins. During Ramadan, limiting food intake for a full month permits the digestive system to reset, rest, and cleanse itself through autophagy and MMC. In addition, several studies of RIF showed anti-inflammatory effects by suppressing several pro-inflammatory cytokines (Interleukin-6 (IL-6), Tumor Necrosis Factor alpha (TNF-α), and IL-1β), reducing oxidative stress, inducing a proteome response associated with increased autophagy, remodeling the gut microbiome, and improving the components of GIT diseases [14, 15]. As discussed below, RIF's positive impact on the gut microbiome may influence the symptomology and clinical course of GI diseases.

9.3 Inflammatory Bowel Disease

Crohn's disease (CD) and ulcerative colitis (UC) are the two main types of inflammatory bowel diseases (IBDs), which encompass a range of conditions causing persistent inflammation of the gastrointestinal tract, resulting in tissue destruction, malabsorption, and systemic consequences [16]. Changes in dietary habits during non-fasting hours can impact individuals with IBDs, influencing the course of the disease [17]. Responses to fasting among individuals with IBDs are diverse, with some experiencing symptom changes while others may not notice significant effects. Tailoring fasting practices to individual needs is crucial to respecting and understanding these variations [2]. Nonetheless, research on 80 IBD patients (60 UC and 20 CD) revealed that RIF did not have any negative impact on inflammatory markers (C-reactive protein (CRP) and calprotectin) [18]. Furthermore, a study that relied on the participants' self-reported symptoms before and after Ramadan revealed no statistically significant differences in their symptoms, and there was no relationship between the number of days fasted and the severity of the disease [19]. In addition, it has been demonstrated that RIF does not impose significant risks on patients with IBD [19]. Careful consideration of food types and meal timing, with a focus on easily digestible, low-fiber options, may be advisable [17]. Medication management is vital for individuals with IBDs, and adjusting the timing of medication administration during Ramadan is crucial to align with fasting and eating schedules [20].

Fasting during Ramadan involves a significant risk of dehydration due to abstaining from food and drinks for an extended period. This risk is heightened for individuals with IBDs, emphasizing the importance of staying well-hydrated during non-fasting hours to prevent the potential worsening of symptoms [5].

9.4 Peptic Ulcer

Disruptions in the mucosal layer of the lining of the gastrointestinal system, often known as open sores or sloughing, are characteristic of peptic ulcers. Their primary locations are in the proximal duodenum (duodenal ulcer) or the stomach (gastric ulcer). A cross-sectional study carried out in Japan found that some foods were linked to a lower likelihood of *Helicobacter pylori* infection, and other foods were linked to a higher risk of atrophic gastritis. Examples of these foods included fruit juice and processed salmon [21]. This implies a relationship between food consumption and the chance of developing peptic ulcer. The diet also modifies the composition of gut microbes, which plays a major role in *H. pylori* infection. Due to the clear correlations between food consumption and peptic ulcer disease, RIF may affect peptic ulcer disease symptoms and the risk of complications.

In summary, the research results were consistent with stomach ulcers, which are associated with a low likelihood of symptom explosions and poor healing because of RIF. However, the study performed by Kocacusak [22] discovered that, in contrast to non-fasting months, more surgical procedures were needed to treat peptic ulcer perforations during fasting months. Research has revealed that the occurrence and symptoms of duodenal ulcers are worse during the Ramadan fast. This is explained by the way that food stimulates the creation of mucus and bicarbonate in the small intestine, hence reducing the pain associated with duodenal ulcers [23].

Moreover, a recent review suggests that there is no correlation between fasting and the risk of getting *H. pylori*–induced peptic ulcers, nor does it affect the incidence of peptic ulcers. This indicates that those with simple ulcers are not in danger of developing more ulcers and can continue to fast [24]. In contrast, a previous study reported that the occurrence of peptic ulcer perforation was significantly high during Ramadan fasting months due to the long fasting periods [22] as well as duodenal ulcers and duodenitis [25]. Another literature review demonstrated that the secretion of gastric acid and pepsin was increased during Ramadan fasting, probably associated with dyspeptic symptoms. However, peptic ulcer complications such as gastrointestinal bleeding and peptic ulcer perforation increase during Ramadan fasting [26].

9.5 Gastroesophageal Reflux Disease (GERD)

The retrograde movement of stomach contents, or GERD, irritates the lining of the esophagus and causes a variety of discomforting symptoms. GERD frequently manifests as dysphagia, regurgitation, retrosternal burning pain, and chest pain. Obesity and advanced age are risk factors and aggravating factors for GERD. Other variables include smoking, alcohol usage, caffeine-containing drinks, painkiller use, and psychological distress [27–29]. Some of these behaviors, like smoking and drinking alcohol, are improved during Ramadan since fasting is regarded as a diet. There may be a reduction in GERD symptoms during Ramadan if these habits are reduced, as they are known to exacerbate symptoms [30]. RIF is believed to be one of the lifestyle modifications that helps minimize GERD symptoms. Based on the gastroesophageal reflux disease questionnaire (GERD-Q) score, the GERD symptoms were milder in the group of RIF than those of the non-fasting group [30]. A six-item assessment called the GERD-Q was created to help diagnose GERD-based symptoms seen in primary care patients. This questionnaire is helpful in the diagnostic process because it can distinguish between symptoms that are related to episodic reflux and persistent symptoms that interfere with an individual's ability to function daily. Additionally, GERD-Q enables tracking of how treatments affect the symptoms of long-term patients [31]. However, another study suggested that RIF also significantly improved gastric fullness, epigastric pain, and heartburn [32]. It is also observed that RIF improves GERD symptoms by decreasing heartburn and regurgitation scores among patients with GERD.

Moreover, there was no relationship between the severity of GERD symptoms before or after fasting and the type of food or the amount of food consumed [33]. According to the results of another trial, RIF does not affect GERD symptoms in people who are using antisecretory drugs such as proton pump inhibitors (PPIs) and H2 blockers [30]. The literature, albeit limited, indicates that there is general agreement that fasting is safe for people with GERD and that medications should only be used in specific circumstances, as they have been shown to reduce symptoms. Other recommendations for GERD patients include adhering to dietary guidelines, modifying eating schedules, and changing medications.

9.6   Colorectal Cancer (CRC)

Considering the multidimensional health benefits of RIF, it has been observed that this regimen has been associated with reducing the severity of CRC. A study examines how RIF affects the acceptability of side effects after chemotherapy and evaluates changes in tumor biomarker levels, specifically lactate dehydrogenase (LDH) and carcinoembryonic antigen (CEA), in 33 CRC patients. After fasting during Ramadan, 27 patients (73%) reported feeling "serenity" and that the adverse effects of their chemotherapy were easier to bear. However, the measured laboratory variables did not show any appreciable differences between pre-fasting values and values after 30 days of Ramadan. The levels of LDH and CEA were lower in 46.9% and 55.6% of patients, respectively, while being statistically insignificant. The fasting group's mean CEA level was significantly lower by over 40%, which was explained by the three patients who saw a highly significant drop in CEA levels ($p = 0.0283$) [34].

In conclusion, this study supports previous results by confirming the safety and tolerability of RIF in CRC patients undergoing chemotherapy. RIF is associated with colorectal, lung, and breast cancers by targeting their metabolic profiles. Recently, a London Ramadan study (LORANS) showed that regardless of changes in body composition, RIF was linked to alterations in 14 metabolites: one inflammatory marker, one amino acid, two glycolysis-related metabolites, two ketone bodies, two triglycerides, and six lipoprotein subclasses. Following the utilization of 117,981 people's data from the UK Biobank, metabolomics-based metabolic scores for lung cancer, breast cancer, and colorectal cancer were produced. They discovered that following Ramadan, there was a decrease in the metabolic scores for breast, colorectal, and lung cancers [35], suggesting that RIF is associated with short-term favorable changes in the metabolic profiles concerning the risk of CRC and other cancers.

9.7   Considerations for Practicing RIF in GI Diseases

In order to inform patients about the dangers of fasting and promote cooperative decision-making, healthcare professionals ought to provide pre-Ramadan counseling. In order to enable more conclusive dialogues between the healthcare provider and the patient, medical professionals must investigate the ways in which Ramadan fasting impacts certain medical issues and provide modifications to diet and medication regimens [2].

Here are some considerations:

1. Impact on GI symptoms: Individuals with GI diseases such as irritable bowel syndrome (IBS), Crohn's disease, or ulcerative colitis may experience exacerbation of symptoms during fasting due to changes in eating patterns, dehydration, or altered gut motility. These individuals need to consult with their healthcare providers before fasting to assess potential risks and develop a management plan.
2. Dehydration: Prolonged fasting without water intake during daylight hours can lead to dehydration, which may worsen symptoms for individuals with GI diseases, such as constipation or hemorrhoids [36, 37]. Adequate hydration before and after fasting hours is crucial to prevent dehydration-related complications.
3. Medication management: Some individuals with GI diseases may require medication or dietary supplements to manage their condition. Fasting may interfere with the timing or effectiveness of drugs. Healthcare providers may need to adjust medication schedules or dosages to accommodate fasting periods while ensuring optimal disease management.
4. Dietary changes: During Ramadan, there may be significant changes in dietary habits, including the types, quality, and timing of food consumed. For individuals with GI diseases, especially those with conditions sensitive to certain foods

(e.g., IBS triggered by specific dietary components), it is essential to maintain a balanced diet and avoid triggering foods during non-fasting hours. Furthermore, following a prolonged period of fasting, binge eating causes the stomach, pancreas, and gallbladder to grow more quickly [38]. Cholangitis and pancreatitis can be brought on by bile reflux, which is caused by the biliary tract being crushed by the stomach and elevated intraduodenal pressure [39]. Furthermore, a stretched stomach causes a significant release of cholecystokinin, which stimulates the biliary and pancreatic systems [40]. A fatty diet also affects the bile system, and high-calorie foods eaten from sunset to sunrise disrupt the balance of cholesterol and triglycerides [36].

5. Gut microbiota: RIF can influence the composition and function of the gut microbiota, which plays a crucial role in maintaining GI health. While short-term fasting may have beneficial effects on gut microbiota diversity and metabolism, prolonged fasting or significant changes in dietary patterns during Ramadan may impact the microbiota composition. It is essential to ensure adequate intake of fiber, prebiotics, and probiotics to support gut health during fasting.

6. Digestive health maintenance: Despite the challenges posed by fasting, individuals with GI diseases can take steps to maintain digestive health during Ramadan. This includes consuming fiber-rich foods during non-fasting hours, staying hydrated, avoiding large meals that may exacerbate symptoms, exercising moderately, and incorporating probiotic-rich foods like yogurt into their diet.

7. Monitoring and follow-up: Regular monitoring and follow-up with healthcare providers are crucial for individuals with GI diseases during Ramadan. This allows for adjustments in treatment plans, monitoring of symptoms, and early intervention if complications arise.

9.8   Conclusion

In summary, individuals with GI diseases should approach Ramadan fasting with caution and consult with their healthcare providers to assess potential risks and develop personalized management plans. Maintaining hydration, balanced nutrition, medication adherence, and monitoring of symptoms are essential for preserving GI health during RIF.

References

1. Zeb F, Wu X, Chen L, Fatima S, Haq IU, Chen A, Li M, Feng Q. Effect of time-restricted feeding on metabolic risk and circadian rhythm associated with gut microbiome in healthy males. Br J Nutr. 2020;123:1216–26.
2. Tibi S, Ahmed S, Nizam Y, Aldoghmi M, Moosa A, Bourenane K, Yakub M, Mohsin H. Implications of Ramadan fasting in the setting of gastrointestinal disorders. Cureus. 2023;15:e36972. https://doi.org/10.7759/CUREUS.36972.

3. Khan MN, Khan SI, Rana MI, Ayyaz A, Khan MY, Imran M. Intermittent fasting positively modulates human gut microbial diversity and ameliorates blood lipid profile. Front Microbiol. 2022;13. https://doi.org/10.3389/FMICB.2022.922727.
4. Ali I, Liu K, Long D, Faisal S, Hilal MG, Ali I, Huang X, Long R. Ramadan fasting leads to shifts in human gut microbiota structured by dietary composition. Front Microbiol. 2021;12. https://doi.org/10.3389/FMICB.2021.642999.
5. Su J, Wang Y, Zhang X, Ma M, Xie Z, Pan Q, Ma Z, Peppelenbosch MP. Remodeling of the gut microbiome during Ramadan-associated intermittent fasting. Am J Clin Nutr. 2021;113:1332–42.
6. Angoorani P, Ejtahed HS, Hasani-Ranjbar S, Siadat SD, Soroush AR, Larijani B. Gut microbiota modulation as a possible mediating mechanism for fasting-induced alleviation of metabolic complications: a systematic review. Nutr Metab (Lond). 2021;18:105. https://doi.org/10.1186/S12986-021-00635-3.
7. Pieczyńska-Zając JM, Malinowska A, Łagowska K, Leciejewska N, Bajerska J. The effects of time-restricted eating and Ramadan fasting on gut microbiota composition: a systematic review of human and animal studies. Nutr Rev. 2023;82:777. https://doi.org/10.1093/NUTRIT/NUAD093.
8. Zeb F, Osaili T, Obaid RS, et al. Gut microbiota and time-restricted feeding/eating: a targeted biomarker and approach in precision nutrition. Nutrients. 2023;15. https://doi.org/10.3390/NU15020259.
9. Mousavi SN, Rayyani E, Heshmati J, Tavasolian R, Rahimlou M. Effects of Ramadan and non-Ramadan intermittent fasting on gut microbiome. Front Nutr. 2022;9:860575. https://doi.org/10.3389/FNUT.2022.860575.
10. Jo YJ, Lee GD, Ahmad S, Son HW, Kim MJ, Sliti A, Lee S, Kim K, Lee SE, Shin JH. The alteration of the gut microbiome during Ramadan offers a novel perspective on Ramadan fasting: a pilot study. Microorganisms. 2023;11:2106. https://doi.org/10.3390/MICROORGANISMS11082106.
11. Zouhal H, Bagheri R, Triki R, Saeidi A, Wong A, Hackney AC, Laher I, Suzuki K, Ben AA. Effects of Ramadan intermittent fasting on gut hormones and body composition in males with obesity. Int J Environ Res Public Health. 2020;17:1–15.
12. Deloose E, Janssen P, Depoortere I, Tack J. The migrating motor complex: control mechanisms and its role in health and disease. Nat Rev Gastroenterol Hepatol. 2012;9:271–85.
13. Bagheriyna M, Butler AE, Barreto GE, Sahebkar A. The effect of fasting or calorie restriction on autophagy induction: a review of the literature. Ageing Res Rev. 2018;47:183–97.
14. Bhatti SI, Mindikoglu AL. The impact of dawn-to-sunset fasting on the immune system and its clinical significance in the COVID-19 pandemic. Metabol Open. 2022;13:100162.
15. Almeneessier AS, BaHammam AA, Alzoghaibi M, Olaish AH, Nashwan SZ, BaHammam AS. The effects of diurnal intermittent fasting on proinflammatory cytokine levels while controlling for sleep/wake pattern, meal composition and energy expenditure. PLoS One. 2019;14:e0226034. https://doi.org/10.1371/JOURNAL.PONE.0226034.
16. Yu YR, Rodriguez JR. Clinical presentation of Crohn's, ulcerative colitis, and indeterminate colitis: symptoms, extraintestinal manifestations, and disease phenotypes. Semin Pediatr Surg. 2017;26:349–55.
17. Yan J, Wang L, Gu Y, Hou H, Liu T, Ding Y, Cao H. Dietary patterns and gut microbiota changes in inflammatory bowel disease: current insights and future challenges. Nutrients. 2022;14. https://doi.org/10.3390/NU14194003.
18. Negm M, Bahaa A, Farrag A, et al. Effect of Ramadan intermittent fasting on inflammatory markers, disease severity, depression, and quality of life in patients with inflammatory bowel diseases: a prospective cohort study. BMC Gastroenterol. 2022;22:203. https://doi.org/10.1186/S12876-022-02272-3.
19. Ramadan fasting and inflammatory bowel disease – PubMed. https://pubmed.ncbi.nlm.nih.gov/19405258/. Accessed 1 Apr 2024.

20. Byron C, Cornally N, Burton A, Savage E. Challenges of living with and managing inflamma-
    tory bowel disease: a meta-synthesis of patients' experiences. J Clin Nurs. 2020;29:305–19.
21. The Risk of Helicobacter Pylori Infection and Atrophic Gastritis from Food and Drink
    Intake: a Cross-sectional Study in Hokkaido, Japan – PubMed. https://pubmed.ncbi.nlm.nih.
    gov/12718682/. Accessed 1 Apr 2024.
22. Does Ramadan fasting contribute to the increase of peptic ulcer perforations? – PubMed.
    https://pubmed.ncbi.nlm.nih.gov/28121343/. Accessed 1 Apr 2024.
23. Peptic ulcer disease – PubMed. https://pubmed.ncbi.nlm.nih.gov/17956071/. Accessed 1
    Apr 2024.
24. Roy YJ, Lyutakov I. The effect of Ramadan and intermittent fasting on the development of
    helicobacter pylori-induced peptic ulcers. Br J Hosp Med (Lond). 2023;84:1. https://doi.
    org/10.12968/HMED.2022.0369.
25. Gokakin AK, Kurt A, Akgol G, Karakus BC, Atabey M, Koyuncu A, Topcu O, Goren E. Effects
    of Ramadan fasting on peptic ulcer disease as diagnosed by upper gastrointestinal endoscopy.
    Arab J Gastroenterol. 2012;13:180–3.
26. Seifi N, Hashemi M, Safarian M, Hadi V, Raeisi M. Effects of Ramadan fasting on common
    upper gastrointestinal disorders: a review of the literature. J Nutr Heal. 2017;5:20–3.
27. Kang JHE, Kang JY. Lifestyle measures in the management of gastro-oesophageal reflux dis-
    ease: clinical and pathophysiological considerations. Ther Adv Chronic Dis. 2015;6:51–64.
28. Saberi-Firoozi M, Khademolhosseini F, Yousefi M, Mehrabani D, Zare N, Heydari ST. Risk
    factors of gastroesophageal reflux disease in shiraz, southern Iran. World J Gastroenterol.
    2007;13:5486–91.
29. Alkhathami AM, Alzahrani AA, Alzhrani MA, Alsuwat OB, Mahfouz MEM. Risk factors for
    gastroesophageal reflux disease in Saudi Arabia. Gastroenterol Res. 2017;10:294–300.
30. The Effects of Ramadhan Fasting on Clinical Symptoms in Patients with Gastroesophageal
    Reflux Disease – PubMed. https://pubmed.ncbi.nlm.nih.gov/27840350/. Accessed 1 Apr 2024.
31. Zavala-Gonzáles MA, Azamar-Jacome AA, Meixueiro-Daza A, de la Medina AR, Job Reyes-
    Huerta J, Roesch-Dietlen F, Remes-Troche JM. Validation and diagnostic usefulness of gastro-
    esophageal reflux disease questionnaire in a primary care level in Mexico. J Neurogastroenterol
    Motil. 2014;20:475–82.
32. Abdallah H, Khalil M, Farella I, JohnBritto JS, Lanza E, Santoro S, Garruti G, Portincasa P,
    Di Ciaula A, Bonfrate L. Ramadan intermittent fasting reduces visceral fat and improves gas-
    trointestinal motility. Eur J Clin Investig. 2023;53:e14029. https://doi.org/10.1111/ECI.14029.
33. Bohamad AH, Aladhab WA, Alhashem SS, Alajmi MS, Alhumam T, Alqattan DJ, Elshebiny
    AM. Impact of Ramadan fasting on the severity of symptoms among a cohort of patients with
    gastroesophageal reflux disease (GERD). Cureus. 2023;15:e36831. https://doi.org/10.7759/
    CUREUS.36831.
34. Alshammari K, Alhaidal HA, Alharbi R, Alrubaiaan A, Abdel-Razaq W, Alyousif G, Alkaiyat
    M. The impact of fasting the holy month of Ramadan on colorectal cancer patients and two
    tumor biomarkers: a tertiary-care hospital experience. Cureus. 2023;15(1):e33920. https://doi.
    org/10.7759/CUREUS.33920.
35. Al-Jafar R, Pinto RC, Elliott P, Tsilidis KK, Dehghan A. Metabolomics of Ramadan fasting and
    associated risk of chronic diseases. Am J Clin Nutr. 2024;119:1007. https://doi.org/10.1016/J.
    AJCNUT.2024.01.019.
36. Drozdinsky G, Agabaria A, Zuker-Herman R, Drescher MJ, Bleetman T, Shiber S. High rate
    of acute pancreatitis during the Ramadan fast. Eur J Gastroenterol Hepatol. 2018;30:608–11.
37. Luckey AE, Parsa CJ. Fluid and electrolytes in older people. Arch Surg. 2003;138:1055–60.
38. Benson JR, Ward MP. Massive gastric dilatation and acute pancreatitis--a case of "Ramadan
    syndrome"? Postgrad Med J. 1992;68:689.
39. Wu BU, Johannes RS, Sun X, Tabak Y, Conwell DL, Banks PA. The early prediction of mortal-
    ity in acute pancreatitis: a large population-based study. Gut. 2008;57:1698–703.
40. The role of cholecystokinin in the pathogenesis of acute pancreatitis in the isolated pancreas
    preparation – PubMed. https://pubmed.ncbi.nlm.nih.gov/1705726/. Accessed 1 Apr 2024.

Chapter 10
Understanding the Link Between Ramadan Intermittent Fasting, Psychiatric Symptoms, and Neurocognitive Function

Hamid A. Alhaj and Meera Alhusaini

Abstract There is an increasing awareness regarding the importance of mental health globally due to the high prevalence of mental disorders associated with a substantial disease burden. Understanding the cultural context is particularly relevant, without which appropriate approaches that combine medical, social, and policy interventions cannot be implemented. Muslims constitute the second-largest religious group worldwide. One of the pillars of Islam is the practice of Ramadan intermittent fasting (RIF), during which healthy adults abstain from consuming food and fluids from dawn to dusk. RIF has been suggested to have beneficial effects on specific psychiatric symptoms, including reduction of anxiety and depressive symptoms. Furthermore, studies have shown that the cumulative impact of RIF may benefit neurocognitive parameters. Mechanisms of these may be related to the enhancement of the neuroplasticity process as well as a reduction of neuroinflammation. RIF may also lead to changes in growth hormone and cortisol production, which could affect mood and neurocognition. While individuals who have severe mental illness (SMI) are typically exempted from the religious duty of fasting, many choose to observe RIF. The evidence regarding the impact of RIF on these individuals' psychiatric conditions is inconclusive. However, studies have suggested a potential adverse effect in patients with schizophrenia and bipolar disorder; hence, prudence should be maintained while advising patients who wish to fast. Taken together, the overall evidence regarding mental health and Ramadan is positive. Yet, further studies are warranted to understand the biological and psychosocial factors that affect mental health and well-being during RIF.

Keywords Ramadan intermittent fasting (RIF) · Mental health · Psychiatry · Neurocognition · Neuroplasticity · Neuroinflammation

H. A. Alhaj (✉) · M. Alhusaini
College of Medicine, University of Sharjah, Sharjah, United Arab Emirates
e-mail: halhaj@sharjah.ac.ae; u22103226@sharjah.ac.ae

© The Author(s), under exclusive license to Springer Nature Singapore Pte Ltd. 2025
M. E. Faris et al. (eds.), *Health and Medical Aspects of Ramadan Intermittent Fasting*, https://doi.org/10.1007/978-981-96-6783-3_10

143

10.1   Introduction

Mental health problems are a significant cause of disease burden and are associated with high rates of morbidity and mortality worldwide [1]. Anxiety and depressive disorders are among the most prevalent conditions globally [2]. The social and economic sequelae of mental problems are substantial, ranging from reduced productivity to increased healthcare costs [3]. Various factors, including socioeconomic inequality, stigma, and limited access to mental health services, contribute to the complexity of this global concern. Addressing the burden of mental health requires comprehensive and integrated culturally appropriate approaches that combine medical, social, and policy interventions.

Dietary and lifestyle behaviors play a fundamental role in determining the development and prognosis of mental health problems [4]. Diets that include unhealthy ingredients, such as a high intake of ultra-processed foods, processed red meats, and high-sugar drinks, have been associated with increased inflammation and disrupted gut microbiota [5]. These effects may result in a higher risk of mental health issues, including depression, anxiety, and cognitive decline [5]. Similarly, inactivity and sedentary lifestyles can worsen negative moods and exacerbate existing mental health conditions.

Intermittent fasting (IF) is a dietary approach involving alternating periods of fasting and eating. While the primary purpose of IF has been related to weight loss and metabolic health, there is a growing interest in its potential effects on psychiatric symptoms and neurocognitive function [6]. Emerging evidence suggests that IF may positively influence brain function and neuroplasticity, potentially mitigating the risk of neurodegenerative disorders [7]. Additionally, these dietary practices could impact mood regulation and stress resilience, with potential implications for conditions such as depression and anxiety [8]. Indeed, a meta-analysis concluded that compared to control groups, IF demonstrated a positive and moderate impact on depression scores [9]. The underlying mechanisms have been postulated to be related to the modulation of neurotrophic factors, neurotransmitter systems, and inflammation, all of which play pivotal roles in mental well-being. Studies have reported that IF can improve learning and memory and may play a neuroprotective role against cognitive decline related to age in animals [10]. Further, it has been shown that IF can improve mood and reduce anxiety-like behavior in rodents. In humans, a small body of evidence suggests that IF may improve attention and executive function in older adults [11].

Ramadan intermittent fasting (RIF) is a specific form of IF observed by adult Muslims and involves abstinence from food and drinks from dawn to dusk. In addition, observing RIF for a month encompasses significant transformation in dietary and lifestyle behaviors, including total energy, macronutrient and food group intakes, physical activity patterns, and sleep duration and quality [12, 13]. While the primary purpose of fasting during Ramadan is spiritual, there has been increasing interest in its potential effects on psychiatric symptoms and neurocognitive function. This chapter aims to critically explore the current literature involving these parameters in health and disease.

10.2 Effects of RIF on Anxiety and Depressive Symptoms

The effects of Ramadan fasting on symptoms of depression, anxiety, and stress have been studied in individuals with diabetes [14]. In this research, a significant reduction of depression and anxiety in the fasting group was identified, as compared to no improvement in the non-fasting group. Furthermore, stress scores demonstrated a substantial fall in the fasting group alone [14]. Similarly, RIF was associated with a significant reduction in both depression and diabetes distress scores in individuals with type 2 diabetes (T2DM) [15]. A study on patients with fibromyalgia demonstrated that RIF has positive effects on neuropsychiatric symptoms. In this cohort, symptoms of anxiety and depression were significantly decreased after 1 week of RIF [16].

A study conducted in Germany that investigated the impact of RIF on mood and quality of life reported a positive effect on within-group comparisons [17]. Stress and depression scores were also shown to be reduced in fasting nurses during Ramadan, although anxiety scores were demonstrated to have a mild, nonsignificant reduction [18]. A study conducted during the COVID-19 global pandemic showed that participation in Ramadan fasting was significantly associated with reduced anxiety levels and better well-being among the study participants [19]. Similarly, individuals who observed RIF reported higher levels of well-being, such as increased life satisfaction, greater positive emotions, and significantly fewer negative emotions [19]. RIF's effect on depression and anxiety symptoms may present as an increase in the ability to adapt to challenging situations, also known as resilience. A study that was designed to examine the effects of RIF on the psychological hardiness of students and resilience collected data using the Ahvaz psychological hardiness questionnaire and the Connor–Davidson resilience questionnaire. The results showed significant differences in the posttest resilience and psychological hardiness scores with an effect size of 0.73 and 0.78, respectively [20].

The positive effect seen in RIF groups may be attributed to changes in neurotransmitter (NT) levels and an increase in the release of factors essential for neuron differentiation and maintaining synaptic integrity, such as brain-derived neurotrophic factor (BDNF) (as demonstrated in Fig. 10.1). A study reported enhanced plasma levels of BDNF, serotonin (5-HT), and nerve growth factor (NGF) in fasting subjects, while dopamine levels remained unchanged [21]. Other studies reported similar results; RIF was shown to increase serum serotonin levels compared to pre-Ramadan levels [22]; similarly, in rats that fasted for 12 h. Daily, there were significant increases in forebrain levels of serotonin [23]. Elevated serotonin (5-HT) levels are related to reduced anxiety symptoms in rodents, and the activation of 5-HT receptor 5-HT1A in the dorsal area of the forebrain produced anxiolytic effects, as shown using optogenetic stimulation [24]. Moreover, $5\text{-}HT_4R$ knockout (KO) mice showed increased anxiety-like behavior and signs of anhedonia and despair [25].

A substantial amount of evidence confirms the significant role of fasting in inducing BDNF expression [26]. Studies in humans [27–29] and animal studies

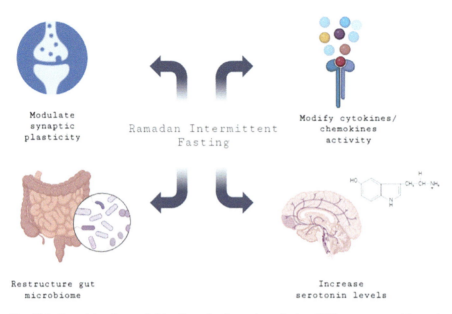

Fig. 10.1 Potential pathways linking Ramadan intermittent fasting (RIF) to neurocognition and mental health

[30, 31] support the effect of fasting on the levels of BDNF. One study investigated the impact of 16 h. of daily fasting for 3 months on levels of BDNF in type 2 diabetes (T2DM) rat model vs. control. Interestingly, BDNF was significantly increased in both groups, and this change in BDNF levels was accompanied by a reduction in anxiety and depression seen in the T2DM group [31]. It is worth noting that this study showed increased levels of serotonin and downregulated serum corticosterone levels.

The mediating antidepressant/anxiolytic role of BDNF in RIF aligns well with the "neurotrophic hypothesis of depression" [32]. This theory suggests that diminished levels of BDNF in the brain might play a role in the shrinkage and loss of cells in the hippocampus and prefrontal cortex, a phenomenon observed in individuals with depression [33]. Conversely, antidepressants may work by boosting BDNF levels, potentially reversing the process of neuronal shrinkage and cell loss, thus exerting their therapeutic effects. Similarly, reduced levels of BDNF were associated with several anxiety and stress-related disorders, including post-traumatic stress disorder (PTSD) and obsessive-compulsive disorder (OCD) [34, 35].

The gut microbiome (GMB) refers to the assortment of microorganisms inhabiting the human body's gastrointestinal (GI) tract. Additionally, the makeup of the GMB is associated with genetic differences in the host's immune-related pathways [36]. For instance, it was revealed that tumor necrosis factor-alpha (TNFα) and interferon gamma (IFNγ) production is related to metabolic activities within the GMB [37].

GMB has recently gained attention for its role in modulating brain activity via the "gut–brain axis," which is a communication channel between the central nervous system, the enteric tract, and the gastrointestinal tract [38]. Indeed, strong evidence from human and animal studies supports the link between GMB and mental disorders [39–41]. The evidence on RIF and GMB changes is present; nonetheless, few studies have found significant changes in the diversity and microbial richness of GMB in fasting subjects [42, 43]. One study compared the composition of GMB in samples taken during and after Ramadan; they found a consequential change in GMB structure, and remarkably, they found a significant upregulation in members of the *Lachnospiraceae* family, an essential source of butyric acid [44]. Decreased levels of operational taxonomic units from the lineages of *Lachnospiraceae* were associated with psychological distress in the Swiss inflammatory bowel disease (IBD) cohort. Specifically, *Lachnospiraceae* was identified to be correlated with anxiety measures and depression [45]. However, the role of RIF in changing GMB and its consequences on brain activity and health requires further investigation.

10.3 Effects of RIF on Neurocognitive Function

A nutritious diet and healthy lifestyle habits, including regular physical activity, are widely recognized for maintaining cognitive function and metabolic health [46–49]. Evidence suggests that RIF is associated with significant improvements in factors that predispose to the development of impaired cognitive functions, such as obesity and overweight [50], metabolic syndrome components [51], inflammatory and oxidative stress markers [52], and disturbed glucose homeostasis [53]. Furthermore, RIF has been associated with upregulation in genes associated with enhanced neuroplasticity and decreased neuroinflammation, such as Nuclear factor erythroid 2-related factor 2 (Nrf2), mitochondrial transcription factor A (TFAM), and superoxide dismutase 2 (SOD2) [54–56]. RIF has been postulated to have a prophylactic role in promoting healthy aging and preventing aging-related neurodegenerative diseases and decreased cognitive functions.

The ability of RIF to reduce pro-inflammatory cytokines, namely Interleukin (IL)-1β, IL-6, TNF-α, and pro-inflammatory ceramides, and alleviate oxidative stress markers suggests a positive impact on improving neurocognitive functions [57, 58].

Under normal conditions (non-fasting state), neurons can produce proteins and lipids by activating the mammalian target of rapamycin (mTOR) pathway, a central control pathway that utilizes signals from different sources to regulate cell metabolism and proliferation [59]. On the other hand, the fasting state inhibits the mTOR pathway and induces autophagy, a housekeeping process that degrades defective proteins [60]; moreover, autophagy enhances the cell's antioxidant abilities and DNA repair [61].

As discussed earlier, RIF is associated with an increase in the concentration of BDNF [21, 28, 29, 31]; BDNF is known to play an integral role in long-term potentiation, a long-term enhancement of synaptic connectivity that underlies memory and learning [62]. A study showed an enhancement in hippocampal-dependent learning tasks parallel to increased serum BDNF levels following aerobic exercise [63]. Serum BDNF levels correlated with poorer performance in the digit symbol substitution task and memory of stories in patients with mild cognitive impairments [64].

However, the evidence regarding the effect of RIF on cognitive abilities has been inconclusive; while limited studies reported enhancement in cognitive functions [65], others reported no effect, and some research groups reported worsening impacts. These discrepancies can be attributed to multiple factors; for example, nicotine suspension and withdrawal seen in individuals observing RIF should be taken into consideration, as it has been found that nicotine withdrawal can affect cognitive functions, and the same goes for caffeine intake. Moreover, the lack of significance in cognitive abilities' enhancement could be due to a ceiling effect when testing young, healthy adults. For a summary of studies investigating cognitive functions in Ramadan-fasting subjects, see Table 10.1.

Table 10.1 Summary of studies investigating the effect of RIF on cognitive functions

References	Method	Country	Findings	Limitations
[66]	Randomized order of completing the Wingate test at different times Cognitive measurements: reaction time (RT), MRT, SAT	Tunisia	RT, the number of correct answers, and SAT were higher in the evening before exercise during the second and third week of Ramadan compared to before Ramadan Cognitive and anaerobic performances were not affected in the morning during RIF	Small sample size (n = 11) No control
[67]	Participants were assigned to sedentary and physically active groups Cognitive measurements: Neurotrack digital cognitive battery, assessed before and during Ramadan	Tunisia	Physically active elderly individuals showed improved cognitive performance during Ramadan Sedentary individuals showed decreased associative learning performance during Ramadan	The study relied on self-reported measures of cognitive performance The study did not consider medications that may interfere with the results, given the subjects' age (>60 years) Dietary intake, caffeine, and nicotine habits were not investigated
[68]	Cognitive measurements: ST and TMT	Malaysia	Subjects showed slower RT in ST during Ramadan fasting Improvement in TMT was seen, compared to scores before Ramadan	Healthy young adults may present a ceiling effect in cognitive testing

(continued)

Table 10.1 (continued)

References	Method	Country	Findings	Limitations
[69]	The cognitive testing was conducted twice daily: pre- and post-Ramadan Cognitive measurements: Cambridge neuropsychological test automated battery (CANTAB), specifically RTI and RVP	Qatar	RTI and movement times remained consistent throughout the study period, while the RVP test demonstrated a decrease in false alarms during Ramadan Accuracy significantly increased at different time points during Ramadan, compared to the baseline	Small sample size ($n = 11$) The study did not have a control group (i.e., non-fasting cyclists) The results may be affected by a shift in participants' locations (from the gulf cooperation council (GCC) to Europe) after the first week of Ramadan

MRT mental rotation test, *SAT* selective attention test, *ST* Stroop color and word test, *TMT* trail-making test, *RTI* reaction time index, *RVP* rapid visual information processing

10.4 RIF in Patients with Severe Mental Illness

Patients with severe mental illness (SMI), such as schizophrenia spectrum and bipolar disorders, have been reported to have a shorter life expectancy of 15–20 years than the general population. Metabolic syndrome and cardiovascular disease (CVD) are common among patients with SMI and have been shown to contribute to shortened life expectancy. Risk factors include unhealthy lifestyles, including poor diet, smoking, and reduced exercise; hence, lifestyle modification and CVD treatments have been demonstrated to have beneficial effects. Although Muslim scholars agree that sick individuals are exempted from fasting, several patients give preference to observing the RIF.

Limited studies have examined RIF in patients with SMI. A study from Egypt demonstrated that RIF is associated with adverse effects in patients with schizophrenia, especially those who have metabolic syndrome. In this particular group, RIF was associated with decreased high-density lipoprotein-C (HDL-C) and BDNF levels; increased glucose, insulin, and insulin resistance; and a worsening of psychiatric symptoms [70]. Another study in bipolar patients showed that RIF is associated with worsening metabolic parameters and psychiatric symptoms [71].

A study investigated the effect of RIF on serum lithium levels and psychiatric symptoms in individuals with bipolar disorder and reported participants' decrease in depression and mania symptoms during the period of fasting [72]. Interestingly, the study found no significant changes in serum electrolyte levels between the three measuring points (1 week before Ramadan, the second week of Ramadan, and 2 weeks after Ramadan).

While the current evidence is not entirely conclusive, the recommendations that patients with SMI should be considered as a group at a particular risk of RIF remain prudent [73].

10.5 Conclusions

The examination of the impact of RIF on mental health and neurocognition reveals a subtle relationship that extends beyond dietary patterns. The potential alleviation of symptoms related to depression and anxiety during RIF presents an attractive non-pharmacological/supportive approach for managing mental health disturbances. However, it is essential to acknowledge the limitations and complexities surrounding this topic, with many studies exhibiting methodological variations and inconsistencies in findings, as seen in the impact of RIF on neurocognitive functions and severe mental illness. As such, more robust and standardized research is warranted to elucidate the underlying mechanisms of RIF and optimize its therapeutic potential.

References

1. Walker ER, McGee RE, Druss BG. Mortality in mental disorders and global disease burden implications: a systematic review and meta-analysis. JAMA Psychiatry [Internet]. 2015 [cited 2024 Mar 25];72(4):334–41. Available from: https://pubmed.ncbi.nlm.nih.gov/25671328/
2. Santomauro DF, Mantilla Herrera AM, Shadid J, Zheng P, Ashbaugh C, Pigott DM, et al. Global prevalence and burden of depressive and anxiety disorders in 204 countries and territories in 2020 due to the COVID-19 pandemic. Lancet [Internet] 2021 [cited 2024 Mar 25];398(10312):1700–1712. Available from: http://www.thelancet.com/article/S0140673621021437/fulltext
3. Donohue JM, Pincus HA. Reducing the societal burden of depression: a review of economic costs, quality of care and effects of treatment. Pharmacoeconomics [Internet]. 2007 [cited 2024 Mar 25];25(1):7–24. Available from: https://pubmed.ncbi.nlm.nih.gov/17192115/
4. Firth J, Solmi M, Wootton RE, Vancampfort D, Schuch FB, Hoare E, et al. A meta-review of "lifestyle psychiatry": the role of exercise, smoking, diet and sleep in the prevention and treatment of mental disorders. World Psychiatry [Internet]. 2020 [cited 2024 Mar 25];19(3):360–380. Available from: https://pubmed.ncbi.nlm.nih.gov/32931092/
5. Juul F, Vaidean G, Parekh N. Ultra-processed foods and cardiovascular diseases: potential mechanisms of action. Adv Nutr [Internet]. 2021 [cited 2024 Mar 25];12(5):1673–80. Available from: https://pubmed.ncbi.nlm.nih.gov/33942057/
6. Gudden J, Arias Vasquez A, Bloemendaal M. The Effects of Intermittent Fasting on Brain and Cognitive Function. Nutrients. 2021;13(9):3166. https://pubmed.ncbi.nlm.nih.gov/34579042/
7. Mattson MP, Moehl K, Ghena N, Schmaedick M, Cheng A. Intermittent metabolic switching, neuroplasticity and brain health. Nat Rev Neurosci 2018 19:2 [Internet]. 2018 [cited 2024 Mar 25];19(2):81–94. Available from: https://www.nature.com/articles/nrn.2017.156
8. Alhaj HA, Selman M, Jervis V, Rodgers J, Barton S, McAllister-Williams RH. Effect of low-dose acute tryptophan depletion on the specificity of autobiographical memory in healthy subjects with a family history of depression. Psychopharmacology (Berl) [Internet]. 2012 [cited 2024 Mar 25];222(2):285–92. Available from: https://pubmed.ncbi.nlm.nih.gov/22286957/
9. Fernández-Rodríguez R, Martínez-Vizcaíno V, Mesas AE, Notario-Pacheco B, Medrano M, Heilbronn LK. Does intermittent fasting impact mental disorders? A systematic review with meta-analysis. https://doi.org/101080/1040839820222088687 [Internet]. 2022 [cited 2023 Feb 23]; Available from: https://www.tandfonline.com/doi/abs/10.1080/10408398.2022.2088687
10. Nasaruddin ML, Syed Abd Halim SA, Kamaruzzaman MA. Studying the relationship of intermittent fasting and β-amyloid in animal model of Alzheimer's disease: a scoping review.

Nutrients 2020 [Internet]. 2020 [cited 2024 Mar 20];12(10):3215. Available from: https://www.mdpi.com/2072-6643/12/10/3215/htm

11. Ooi TC, Meramat A, Rajab NF, Shahar S, Ismail IS, Azam AA, et al. Intermittent fasting enhanced the cognitive function in older adults with mild cognitive impairment by inducing biochemical and metabolic changes: a 3-year progressive study. Nutrients 2020 [Internet]. 2020 [cited 2024 Mar 20];12(9):2644. Available from: https://www.mdpi.com/2072-6643/12/9/2644/htm

12. Alkurd R, Mahrous L, Zeb F, Khan MAB, Alhaj H, Khraiwesh HM, et al. Effect of calorie restriction and intermittent fasting regimens on brain-derived neurotrophic factor levels and cognitive function in humans: a systematic review. Medicina (Kaunas) [Internet]. 2024 [cited 2024 Mar 25];60(1). Available from: https://pubmed.ncbi.nlm.nih.gov/38276070/

13. Body composition, nutrient intake and physical activity patterns in young women during Ramadan – PubMed [Internet]. [cited 2024 Mar 25]. Available from: https://pubmed.ncbi.nlm.nih.gov/17909674/

14. Yousuf S, Syed A, Ahmedani MY. To explore the association of Ramadan fasting with symptoms of depression, anxiety, and stress in people with diabetes. Diabetes Res Clin Pract [Internet]. 2021 [cited 2024 Mar 21];172. Available from: https://pubmed.ncbi.nlm.nih.gov/33227360/

15. Al-Ozairi E, AlAwadhi MM, Al-Ozairi A, Taghadom E, Ismail K. A prospective study of the effect of fasting during the month of Ramadan on depression and diabetes distress in people with type 2 diabetes. Diabetes Res Clin Pract. 2019;153:145–9.

16. Hussein M, Fathy W, Abdelghaffar M, Hegazy MT, Teleb DA, Adel S, et al. Effect of first week-intermittent fasting during Ramadan on the severity of neuropsychiatric symptoms in patients with fibromyalgia: a prospective study. Egypt Rheumatol. 2024;46(1):47–50.

17. Nugraha B, Ghashang SK, Hamdan I, Gutenbrunner C. Effect of Ramadan fasting on fatigue, mood, sleepiness, and health-related quality of life of healthy young men in summer time in Germany: a prospective controlled study. Appetite [Internet]. 2017 [cited 2024 Mar 21];111:38–45. Available from: https://pubmed.ncbi.nlm.nih.gov/28027907/

18. Koushali AN, Hajiamini Z, Ebadi A, Bayat N, Khamseh F. Effect of Ramadan fasting on emotional reactions in nurses. Iran J Nurs Midwifery Res [Internet] 2013 [cited 2024 Mar 21];18(3):232. Available from: /PMC/articles/PMC3748544/. https://journals.lww.com/jnmr/fulltext/2013/18030/effect_of_ramadan_fasting_on_emotional_reactions.12.aspx

19. Akbari HA, Yoosefi M, Pourabbas M, Weiss K, Knechtle B, Vancini RL, et al. Association of Ramadan participation with psychological parameters: a cross-sectional study during the COVID-19 pandemic in Iran. J Clin Med [Internet]. 2022 [cited 2024 Mar 21];11(9). Available from: https://pubmed.ncbi.nlm.nih.gov/35566470/

20. Nasiri M. Effects of Ramadan fasting on the resilience and psychological hardiness of students. J Nutr Fasting Health [Internet]. 2021 [cited 2024 Mar 21];9(3):207–11. Available from: https://jnfh.mums.ac.ir/article_17121.html

21. Bastani A, Rajabi S, Kianimarkani F. The effects of fasting during Ramadan on the concentration of serotonin, dopamine, brain-derived neurotrophic factor and nerve growth factor. Neurol Int 2017 [Internet]. 2017 [cited 2024 Mar 19];9(2):7043. Available from: https://www.mdpi.com/2035-8377/9/2/7043

22. Şentürk E, Yıldız M, Şentürk M, Varol E, Yildirim MS, Yilmaz DA, et al. Investigation of the effect of Ramadan fasting on serum levels of melatonin, cortisol, and serotonin: the case of Turkey. Ir J Med Sci [Internet]. 2023 [cited 2024 Mar 19];1–5. Available from: https://link.springer.com/article/10.1007/s11845-023-03532-1

23. Shawky S, Anis A, Orabi S, Shoghy K, Hassan W. Effect of intermittent fasting on brain neurotransmitters, neutrophils phagocytic activity, and histopathological findings in some organs in rats. Int J Res Stud Biosci. 2015;3:38–45.

24. Garcia-Garcia AL, Canetta S, Stujenske JM, Burghardt NS, Ansorge MS, Dranovsky A, et al. Serotonin inputs to the dorsal BNST modulate anxiety in a 5-HT1A receptor-dependent manner. Mol Psychiatry 2018 [Internet]. 2017 [cited 2024 Mar 19];23(10):1990–7. Available from: https://www.nature.com/articles/mp2017165

25. Karayol R, Medrihan L, Warner-Schmidt JL, Fait BW, Rao MN, Holzner EB, et al. Serotonin receptor 4 in the hippocampus modulates mood and anxiety. Mol Psychiatry 2021 [Internet]. 2021 [cited 2024 Mar 19];26(6):2334–49. Available from: https://www.nature.com/articles/s41380-020-00994-y

26. Seidler K, Barrow M. Intermittent fasting and cognitive performance—targeting BDNF as a potential strategy to optimize brain health. Front Neuroendocrinol. 2022;65:100971.

27. Araya AV, Orellana X, Espinoza J. Evaluation of the effect of caloric restriction on serum BDNF in overweight and obese subjects: preliminary evidence. Endocrine [Internet] 2008 [cited 2024 Mar 19];33(3):300–4. Available from: https://link.springer.com/article/10.1007/s12020-008-9090-x

28. Ghashang SK, Hamdan I, Lichtinghagen R, Gutenbrunner C, Nugraha B. Alterations of brain-derived neurotrophic factor and creatinine during Ramadan fasting: a prospective, controlled clinical trial. Iran Red Crescent Med J. 2019;21(5):88324.

29. Jamshed H, Beyl RA, Manna DLD, Yang ES, Ravussin E, Peterson CM. Early time-restricted feeding improves 24-hour glucose levels and affects markers of the circadian clock, aging, and autophagy in humans. Nutrients 2019 [Internet]. 2019 [cited 2024 Mar 19];11(6):1234. Available from: https://www.mdpi.com/2072-6643/11/6/1234/htm

30. Cui R, Fan J, Ge T, Tang L, Li B. The mechanism of acute fasting-induced antidepressant-like effects in mice. J Cell Mol Med [Internet]. 2018 [cited 2024 Mar 19];22(1):223–9. Available from: https://onlinelibrary.wiley.com/doi/full/10.1111/jcmm.13310

31. Sacco RL, Kasner SE, Broderick JP, Caplan LR, Connors J, Culebras A, et al. The impact of intermittent fasting on brain-derived neurotrophic factor, neurotrophin 3, and rat behavior in a rat model of type 2 diabetes mellitus. Brain Sci 2021 [Internet]. 2021 [cited 2024 Mar 19];11(2):242. Available from: https://www.mdpi.com/2076-3425/11/2/242/htm

32. Duman RS, Monteggia LM. A neurotrophic model for stress-related mood disorders. Biol Psychiatry. 2006;59(12):1116–27.

33. Alhaj HA, Massey AE, McAllister-Williams RH. Effects of cortisol on the laterality of the neural correlates of episodic memory. J Psychiatr Res [Internet]. 2008 [cited 2024 Mar 25];42(12):971–81. Available from: https://pubmed.ncbi.nlm.nih.gov/18187154/

34. dos Santos IM, Ciulla L, Braga D, Cereser KM, Gama CS, Kapczinski F, et al. Symptom dimensional approach and BDNF in unmedicated obsessive-compulsive patients: an exploratory study. CNS Spectr [Internet] 2011 [cited 2024 Mar 19];16(9):179–89. Available from: https://www.cambridge.org/core/journals/cns-spectrums/article/abs/symptom-dimensional-approach-and-bdnf-in-unmedicated-obsessivecompulsive-patients-an-exploratory-study/20DF979A65040E6A81FB5B7EA7A9CCD3

35. Dell'Osso L, Carmassi C, Del Debbio A, Dell'Osso MC, Bianchi C, da Pozzo E, et al. Brain-derived neurotrophic factor plasma levels in patients who have post-traumatic stress disorder. Prog Neuro-Psychopharmacol Biol Psychiatry. 2009;33(5):899–902.

36. Blekhman R, Goodrich JK, Huang K, Sun Q, Bukowski R, Bell JT, et al. Host genetic variation impacts microbiome composition across human body sites. Genome Biol [Internet] 2015 [cited 2024 Mar 19];16(1):1–12. Available from: https://genomebiology.biomedcentral.com/articles/10.1186/s13059-015-0759-1

37. Schirmer M, Smeekens SP, Vlamakis H, Jaeger M, Oosting M, Franzosa EA, et al. Linking the human gut microbiome to inflammatory cytokine production capacity. Cell [Internet] 2016 [cited 2024 Mar 19];167(4):1125–36.e8. Available from: http://www.cell.com/article/S0092867416314039/fulltext

38. Mayer EA, Tillisch K, Gupta A. Gut/brain axis and the microbiota. J Clin Invest. 2015;125(3):926–38.

39. Bastiaanssen TFS, Cowan CSM, Claesson MJ, Dinan TG, Cryan JF. Making sense of the microbiome in psychiatry. Int J Neuropsychopharmacol [Internet] 2019 [cited 2024 Mar 19];22(1):37. Available from: /PMC/articles/PMC6313131/. https://pubmed.ncbi.nlm.nih.gov/30099552/.

40. Jiang HY, Zhang X, Yu ZH, Zhang Z, Deng M, Zhao JH, et al. Altered gut microbiota profile in patients with generalized anxiety disorder. J Psychiatr Res [Internet]. 2018 [cited 2024 Mar 19];104:130–6. Available from: https://pubmed.ncbi.nlm.nih.gov/30029052/

41. Limbana T, Khan F, Eskander N. Gut microbiome and depression: how microbes affect the way we think. Cureus [Internet]. 2020 Available from: /PMC/articles/PMC7510518/. https://pubmed.ncbi.nlm.nih.gov/32983670/.

42. Saglam D, Colak GA, Sahin E, Ekren BY, Sezerman U, Bas M. Effects of Ramadan intermittent fasting on gut microbiome: is the diet key? Front Microbiol. 2023;14:1203205. https://doi.org/10.3389/fmicb.2023.1203205. PMID: 37705730; PMCID: PMC10495574. https://pubmed.ncbi.nlm.nih.gov/37705730/

43. Ozkul C, Yalinay M, Karakan T. Structural changes in gut microbiome after Ramadan fasting: a pilot study [Internet]. 2020 [cited 2024 Mar 19];11(3):227–33. https://doi.org/10.3920/BM2019.0039. Available from: https://www.wageningenacademic.com/doi/10.3920/BM2019.0039

44. Su J, Wang Y, Zhang X, Ma M, Xie Z, Pan Q, et al. Remodeling of the gut microbiome during Ramadan-associated intermittent fasting. Am J Clin Nutr. 2021;113(5):1332–42.

45. Humbel F, Rieder JH, Franc Y, Juillerat P, Scharl M, Misselwitz B, et al. Association of alterations in intestinal microbiota with impaired psychological function in patients with inflammatory bowel diseases in remission. Clin Gastroenterol Hepatol. 2020;18(9):2019–2029.e11.

46. Mistretta A, Marventano S, Platania A, Godos J, Galvano F, Grosso G. Metabolic profile of the Mediterranean healthy eating, lifestyle and aging (MEAL) study cohort. Med J Nutr Metab. 2017;10(2):131–40.

47. Taetzsch A, Roberts SB, Bukhari A, Lichtenstein AH, Gilhooly CH, Martin E, et al. Eating timing: associations with dietary intake and metabolic health. J Acad Nutr Diet. 2021;121(4):738–48.

48. Cohen JFW, Gorski MT, Gruber SA, Kurdziel LBF, Rimm EB. The effect of healthy dietary consumption on executive cognitive functioning in children and adolescents: a systematic review. Br J Nutr [Internet]. 2016 [cited 2023 Dec 12];116(6):989–1000. Available from: https://www.cambridge.org/core/journals/british-journal-of-nutrition/article/effect-of-healthy-dietary-consumption-on-executive-cognitive-functioning-in-children-and-adolescents-a-systematic-review/5B4903E20D46E00D57E29FD7A6BEDB41

49. Ye X, Scott T, Gao X, Maras JE, Bakun PJ, Tucker KL. Mediterranean diet, healthy eating index 2005, and cognitive function in middle-aged and older Puerto Rican adults. J Acad Nutr Diet. 2013;113(2):276–81.e3.

50. Jahrami HA, Alsibai J, Clark CCT, Faris ME. A systematic review, meta-analysis, and meta-regression of the impact of diurnal intermittent fasting during Ramadan on body weight in healthy subjects aged 16 years and above. Eur J Nutr [Internet] 2020 [cited 2023 Dec 12];59(6):2291–316. Available from: https://link.springer.com/article/10.1007/s00394-020-02216-1

51. Faris ME, Alsibai J, Jahrami HA, Obaideen AA, Jahrami HA, Obaideen AA. Impact of Ramadan diurnal intermittent fasting on the metabolic syndrome components in healthy, non-athletic Muslim people aged over 15 years: a systematic review and meta-analysis. Br J Nutr [Internet] 2020 [cited 2023 Dec 12];123(1):1–22. Available from: https://www.cambridge.org/core/journals/british-journal-of-nutrition/article/impact-of-ramadan-diurnal-intermittent-fasting-on-the-metabolic-syndrome-components-in-healthy-nonathletic-muslim-people-aged-over-15-years-a-systematic-review-and-metaanalysis/390F52CFFD34278113368A64787DC14A

52. Faris ME, Jahrami HA, Obaideen AA, Madkour MI. Impact of diurnal intermittent fasting during Ramadan on inflammatory and oxidative stress markers in healthy people: systematic review and meta-analysis. J Nutr Intermed Metab. 2019;15:18–26.

53. Faris ME, Jahrami H, BaHammam A, Kalaji Z, Madkour M, Hassanein M. A systematic review, meta-analysis, and meta-regression of the impact of diurnal intermittent fasting during Ramadan on glucometabolic markers in healthy subjects. Diabetes Res Clin Pract [Internet].

2020 [cited 2023 Dec 12];165. Available from: http://www.diabetesresearchclinicalpractice. com/article/S0168822720304769/fulltext

54. Vasconcelos AR, Orellana AMM, Paixão AG, Scavone C, Kawamoto EM. Intermittent fasting and caloric restriction: neuroplasticity and neurodegeneration. In: Handbook of famine, starvation, and nutrient deprivation [Internet]. 2018 [cited 2023 Dec 12];1–18. Available from: https://link.springer.com/referenceworkentry/10.1007/978-3-319-40007-5_99-1

55. Mattson MP, Moehl K, Ghena N, Schmaedick M, Cheng A. Intermittent metabolic switching, neuroplasticity and brain health. Nat Rev Neurosci [Internet] 2018;19(2):63. Available from: / PMC/articles/PMC5913738/. https://pubmed.ncbi.nlm.nih.gov/29321682/.

56. Madkour MI, El-Serafi AT, Jahrami HA, Sherif NM, Hassan RE, Awadallah S, et al. Ramadan diurnal intermittent fasting modulates SOD2, TFAM, Nrf2, and sirtuins (SIRT1, SIRT3) gene expressions in subjects with overweight and obesity. Diabetes Res Clin Pract [Internet] 2019 [cited 2023 Dec 12];155. Available from: http://www.diabetesresearchclinicalpractice.com/ article/S0168822719302177/fulltext

57. Madkour MI, Islam MT, Tippetts TS, Chowdhury KH, Lesniewski LA, Summers SA, et al. Ramadan intermittent fasting is associated with ameliorated inflammatory markers and improved plasma sphingolipids/ceramides in subjects with obesity: lipidomics analysis. Sci Rep 2023 [Internet]. 2023 [cited 2024 Mar 25];13(1):1–12. Available from: https://www. nature.com/articles/s41598-023-43862-9

58. Cherif A, Roelands B, Meeusen R, Chamari K. Effects of intermittent fasting, caloric restriction, and Ramadan intermittent fasting on cognitive performance at rest and during exercise in adults. Sports Med [Internet]. 2016 [cited 2024 Mar 25];46(1):35–47. Available from: https:// pubmed.ncbi.nlm.nih.gov/26438184/

59. LiCausi F, Hartman NW. Role of mTOR Complexes in Neurogenesis. Int J Mol Sci. 2018;19(5):1544. https://doi.org/10.3390/ijms19051544. PMID: 29789464; PMCID: PMC5983636. https://pubmed.ncbi.nlm.nih.gov/29789464/.

60. Bagherniya M, Butler AE, Barreto GE, Sahebkar A. The effect of fasting or calorie restriction on autophagy induction: a review of the literature. Ageing Res Rev. 2018;47:183–97.

61. Giordano S, Darley-Usmar V, Zhang J. Autophagy as an essential cellular antioxidant pathway in neurodegenerative disease. Redox Biol. 2014;2(1):82–90.

62. Lu B, Nagappan G, Lu Y. BDNF and synaptic plasticity, cognitive function, and dysfunction. Handb Exp Pharmacol [Internet]. 2015 [cited 2024 Mar 20];220:223–50. Available from: https://link.springer.com/chapter/10.1007/978-3-642-45106-5_9

63. Griffin ÉW, Mullally S, Foley C, Warmington SA, O'Mara SM, Kelly ÁM. Aerobic exercise improves hippocampal function and increases BDNF in the serum of young adult males. Physiol Behav. 2011;104(5):934–41.

64. Shimada H, Makizako H, Doi T, Yoshida D, Tsutsumimoto K, Anan Y, et al. A large, cross-sectional observational study of serum BDNF, cognitive function, and mild cognitive impairment in older people. Front Aging Neurosci. 2014;6:81980.

65. Amin DA, Kumar Sai DS, Mishra DS, Kumar Reddy DU, Sriram N, Mukkadan JK. Effects of fasting during Ramadan month on depression, anxiety, stress, and cognition. Int J Med Res Rev [Internet] 2016 [cited 2024 Mar 20];4(5):771–4. Available from: https://ijmrr.medresearch.in/index.php/ijmrr/article/view/555

66. Khemila S, Romdhani M, Farjallah MA, Abid R, Bentouati E, Souissi MA, et al. Effects of Ramadan fasting on the diurnal variations of physical and cognitive performances at rest and after exercise in professional football players. Front Psychol [Internet]. 2023 [cited 2024 Mar 21];14:1148845. Available from: https://data.bnf.fr/fr/11864527/ institut_national_de_la_statistique_

67. Boujelbane MA, Trabelsi K, Jahrami HA, Masmoudi L, Ammar A, Khacharem A, et al. Time-restricted feeding and cognitive function in sedentary and physically active elderly individuals: Ramadan diurnal intermittent fasting as a model. Front Nutr. 2022;9:1041216.

68. Norlis Dalisa T, Omar T, Suhaili C, Taha C. The relationship between dietary intake and cognitive performance before and during Ramadan fasting among healthy adult population in Kuala

Nerus, Terengganu. Asian J Med Biomed [Internet] 2022 [cited 2024 Mar 21];6(S1):121–2. Available from: https://journal.unisza.edu.my/ajmb/index.php/ajmb/article/view/555

69. Chamari K, Briki W, Farooq A, Patrick T, Belfekih T, Herrera CP. Impact of Ramadan intermittent fasting on cognitive function in trained cyclists: a pilot study. Biol Sport [Internet] 2016 [cited 2024 Mar 21];33(1):49. Available from: /PMC/articles/PMC4786586/. https://pubmed.ncbi.nlm.nih.gov/26985134/.

70. Fawzi MH, Fawzi MM, Said NS, Fawzi MM, Fouad AA, Abdel-Moety H. Effect of Ramadan fasting on anthropometric, metabolic, inflammatory and psychopathology status of Egyptian male patients with schizophrenia. Psychiatry Res [Internet] 2015 [cited 2024 Mar 21];225(3):501–8. Available from: https://pubmed.ncbi.nlm.nih.gov/25529262/

71. Eddahby S, Kadri N, Moussaoui D. Fasting during Ramadan is associated with a higher recurrence rate in patients with bipolar disorder. World Psychiatry [Internet] 2014 [cited 2024 Mar 21];13(1):97. Available from: https://pubmed.ncbi.nlm.nih.gov/24497261/

72. Farooq S, Nazar Z, Akhter J, Irafn M, Subhan F, Ahmed Z, et al. Effect of fasting during Ramadan on serum lithium level and mental state in bipolar affective disorder. Int Clin Psychopharmacol [Internet] 2010 [cited 2023 Dec 9];25(6):323–7. Available from: https://pubmed.ncbi.nlm.nih.gov/20827213/

73. Wilhelmi De Toledo F, Buchinger A, Burggrabe H, Hölz G, Kuhn C, Lischka E, et al. Fasting therapy – an expert panel update of the 2002 consensus guidelines. Forsch Komplementmed [Internet]. 2013 [cited 2024 Mar 21];20(6):434–43. Available from: https://pubmed.ncbi.nlm.nih.gov/24434758/

Chapter 11
Immunomodulatory Effects of Intermittent Fasting and Its Implication on Cancer: Ramadan Fasting Perspective

Mohamed Labib Salem, Saleh Alwasel, MoezAlIslam E. Faris,
Walid Al-Dahmash, Noura E. Sanoh, Hager A. Elkomy, Esraa M. Khallaf,
Amro A. Shaheraldin, Toqa Solaiman, Nada Mostafa, Mai Alalem,
and Sohaila M. Khalil

Abstract Intermittent fasting (IF), which is also called fasting on a schedule or a fasting-mimicking diet (FMD), has been found to be beneficial for health by reducing risk factors and reversing symptoms of serious health conditions, including cancer. Although the mechanisms behind these beneficial effects of IF are not clearly understood, several potential mechanisms have been suggested. Overall, IF is associated with the conversion of the energy metabolic response from glucose to ketone bodies as an energy source, enhancing ketone body production, autophagy, DNA repair, anti-stress abilities, and antioxidant defense. In tumor cells, these events result in the inhibition of the IGF-1/AKT and the mammalian target of rapamycin (mTORC1)

M. L. Salem (✉) · A. A. Shaheraldin · T. Solaiman · S. M. Khalil
Immunology & Parasitology Unit, Department of Zoology, Faculty of Science,
Tanta University, Tanta, Egypt

Center of Excellence in Cancer Research, Tanta University, Tanta, Egypt
e-mail: Mohamed.labib@science.tanta.edu.eg

S. Alwasel · W. Al-Dahmash
Zoology Department, College of Science, King Saud University, Riyadh, Saudi Arabia

M. E. Faris
Department of Clinical Nutrition and Dietetics, Faculty of Allied Medical Sciences,
Applied Science Private University, Amman, Jordan

N. E. Sanoh
Center of Excellence in Cancer Research, Tanta University, Tanta, Egypt

Chemistry Department, Faculty of Science, Tanta University, Tanta, Egypt

157

M. E. Faris et al. (eds.), *Health and Medical Aspects of Ramadan Intermittent Fasting*, https://doi.org/10.1007/978-981-96-6783-3_11

pathways and increase adenosine monophosphate (AMP)-activated protein kinase (AMPK), which is dependent on the sirtuin-1 (SIRT1) and SIRT3 pathways. These molecular cascades can hinder tumor cell growth. Furthermore, in cancer cells, IF alters autophagy, which is a conserved lysosomal degradation pathway for the intracellular recycling of macromolecules and clearance of damaged organelles and misfolded proteins to ensure cellular homeostasis. IF can also increase the sensitivity of cancer cells to chemotherapy and radiotherapy; it can also reduce the side effects of conventional anticancer treatments. Further, IF can influence gene expression regulation by acting on certain types of microRNAs (miRNAs). Most importantly, IF can enhance the quality and quantity of both innate and adaptive immune cells by triggering stem cells to regenerate the immune system, as well as by increasing the production of tumor-killing immune cells, thereby inhibiting tumor growth and improving antitumor immune responses. Given these beneficial effects of IF, it is recommended to use fasting as an adjuvant therapy for cancer treatment, including immunotherapy.

Keywords Apoptosis · Autophagy · Cancer · Immune cells · Intermittent fasting · Lysosome · Metabolism · Microbiota · microRNA · Mitochondria · Tumor

11.1 Introduction

Fasting refers to refraining from consuming food and/or drinks for varying durations [1]. Calorie restriction (CR) differs from fasting and is described as limiting daily calorie consumption over a particular period without producing malnutrition [2]. Intermittent fasting (IF) is a method of dietary energy restriction that involves various protocols aimed at limiting the time window for eating. IF encompasses different subtypes based on the duration of the fasting period [3]. One common type is time-restricted feeding (TRF), in which fasting occurs within 24 hours, usually

H. A. Elkomy
Biochemistry Division, Chemistry Department, Faculty of Science, Tanta University, Tanta, Egypt

E. M. Khallaf
Center of Excellence in Cancer Research, Tanta University, Tanta, Egypt

Immunology Unit, Department of Zoology, Faculty of Science, Cairo University, Giza Governorate, Egypt

Healthcare, Saxony Egypt University, Cairo, Egypt

N. Mostafa
Center of Excellence in Cancer Research, Tanta University, Tanta, Egypt

Biotechnology Department, Faculty of Science, Tanta University, Tanta, Egypt

M. Alalem
Department of Molecular Biology, Genetic Engineering and Biotechnology Research Institute, University of Sadat City, El Sadat, Egypt

lasting 12–18 hours per day. An example of TRF is followed during the fasting traditions of Ramadan in the Islamic faith [4]. There are different types of IF methods. One of the most popular IF methods is the lean gains [16/8 h] method [5], which involves fasting for 16 hours of the day and an 8-hour eating window. The 16-hour fast has been proven to activate autophagy, which is responsible for cleaning out damaged cells and helping regenerate newer, healthier cells. Another fasting method is the warrior diet, which includes fasting for 20 hours each day and eating in a 4-hour window [6]. Another form of the IF method is the 5:2 [7]. The diet consists of regularly eating five days a week with no CR and consuming 500–600 calories on the other two days. Another option is the eat-stop-eat strategy, which entails fasting for 24 hours once or twice a week and drinking noncaloric liquids during the fasting period [8]. Choosing either of these methods depends on individual needs and health performance [9]. Results of studies in humans revealed that IF can decrease body weight and fat mass while also preserving muscle mass. It can also lower triglycerides and improve factors associated with heart health, including improved insulin sensitivity and reduced blood pressure [10]. However, the results vary greatly in terms of the effects of IF on blood markers of inflammation and other factors associated with age-related metabolic diseases. Indeed, there is less evidence for actual metabolic benefits since there are few studies on the effect of IF on young, healthy, lean individuals [11]. Results of studies in animals demonstrate that IF can lower insulin and glucose levels, lower the levels of blood lipids such as cholesterol and triglycerides, decrease blood pressure, reduce markers of inflammation, decrease body fat, lower body weight, and maintain lean muscle mass. Increased autophagy, an evolutionary mechanism for nutrient trimming and recycling, is also a result of IF-α. Despite these metabolic improvements, which are seen after IF in animals, reproducing these results in humans needs to be confirmed through randomized controlled trials [12]. It is also unclear whether people would be able to tolerate the typically severe CR required to promote weight loss for the duration needed to achieve health benefits from IF [13].

11.2 Fasting and Metabolism

The fasting-to-fed switch at the cellular level is signaled by the intracellular levels of energy metabolites [14]. Some processes build cells and tissue in the body for repair and growth [anabolic]. In contrast, others tend to break down tissue, release energy [catabolic], or remove metabolic waste [15]. The human body stores excess energy in adipocytes (fat cells). In fasting states, when food is not readily available, other sources of energy are utilized, such as proteins and lipids in tissues and cells. For the body to repair and grow, the cells transit from a catabolic state back to an anabolic state. In everyday situations, where there is a constant feeling of hunger, that switch rarely happens, and the body keeps breaking down tissues and cells, using proteins and fats. It has also been suggested that stress is caused by fasting periods might stimulate the production of proteins that are beneficial for metabolic health through a mechanism called hormesis [16].

Numerous studies have investigated the effects of IF on metabolism, shedding light on its potential benefits [17]. These studies have demonstrated that IF can lead to improvements in various metabolic parameters, including insulin sensitivity, lipid profiles, and inflammatory indicators, as well as an increase in fat oxidation and the preservation of lean muscle mass [18]. Additionally, IF has been shown to increase levels of growth hormone, which can have a positive effect on metabolism and muscle growth [19]. Both human and animal research studies have indicated that IF benefits the health and metabolic system. IF has such a positive impact on metabolism and physiology that it can help with a variety of lifestyle disorders, like obesity and hyperglycemia. IF's positive benefits are mediated by glucose control, which increases insulin sensitivity in the liver and other tissues, high-density lipoprotein (HDL) levels, and cardiovascular and pulmonary functioning. On the other hand, it reduces blood lipid profiles, fat mass, oxidative stress, and inflammation [20].

Many studies have revealed the positive effects of IF on fat loss and metabolism [21]. IF can increase fat oxidation, where daily feeding interventions for 6 h for eight weeks increase fat oxidation in young, nonobese women, compared to consuming three meals within 12 hours. On the other hand, the same effects of 8 weeks of time-restricted feeding on fat oxidation were significantly found in other healthy people [22]. IF regulates the levels of energy metabolites and hormones in the blood, enhances metabolic switching, and offers protection to the cells and tissues [23]. The breaking of the fast is characterized by a decrease in insulin levels, a rise in glucagon, and the activation of the mTOR signaling pathway, which initiates protein synthesis and the building of cells and tissues by switching the metabolic signaling from a catabolic to an anabolic state [24], improving insulin sensitivity, immune response, neuroprotection, and cardiovascular health [25]. While it might sound counterintuitive that longer periods of not eating improve insulin sensitivity, it has also been shown that a longer overnight fast triggers increased adiponectin secretion the next day, which helps increase glucose uptake in muscles [26].

Although fat oxidation is utilized as an energy source during fasting, fatty acid (FA) production in the liver is discouraged via death-associated protein kinase (DAPK) through the interplay of the PP–AMP-activated protein kinase (AMPK)/NO-AMPK pathway [27]. Recent studies investigated whether there is a link between DAPK, eukaryotic translation elongation factor 2 (EEF2), and liver FA mobilization. While FA consumption does not occur in the liver, muscle cells are dependent on circulating FA for energy metabolism. However, during IF, muscle cells consume less fat. This study exhibited markers of glucose metabolism and energy consumption in 60-year-old male volunteers and identified the lowered fat oxidation rate attributable to a lower expression of the lipolysis activator, peroxisome proliferator–activated receptor (PPAR), a coactivator-1 alpha in muscle cells [28].

IF can increase levels of norepinephrine, a hormone that helps break down fat cells for energy. Studies have shown that fasting can increase norepinephrine levels by up to three to five times, which can lead to greater weight loss [29] by improving insulin sensitivity, reducing fat storage, and promoting fat burning [30]. Another way that IF can increase fat burning is by boosting the levels of human growth hormone (HGH), which plays a key role in metabolism, fat burning, and muscle growth. Since IF can increase HGH levels by up to five times, it can help preserve muscle mass while promoting fat loss [31]. On the other hand, during fasting, the body starts to use stored fat as a source of energy. This process is known as ketosis, where the body produces fat stores to fuel the brain and muscles [5].

Insulin sensitivity is a crucial factor in maintaining a healthy metabolism and preventing the development of chronic diseases, such as type 2 diabetes. When cells become resistant to the effects of insulin, it can lead to elevated blood sugar levels and ultimately result in a range of health issues [7]. One key mechanism by which IF improves insulin sensitivity is by reducing insulin levels in the body [32]. This can help with weight loss and avoid obesity, which is a risk factor for developing metabolic disorders [33].

In conclusion, IF can increase fat burning through a variety of metabolic changes, including ketosis, increased norepinephrine levels, improved insulin sensitivity, and higher HGH levels. These changes can help promote weight loss, improve metabolic health, and enhance overall well-being.

11.3   IF Increases Mitochondrial Biogenesis and Function

IF, through different mechanisms, can induce recycling of the dysfunctional mitochondria and repair the damage in the mitochondrial system. These mechanisms include different signaling pathways, such as insulin/insulin-like growth factor (IGF) resistance Insulin/Insulin Signaling (IIS) and the target of rapamycin (TOR) [34]. In addition, IF increases the resistance of mitochondria to oxidative stress damage by increasing the antioxidant defense mechanisms and decreasing the production of free radicals [35].

Mitochondrial function declines with age and influences many age-related diseases, including neurodegenerative diseases, cancer, heart diseases, and diabetes. Many factors, such as the accumulation of mitochondrial DNA (mtDNA) mutations, decline in mitochondrial function, enhanced reactive oxygen species (ROS) production, decline in mitochondrial turnover, and greater accumulation of dysfunctional mitochondria, drive aging [36]. Interventions that improve mitochondrial health and function are, therefore, an important area of research in developing therapeutics to delay the onset of age-related diseases and promote healthy aging. Importantly, studies have shown that IF can promote longevity in a variety of model organisms, including worms, flies, and mice [37].

IF has been shown to have several beneficial effects on mitochondria through a process called mitochondrial biogenesis, which refers to the creation of new mitochondria within cells, which helps increase the overall number and function of these organelles. By promoting mitochondrial biogenesis, IF can enhance the efficiency of energy production within cells, leading to improved cellular function and overall health [38]. IF has also been shown to improve mitochondrial quality control mechanisms. Mitochondria are constantly under threat from oxidative stress and damage, which can impair their function and lead to cellular dysfunction. IF has been shown to upregulate various cellular pathways that help protect and repair damaged mitochondria, thereby improving mitochondrial function and overall cellular health [38].

One of the main ways by which IF promotes mitochondrial biogenesis is by stimulating multiple signaling pathways within the cell. During fasting, the body's metabolic changes activate AMP-activated protein kinase (AMPK) and sirtuins, which are important regulators of mitochondrial biogenesis. These signaling pathways contribute to the development of new mitochondria within the cell, which improves energy output and general cellular function [39]. One of the lesser-known benefits of IF is its ability to enhance mitochondrial function through the stimulation of mitochondrial biogenesis, leading to improved energy production and overall cellular function. In addition, IF has been shown to increase the efficiency of mitochondrial energy production, resulting in less oxidative stress and improved cellular health [40]. Studies have also shown that IF can increase levels of mitochondrial biogenesis factors such as PGC-1α, a master regulator of mitochondrial biogenesis. By upregulating the expression of PGC-1α, IF can stimulate the production of new mitochondria and improve mitochondrial function within the cell [41]. IF improves mitochondrial activity by activating a cellular stress response pathway and inducing autophagy. It helps eliminate old and damaged mitochondria, facilitating the production of new, healthy mitochondria. During fasting, the body uses fatty acids and ketones rather than glucose as its primary fuel source. This metabolic shift has been found to increase mitochondrial efficiency and minimize oxidative stress, resulting in better mitochondrial function.

Furthermore, IF has been shown to enhance mitochondrial quality control mechanisms, such as mitochondrial fusion and fission. These processes help maintain the integrity of mitochondria and ensure their optimal function. By promoting mitochondrial quality control, IF helps prevent the accumulation of damaged mitochondria and maintain a healthy mitochondrial population within cells [42].

In conclusion, IF can be considered a promising strategy for enhancing mitochondrial function and promoting overall cellular health by helping optimize energy production and reducing oxidative stress within cells. Further research is needed to fully understand the mechanisms underlying the effects of IF on mitochondrial function and explore its potential therapeutic applications.

11.4   Fasting and Autolysis of Fats

Lysosomes are a type of cytoplasmic vesicles that have a single membrane and a diameter of 0.1–1.2 μm. Digestive enzymes are found in membrane-bound lysosomal cell organelles. They have lysosomal hydrolases, which are capable of degrading proteins, carbohydrates, lipids, and nucleic acids. Approximately 50 distinct degradative enzymes that may hydrolyze proteins, lipids, polysaccharides, DNA, and RNA are found in lysosomes, according to Minchew et al. (2017). All lysosomal enzymes are acid hydrolases, which means they are active at the acidic pH of around five and are maintained within lysosomes but are inactive at the neutral pH of roughly 7.2, which is typical of the remaining cytoplasm [43]. These lysosomal hydrolases need to provide a twofold defense against unchecked digestion of the cytosol's contents for an acidic pH; even if the lysosomal membrane were to break down, the released acid hydrolases would be inactive at the neutral pH of the cytosol [44].

Lysosomes need to actively concentrate on H+ ions [protons] to maintain their internal acidic pH. This is achieved by a proton pump in the lysosomal membrane, which actively transports protons into the lysosome from the cytosol. This pumping requires the expenditure of energy in the form of ATP hydrolysis since it maintains an approximately 100-fold higher H+ concentration inside the lysosome [45]. Lysosomes are involved in a variety of cell processes, including breaking down excess or worn-out cell parts and destroying invasive viruses and bacteria. If the cell is damaged beyond repair, lysosomes can assist it in self-destructing, a process known as programmed cell death or apoptosis [46].

Most of these enzymes function optimally at an acidic pH [4.5–5.5] that is reached within lysosomes after fusion with other intracellular vehicles. Lysosomes have a central role in the degradation of intracellular components via autophagy [44]. They are also involved in the breakdown of extracellular material by endocytosis, phagocytosis, or micropinocytosis. They are central contributors to plasma membrane repair and the formation of extracellular vesicles.

Lysosomes serve as hubs for signaling and degradation and are crucial for aging, development, and cellular homeostasis. Lysosome function alterations are necessary to facilitate cellular adaptability to various signals and stimuli. They are synthesized in the Endoplasmic Reticulum (ER) and transported to the trans-Golgi network, where they are decorated with mannose-6-phosphate (M6P) and targeted to the M6P receptor. The resulting complexes are transported through clathrin-coated vesicles or via alternative clathrin-independent mechanisms to early endosomes. Some lysosomal hydrolases can also be delivered to lysosomes via M6P-independent targeting mechanisms. More than 60 lysosomal hydrolases have been identified.

The fasting-induced hormone FGF21 mobilizes calcium from the ER in a PLCγ1- and InsP3R-dependent manner, shuttling downstream regulatory element antagonist modulator (DREAM) to the nucleus. DREAM then inhibits the expression of the MID1 gene, leading to the stabilization and accumulation of PP2A, which enhances the transcription of genes involved in lysosome biogenesis, autophagy, and lipid metabolism. Adaptation to fasting or starvation has evolved in animals to ensure the availability and conservation of energy when nutrients are scarce [42].

The lysosomal-autophagic pathway plays a critical role in maintaining energy homeostasis during nutrient deprivation. Acute regulation of this pathway by signaling mechanisms linked to nutrient sensing has been well-described, and mTOR is a master regulator of this pathway. Previous studies show that mTOR inhibition is sufficient to induce nuclear shuttling of transcription factor EB (TFEB) without the inhibition of phosphatase activity, whereas our results demonstrate that PP2A modulates the FGF21-TFEB signaling axis during fasting [47]. As the nuclear-localized

TFEB is dephosphorylated, both phosphatase activation and kinase inactivation may be necessary to induce the rapid and maximal nuclear shuttling of TFEB and, thereby, mediate the lysosomal-autophagic pathway in response to different environmental cues.

Weight loss and maintenance are two key factors in achieving a healthy lifestyle, and IF has gained popularity as an alternative therapy for obesity [48]. Although fasting experience and substantial human consumption with fasting weight control are not novel, with the increasing number of obese patients, IF has been refocused on the attention of clinical advances [49]. IF allows for restrictive energy consumption without food restrictions through the fasting period [50]. The advantages of an IF diet may be expected to lower the risk of obesity and associated diseases, including endothelial cell dysfunction and metabolic disorders, such as hyperglycemia, insulin resistance, and inappropriate fatty metabolism connected to fat accumulation [20].

In line with the above notion, IF has been found to induce changes in hunger hormones, including ghrelin and leptin levels, over other strategies for calorie reduction. Because hormones play a significant role in weight management methods, endocrine signals such as hunger and satiety play an important part in establishing body fat stores and might be particularly necessary to preserve fat reduction by the energy-stabilizing endocrine system. This can indeed be seen in individuals exposed to continuous CR, as hunger hormones are modified. However, in leaner, unhealthy individuals, dissimilar changes in hunger and satiety hormones appear during the per-day isocaloric fasting intervention, probably reducing the chances of weight loss.

The crucial function of fibroblast growth factor 21 (FGF21) was studied in relation to lysosome homeostasis in mice, where it was found that a deficiency in FGF21 impairs hepatic lysosomal function by blocking transcription factor EB (TFEB), a master regulator of lysosome biogenesis and autophagy. FGF21 causes the mobilization of calcium from the endoplasmic reticulum, which activates the transcriptional repressor downstream regulatory element antagonist modulator (DREAM), which, in turn, causes the expression of MID1 (which encodes the E3 ligase midline-1) to be inhibited [51]. As a substrate of MID1, protein phosphatase PP2A accumulates and dephosphorylates TFEB, upregulating genes involved in lysosome biogenesis, autophagy, and lipid metabolism [52].

11.5   Fasting and Autophagy

An intercellular degradation mechanism called autophagy enables cells to recycle broken intercellular components to produce energy and serve as building blocks for the formation of new cellular structures [53]. Indeed, stress, oxidation, lack of sleep, bad eating habits, and bad behavior lead to a significant accumulation of fats and proteins in all cells, albeit in different proportions. In addition to these exogenous biological and non-biological wastes, the endogenous biological wastes from metabolic products also accumulate in cells and harm them. Under this setting, the role of the self-eating process becomes of paramount significance, as they recycle all these accumulated exogenous and endogenous wastes and turn them into useful materials for the cell itself to make energy and new proteins [54].

The process of recycling biological waste, especially proteins and fats, is called autophagy, meaning self-eating, and here, "self" means parts of the cell are eaten by the cell itself. Autophagy is a Latin term made up of two parts: "auto," which means "self," and "phagy," which means "to eat." The term "autophagy" has been around and used often since the mid-nineteenth century. In its current form, the term autophagy was developed in 1963 by Belgian scientist Christian de Duve based on his discovery of the functions of the lysosome.

Autophagy is a cellular process that degrades and recycles damaged or defective cellular components. It is essential for cellular balance and health. Mitophagy is a type of autophagy that targets damaged or defective mitochondria for destruction. Autophagy helps remove inflammatory cells and reduce oxidative stress in the body. By promoting autophagy through IF, inflammation was reduced, and overall cellular health improved [55].

Autophagy, or self-eating, is a natural and continuous cellular process that occurs in every cell of the body including during the embryonic stage in both humans and animals. Its primary function is to maintain a balance between the breakdown and renewal of cellular components, helping to preserve the body's overall size, shape, and weight once maturity is reached. Before birth and during the early fetal stage, before the cells are formed into a body, the process of "self-eating" occurs quickly and continuously but for the purpose of differentiating the cells into specific tissues [56]. During this process, some embryonic cells die and are decomposed through autophagy to make way for neighboring cells to form into tissues in their functional form; that is, they sacrifice themselves so that other cells can feed on them.

The identification of autophagy-related genes in yeast during the 1990s enabled researchers to unravel the mechanisms underlying autophagy. This groundbreaking work ultimately led to the awarding of the 2016 Nobel Prize in Physiology or Medicine to Japanese scientist Yoshinori Ohsumi, in recognition of his discovery of how autophagy is precisely regulated within cells [57]. During autophagy, defective or senescent cytoplasmic components [such as mitochondria] are targeted and isolated from the rest of the cell within a double-membrane vesicle, known as an autophagosome. Over time, the autophagosome fuses with the lysosome, leading to a process of specializing in the elimination of autophagosomes, waste management, and disposal. Eventually, the contents of the vehicle, now called the autolysosome, are degraded, and its components are recycled.

Because the incidence of most diseases is due to the accumulation of biological and non-biological waste or the malfunction or damage that has occurred to certain proteins, self-eating is the ideal way to get rid of the excess and the defect to create a new protein that is fit, healthy, and strong, as the cells have learned and trained to do. Indeed, this self-repair method is much better than giving medications, which themselves may cause major adverse effects. This has been proven in many diseases, such as Alzheimer's disease, atherosclerosis, heart disease, diabetes, and hormonal imbalance. This notion would explain why IF benefits the health performance of patients suffering from these diseases [58].

Nowadays, there are many IF programs (fasting one day and breakfast the other day), which last for at least 17 hours, that are applied with the aim of awakening the process of self-recycling of biological waste and gradually returning the body to its normal state, away from satiety, aging, and silent and glaring diseases. Indeed, awakening autophagy through fasting leads to improving the functions of the liver, pancreas, immune cells, and brain, increasing human memory [59]. IF has been shown to increase the levels of autophagy and mitophagy in the body. During fasting periods, when the body is deprived of nutrients, cellular energy levels decrease, leading to the activation of various signaling pathways that stimulate autophagy. This process helps clear out damaged proteins and organelles, promoting cellular renewal and rejuvenation.

Furthermore, IF has been shown to promote autophagy [60]. Previous research has shown that IF or CR can induce adaptive autophagy, increasing cell lifespan. However, prolonged CR with an intensive autophagy response can be harmful and increase type II autophagic cell death [61]. The precise molecular mechanisms associated with this phenomenon remain unclear. The detailed mechanisms governing the effect of CR and IF on autophagy and its impact on tumor cells have been discussed in detail recently [61].

Emerging research highlights the multifaceted effects of fasting on health, including potential implications for cancer prevention and immune modulation. This study investigated the impact of Ramadan IF (RIF), a form of time-restricted feeding, on autophagy gene expression in overweight and obese individuals, a population often at increased risk for various cancers and immune dysregulation. Fifty-one participants [36 men and 15 women] underwent four weeks of RIF, with measurements of autophagy gene expression (LAMP2, LC3B, ATG5, and ATG4D) taken before and after, alongside a control group of six healthy normal-weight individuals. The results showed significant upregulation of LAMP2, LC3B, and ATG5 genes post-RIF in the overweight/obese group, suggesting enhanced autophagy. Simultaneously, RIF led to improvements in metabolic parameters [decreased weight, BMI, fat mass, low-density lipoprotein (LDL) cholesterol, and inflammatory markers 6 and tumor necrosis factor alpha (TNF-α) and increased HDL cholesterol and IL-10], potentially beneficial for cancer prevention and immune function [62].

The observed upregulation of autophagy genes in conjunction with metabolic and inflammatory improvements suggests that RIF might contribute to a healthier cellular environment less conducive to cancer development. Furthermore, the modulation of inflammatory markers by RIF may favorably impact immune responses, potentially enhancing the body's ability to combat cancerous cells. Although this study focused on overweight/obese individuals and did not directly assess cancer prevention or immune cell function, the findings suggest that RIF's influence on autophagy and metabolic health warrants further investigation in the context of cancer and immune system modulation. Future studies directly exploring RIF's impact on cancer cell growth and immune cell activity are necessary to elucidate these potential benefits fully.

In conclusion, autophagy and mitophagy play a crucial role in the health benefits of IF. By promoting cellular renewal, improving metabolism, and reducing inflammation, these processes help protect against age-related diseases and promote overall health and well-being. Incorporating IF into the lifestyle can help harness the power of autophagy and mitophagy to optimize health and longevity.

11.6   Fasting and Microbiota

The human gut harbors a diverse ecosystem of microbes crucial for health, with Firmicutes and Bacteroidetes dominating its composition. Dietary patterns profoundly affect this microbiota, and IF has gained attention as a promising approach. Unlike CR, IF focuses on timing rather than just reducing calories. Research indicates that IF can enhance microbial diversity, increase beneficial metabolites like short-chain fatty acids (SCFAs), and improve metabolic health markers such as obesity and insulin sensitivity. It also influences circadian CLOCK genes, impacting the body's internal rhythm [63].

The human body harbors a vast array of microbiota, with the largest concentration residing in the intestines, forming what is called the gut microbiota. This microbial community comprises bacteria, fungi, and viruses. In the realm of bacterial phyla detected in the intestinal microbiota, Firmicutes [gram-positive] [64] and Bacteroidetes [gram-negative] make up 90% of the gut microbiota community [65]. These organisms are crucial for breaking down cellulose and providing raw materials for producing glucose and fats within the cells lining the intestine. Butyrate, propionate, and acetate are examples of SCFAs that are synthesized through the fermentation of food fibers and play a substantial role in liver function through diverse mechanisms. Additionally, the gut microbiota aids in fermenting amino acids, modifying bile acids, synthesizing vitamins, and regulating both the movement and immune functions of the gastrointestinal tract [66].

Dietary restrictions have the potential to cause alterations in the variety and makeup of the gut microbiota, as well as metabolic changes. Fasting or reducing calorie intake can modify nutritional availability and energy sources, which may impact the gut ecology, leading to changes in the growth of specific microbial groups and influencing the process of generating SCFAs. One element influencing the gut microbiota is diet [67]. IF has been shown to cause notable alterations in the microbiota of the gut, boost the synthesis of SCFAs, decrease lipopolysaccharide levels in the blood, and reduce the risk of obesity and metabolic diseases [49].

In a colitis-induced mouse model, two intermittent IF programs, one short-term and the other long-term, resulted in distinct alterations in the composition of the gut microbiota. *Ruminiclostridium* decreased by short-term IF, while *Muribaculum*, *Bacteroides*, and *Akkermansia* increased. Conversely, long-term IF reduced *Akkermansia* but increased *Lactobacillus*. IF, over the long run, was linked to a reduction in colitis severity, potentially mediated through the action of SCFAs. Additionally, the bile acids and inosine from *Akkermansia* probably enhance the anti-colitis properties of IF [68].

Su et al. investigated the impact of a 30-day Ramadan fast on the microbiota in the gut of young and middle-aged people in a cohort study. Fasting resulted in notable alterations in the gut microbiota, with increased diversity observed among the younger cohort. This increase was connected to higher levels of the *Lachnospiraceae* and *Ruminococcaceae* families, which are known for their production of butyrate and their positive influence on blood glucose levels, body weight, and fat mass. Conversely, the *Prevotellaceae* family became less abundant. But following the fasting phase, the composition of the microbiome restored to baseline levels [69].

Ozkul et al. examined how nine volunteers' microbiota changed over Ramadan IF (RIF). Following fasting, they discovered that microbial richness rose, along with higher concentrations of microorganisms that make SCFAs, including *Roseburia*, *Faecalibacterium prausnitzii*, *Akkermansia*, and *Eubacterium*. However, *Butyricicoccus pullicaecorum*, a significant butyrate producer, was notably affected. Although the Firmicutes/Bacteroidetes ratio remained high, there was an increase in Bacteroidetes abundance compared to the baseline. These findings are consistent with another study conducted by the same researchers during Ramadan-based fasting, which similarly found elevated levels of the *Bacteroides fragilis* group and *Akkermansia muciniphila* [49].

Obese mice subjected to a 12-week time-restricted feeding (TRF) program exhibited alterations in their gut microbiota, including heightened levels of *Lactobacillus* and *Verrucomicrobiaceae*, such as *Akkermansia muciniphila*, alongside reduced lipid absorption. These changes were linked to the inhibition of the PI3K/AKT signaling pathway [55]. Favorable results are associated with increased *Lactobacillus* abundance through several pathways, including bile salt hydrolase activity and lactate production [70].

Time-restricted feeding (TRF) has been shown by Zeb et al. to improve metabolic regulation and increase circadian CLOCK gene activity [71]. According to their research, TRF significantly raised the BMAL1 and CLOCK genes' mRNA levels in comparison to groups that did not have TRF. All individuals in the early time-restricted feeding (eTRF) group exhibited higher MESOR values that is, mean expression levels over the circadian cycle for BMAL1, Per2, and SIRT1 mRNA compared to control groups'. The activation of SIRT1 influences the circadian rhythm, with elevated mRNA levels observed both before and after fasting, as well as in non-TRF groups. The eTRF group demonstrated an increased amplitude in SIRT1 mRNA expression for all subjects. Moreover, SIRT1 expression, which has a strong positive connection with the CLOCK gene, was correlated with the relative abundance of *Prevotella*, *Prevotellaceae*, and *Bacteroidia* [71].

Previous studies suggest that changes in gut bacteria may contribute to the benefits of time-restricted feeding [TRF]. Short-chain fatty acids (SCFAs) initiate feelings of fullness by stimulating gut surface proteins, such as G-protein-coupled receptors GRP41 and GRP43. When GRP41 is activated, enteroendocrine cells create more peptide YY, a type of hormone that lowers the body's absorption of energy from food and affects how well the body uses glucose. By stimulating enteroendocrine cells and encouraging the manufacture of hormones like GLP1, peptide YY, and cholecystokinin, SCFAs and neurotransmitters like gamma-aminobutyric acid (GABA) and serotonin [5-HT] generated during food digestion by gut flora affect eating behavior [72]. In db/db mice, IF was shown to raise 5-HT levels and reduce anxiety in another investigation [40].

Food-allergic mice's intestinal microbiota was affected by IF. *Alistipes* and *Rikenella* were shown to be more abundant in 24/24IF mice, whereas *Odoribacter* was more abundant in 16/8 IF animals. These bacteria are resilient to bile and are typically found in the ileocecal region. *Rikenella* mostly produces propionic acid and succinic acid, whereas *Alistipes* primarily generates indole, succinic acid, acetic acid, and propionic acid. Deficiency in *Rikenella* has been associated with premature aging. *Odoribacter* increases SCFAs and exhibits protective effects against colitis and colon cancer. It promotes the production of T helper 17 (Th17) cells and possess anti-inflammatory properties by increasing IL-10 production [73].

The intricate relationship between IF, gut microbiota, and metabolic health unfolds a promising frontier in the quest for improved well-being. IF emerges as a potent modulator of gut microbial composition, driving shifts toward a profile associated with enhanced metabolic resilience. Through mechanisms such as increased production of short-chain fatty acids, modulation of circadian CLOCK gene activity, and promotion of anti-inflammatory responses, IF orchestrates a symphony of physiological changes conducive to metabolic optimization [74]. As evidenced across diverse studies, IF induces alterations in gut microbiota composition, fostering the proliferation of beneficial taxa while suppressing detrimental ones [75].

This microbial remodeling, coupled with metabolic adaptations, holds the key to mitigating conditions ranging from obesity and metabolic disorders to food allergies and inflammatory bowel diseases. The bidirectional interaction between IF and gut microbiota underscores the pivotal role of dietary interventions in shaping host–microbiome symbiosis, thereby opening avenues for novel therapeutic strategies. Harnessing the potential of IF-driven microbiota modulation may pave the way toward personalized approaches for optimizing metabolic health and combating a spectrum of chronic diseases [76].

In conclusion, the convergence of IF, gut microbiota, and metabolic health heralds a transformative paradigm in preventive and therapeutic medicine, offering hope for a healthier future through the power of dietary modulation.

11.7 Fasting Speeds Up the Healing Process and Delays Aging

Cellular repair is a crucial aspect of maintaining optimal health and functioning of the body. Our cells are constantly exposed to various stressors and damage from factors such as toxins, pollutants, and even normal metabolic processes. Over time, this damage can accumulate and lead to cellular dysfunction, which, in turn, can contribute to the development of various chronic diseases and conditions [37]. During the fasting period, the body undergoes a series of metabolic changes in cellular repair mechanisms. One of the keyways in which IF enhances cellular repair is through a process called autophagy. As mentioned in the previous section, autophagy is a cellular process in which damaged or dysfunctional components within the cell are broken down and recycled to generate new building blocks for cellular repair and maintenance. Fasting has been shown to upregulate autophagy, leading to improved cellular function and increased longevity [61].

The benefit of fasting for the body is enormous because it stimulates all the body's cells to recycle damaged, defective, and old proteins and utilize them to restore, repair, and even completely renew themselves. On the one hand, the cells get rid of the biological waste accumulated throughout the year; they benefit from rejuvenating the entire body. Although the process of renewing cells in the body takes place daily, it is sometimes slowed down or disrupted due to the poor diet that some people follow.

Moreover, IF has been found to increase the production of ketone bodies, which are molecules produced by the liver during periods of fasting or low carbohydrate intake. Ketones have been shown to have numerous health benefits, including reducing inflammation, improving cognitive function, and promoting cellular repair. By increasing ketone production, IF provides an additional mechanism through which cellular repair can be enhanced. Furthermore, IF has been shown to reduce oxidative stress, which is a major contributor to cellular damage and dysfunction. By lowering these harmful processes, fasting creates a more favorable environment for cellular repair to take place [77].

Triggering of the endogenous growth hormone, also known as somatotropin, plays a crucial role in growth, metabolism, and overall health [78], which helps preserve muscle mass, promote fat loss, and increase energy levels. Growth hormones also help regulate insulin levels, improve immune function, and repair damaged tissues. Interestingly, fasting for just 24 hours has been found in a recent study to increase growth hormone levels by up to 2000% [79]. This spike in growth hormones helps promote fat burning, muscle growth, and overall health. Another study found that IF can increase growth hormone levels by up to 300%, improving metabolism, reducing inflammation, and improving cognitive function [48].

Continuous cleaning of cells using fasting leads to enhanced cell renewal and prolongs life expectancy, thus delaying aging in those who regularly fast. As the body's need for protein decreases to one-fifth during fasting, this gives a degree of rest to the cells and enhances the renewal process of the body's cells safely and correctly by strengthening the endogenous level of the growth hormone, which is an antiaging hormone [80]. The better antioxidant function of endogenously produced enzymes reduces the level of oxidative damage and improves the lifespan of flies and rodents. Therefore, IF increases an organism's health span by improving energy metabolism and mitochondrial function in various organisms [25].

Previous studies have indicated that the most reliable way to extend the lifespan of mammals is through undernutrition without malnutrition. In line with this notion, some studies have shown that fasting in animals can double their life expectancy. For instance, a study conducted on earthworms found that their lifespan was extended due to fasting. The experiment was conducted in 1930 AD by isolating a single worm and raising it in repeated cycles of fasting and feeding. The isolated worm outgrew its relatives by 19 generations while maintaining the physiological parameters of a young age. The worm was able to survive on its tissue for months. Nutrition scientists said that extending the lifespan of these worms is equivalent to keeping a man alive for 600–700 years [81].

11.8   IF and Innate Immunity

The immune system's defense can be categorized into two categories: immune responses that are innate as well as adaptive and are specifically designed to safeguard the body from disease-causing microorganisms. The innate immune system serves as the initial barrier against infections and can mount a rapid reaction without any delay. The innate immune reaction appears predominantly nonspecific. The type of adaptive immunity is much more targeted and protects against pathogens for a long time. Studies have indicated that fasting has multiple effects on the immune system. By altering leukocyte expression patterns, brief periods of intense fasting might strengthen the immune response, especially the innate immune response.

Effects of IF on Neutrophils Since neutrophils, macrophages/monocytes, and lymphocytes make up the majority of the CD45$^+$ population, earlier research has determined the molecular markers unique to each cell lineage. A substantial increase in Differentially Expressed Genes/ Differentially Expressed Proteins (DEGs/DEPs) linked to neutrophil degranulation was found in the leukocyte-mediated immunity-derived enrichment [82]. Neutrophils play a key part in the removal of pathogens by phagocytosis, degranulation, and the release of neutrophil extracellular traps. However, by interacting with other immune cells like lymphocytes or antigen-presenting cells, neutrophils can potentially affect the immune response [83]. Significantly, IF was found to induce higher enrichment in neutrophil degranulation, as seen by both transcriptomic and proteomic profiling, indicating that neutrophils had been activated during an extended period of fasting. Pro-platelet basic protein was not significantly upregulated and was involved in neutrophil degranulation. On the other hand, phagocytosis and neutrophil extracellular traps did not exhibit any discernible alterations [82].

Effects of IF on Dendritic Cells (DCs) The digestive system is the primary organ that is directly impacted by fasting. However, little is known about how fasting affects the immune system in the stomach. Dendritic cells (DCs) gather antigens in the intestines, go to secondary lymphoid organs, and trigger the immune system. In a recent study, the effects of fasting for brief periods on the changes in the intestinal DCs and their influence on the protective immunity against *Listeria monocytogenes* (LM) were evaluated in mice [84]. The number of CD103$^+$CD11b$^-$ DCs was higher in the small intestine lamina propria (SILP) and mesenteric lymph nodes (MLNs) of the mice on fasting.

Further, the proliferation and migration of SILP CD103$^+$CD11b$^-$ DCs were also observed, which correlated with elevated levels of GM-CSF and C-C chemokine receptor type 7 compared to freely fed mice. Within 24 hours of the LM infection, the mice on short-term fasting showed increased survival after LM infection compared with freely fed mice. As stated in this study, LM infection raised the high TGF-β2 and Aldh1a2 expression levels that LM produced in CD103⁺CD11b⁻ DCs, which, in turn, raised the quantity and activity of Foxp3⁺ regulatory T cells. Following a short fast, the DCs became CD103⁻ rather than CD103⁺, which caused a rise in IFN-producing cells and produced an environment that was biased toward Th1 [84]. Hence, the majority of intestinal DCs shift from tolerogenic to Th1 immunogenic, which has an impact on protection against LM infection when short-term fasting occurs.

Effects of IF on Natural Killer [NK] Cells The initial defense mechanism of the immune system, known as natural killer (NK) cells, can attack neoplastic cells, altered cells, and invasive pathogenic microorganisms without the need for priming to exert their effector function [85]. In clinical practice, acute fasting is often shown to increase NK cells' cytolytic action against malignant cells. The molecular mechanisms by which fasting in mice enhances the function of NK cells were studied by Dang VT et al., reported that [86]. After a three-day fast, the total number of liver-resident NK cells in a unit weight of liver tissue from C57BL/6 J mice remained unchanged. In fasting animals, however, a significant increase in the proportions of CD69⁺ and tumor necrosis factor–related apoptosis-inducing ligand (TRAIL) + was observed in NK cells. This study also showed that adoptively transferring TRAIL− NK cells into Rag-2−/− γ chain−/− mice increased their ability to transform into TRAIL+ NK cells in fasting animals. In response to a 3-day fast, liver NK cells also demonstrated strong TRAIL-mediated anticancer activity.

NK cells in starved mice also showed an increased expression of heat shock protein 70 (HSP70) protein in their liver tissues, as determined by western blotting. The administration of 50 mg/mL recombinant heat shock protein 70 to liver lymphocytes resulted in the overexpression of CD69 and TRAIL in the liver natural killer cells. Furthermore, downregulating TRAIL expression was a result of HSP70 neutralization, which was achieved by intraperitoneally injecting mice with an anti-heat shock protein 70 monoclonal antibody before they fasted. According to this study, heat shock protein 70 overexpression during acute fasting increased TRAIL-mediated liver natural killer cell activity against cancerous cells [86, 87].

Effects of IF on Macrophages Given the pivotal role macrophages play in several diseases, their response to energy limitation might influence the outcome of the disease. However, the various metabolic profiles and roles of macrophages can result in variations in how energy restriction affects macrophages in multiple tissues and disease conditions. Previous studies have demonstrated that fasting for a night or on alternate days in obese rodents can trigger adipocyte lipolysis. This can lead to the synthesis of prostaglandin E2 (PGE2) and cyclooxygenase 2 (COX-2), which can cause mice to infiltrate their subcutaneous adipose tissue through adipose tissue macrophage (ATM) [88].

Previous studies have also revealed that a one-day fast followed by two days of eating could reduce ATM's inflammatory response in mice. Adipose thermogenesis plays a major role in improving metabolic homeostasis against diet-induced obesity and metabolic dysfunction, and fasting-induced adipose-VEGF is a key factor in the anti-inflammatory activation of ATM. White adipose tissue (WAT) macrophage anti-inflammatory activity was elevated in mice that were fed a high-fat diet (HFD) after they fasted for 36 hours [28]. Furthermore, age-related infiltration of pro-inflammatory ATM in the aorta and mesentery lymph nodes can be reduced in aged mice by 25–40% CR [89]. In addition, short-term fasting in mice and healthy humans may suppress the generation of CCL2, which would reduce the number of inflammatory macrophages in the peripheral tissues and circulation [90].

Effect of IF on T Cells Lymphocytes are the cells that make adaptive immune responses possible. There are two types of lymphocytes: B lymphocytes and T lymphocytes. The B cells make humoral immune responses happen, and T lymphocytes make cell-mediated immune responses happen. T lymphocytes, also known as T cells, originate inside the bone marrow (BM) and then undergo maturation within the thymus. These types of cells are divided into two primary groups, CD8 $^+$ and CD4 $^+$ cells, depending on their ability to carry out certain activities and their ability to recognize distinct types of major histocompatibility complex (MHC) molecules [91].

CD4 T cells are essential for adaptive immunological responses. Five helper CD4 T cells (Th) lymphocyte subsets, including Th1, Th2, Th17, Treg (T regulatory), and follicular helper T cells (Tfh), have been reported. Cells of Th1 type are identified via activation of the protein transcription factor T-bet and the expression of interferon-gamma (IFN-γ). They have a role in the immunological responses of type 1 pathogens that are intracellular, like virus types and the species of *Mycobacteria*. Cells with Th2 function, on the other hand, are characterized by the expression of the IL-4, IL-5, and IL-13 cytokines, as well as the transcription protein activator GATA is DNA sequence. They are involved in the immunological responses of Th2 against helminths and other larger extracellular pathogens [92]. Th17 cells express the IL-17/IL-22 cytokines plus the RORγt transcription factor, and they engage in immunological responses of the third type against extracellular infections, which include both certain fungi and bacteria. Cells that are T follicular helper cells (Tfh) produce IL-2 and express Bcl-6 protein, which helps the B cells make specific types of antibodies. In contrast, Tregs express Foxp3 and serve as a regulator for immune responses, holding immune cell balance and preventing immunopathology, as opposed to effector-functioning Th1/Th2/Th17/Tfh cells [93].

CD8$^+$ T lymphocytes are essential for immunological responses, defending against external threats like infections, viruses, and bacteria, as well as internal dangers like cancer cells. Following antigen stimulation, CD8$^+$ T cells that have not been previously exposed to an antigen undergo a significant spike in numbers, resulting in the development of effector and memory T cells [94]. CD8$^+$ Cytotoxic T Lymphocyte (CTLs), also called CD8$^+$ T lymphocyte cells with effector function, can cause death to target cells by two mechanisms. First, they engage with the Fas/Fas ligand, which leads to target cell death. Second, they release a cytolytic mediator called perforin, which produces pores in the target cells. These pores allow the transport of granule serine proteases and granzymes that trigger apoptosis [95]. To keep lymphocytes activating, multiplying, and differentiating, they need complex and coordinated messages. The body's metabolism affects these messages, which are known to decide what T cells do and how they work. Recent studies also show that the amount and type of nutrients can affect how lymphocytes are made, how long they live, and how well they work. This means that these nutrients can affect many different types of autoimmune disorders [96].

It is not clear how fasting reduces inflammation. However, the process of fasting has been observed to have a significant impact on the body's immune system capabilities for the leukocytes, mainly by controlling the movement they make, along with the distribution among bone marrow and peripheral tissues and circulation. As an example, calorie restriction in animals triggers the migration of T lymphocytes from secondary lymphoid organs to the bone marrow, where they take up long-term residence. In a study by Collins et al., mice subjected to a dietary restriction (DR) regimen receiving 50% fewer calories exhibited this immune shift. After three to four weeks, the DR mice showed reduced numbers of antigen-experienced T lymphocytes, B cells, and natural killer (NK) cells in peripheral tissues, indicating a significant redistribution and potential modulation of immune surveillance. Upon closer inspection, it was found that there was an increase in the population of memory T cells throughout the bone marrow (BM) during DR. In contrast, the number of additional lymphocyte groups stayed the same and failed to grow. Although the DR increased the number of effectors and central memory T cells present in the bone marrow, it did not increase their normal proliferation. In fact, during DR, these cells became less proliferative [46].

Other findings indicate that fasting for 48 hours has a stronger impact on genes that regulate the immune system than fasting for 24 hours. The study used both RNA-seq and flow cytometry to look at human peripheral blood mononuclear cells (PBMC) and then potential pathways in human and mouse $CD4^+$ T cells. The FOXO4-FKBP5 axis was found to be a regulatory pathway that helps $CD4^+$ T cells become less responsive when people are fasting [97]. Another investigation examined the effects of sixteen-hour IF on the advancement of mice's epithelial ovarian cancer (EOC), specifically the impact on immune responses that fight against tumor growth during fasting.

IF consistently reduces tumor-promoting growth factors involved in metabolism as well as pro-inflammatory cytokines, replicating modifications that establish an environment that opposes tumor growth. Immune profile analysis demonstrated that IF significantly alters the immune response to cancer by promoting a rise in cells with $CD4^+$ and $CD8^+$. This is accompanied by improved cytotoxic and antitumor Th1 responses, which are further boosted by improving the metabolic fitness of these cells [98]. Another study recruited 50 healthy volunteers (29 women, and 21 men). IL-6, IL-1β, and TNF-α, as well as immune cell types (lymphocytes and overall leukocyte frequency) in circulation, such as the monocytes and granulocytes, were measured prior to, during, and additionally, one month after Ramadan. The pro-inflammatory mediator serum levels of IL-6, IL-1β, and TNF-α decreased significantly. Throughout the entire month of Ramadan, certain behaviors or interventions were stopped, unlike the periods before or after Ramadan intermittent fasting (RIF). However, immune cell counts decreased dramatically but stayed within typical ranges throughout Ramadan. Time-restricted feeding [TRF], a Ramadan-like fast, was tested on 40 adult and young adult participants. It showed fewer CD56+ and CD15+ NK cells. These findings suggest that TRF can reduce age-related immune senescence abnormalities [99].

According to a recent study, there was a decline in the number of CD3+, CD4-positive T lymphocytes, and CD19+ B lymphocytes throughout the time of fasting. In contrast, the number of T lymphocytes with CD8+ remained unchanged. Conversely, fasting led to an increased frequency of TCRγ/δ+ T cells and monocytes characterized as CD14+ CD11c+ CD19− CD3−. Distinctively activated T cells were also affected by fasting. Fasting resulted in a higher percentage of terminally differentiated effector (Teff) CD8+ T cells, along with an increased proportion of fully mature or activated T cells, whereas memory T cells were unaffected. Refeeding somewhat reversed these alterations. There was no change in the CD161+Vα7.2+CD3+ mucosa-associated atypical cell frequencies after fasting or refeeding. However, mucosa-associated lymphoid tissues (MALTs) that are pro-inflammatory, generating TNFα as well as IFNγ, reduced considerably during fasting and seemed barely changed by the refeeding [100]. The results of recent studies indicate that fasting can decrease the accumulation of certain suppressor cells in the spleen [101]. There is also evidence that short-term fasting lowers immunosuppression and enhances antitumor immunity, making it a potential ally in cancer therapy. Dietary measures, including CR, fasting, and time-restricted feeding, can change how immune cells function. Fasting has also been found to stimulate the various forms of cancer cells to be attacked by immune cells. It can impact the energy metabolism of cancerous cells, prevent the growth of tumor cells, enhance the functionality of immune cells, and stimulate an immunological response to tumors [102].

Engagement in exercise, combined with energy limitation, may lead to a decrease in immunosuppressive cells, an increase in effector cell quantity and function, and a change in the immune response. Dietary restriction can delay or stop the deterioration of T cell immunity and enhance T cell responses. A three-day fast can essentially "reset" the immune system, turning on the production of new and more powerful immune cells. Fasting cycles can promote immune cell invasion and prevent the growth of tumors in both breast cancer and melanoma cells, potentially enhancing the efficacy of immunotherapy [103].

Studies have shown that IF lowers inflammatory markers, and fasting lowers them, as well as IL-2 and IL-6. Furthermore, calorie intake plays a major role in determining whether immune cells adopt a pro-inflammatory or anti-inflammatory polarization. IF has also been shown to ameliorate the clinical progression and pathological characteristics of the experimental autoimmune encephalomyelitis (EAE) model, which is used to study multiple sclerosis (MS), which will be discussed. Fast protocols can enhance well-being, alleviate chronic immunological conditions, and enhance age-related physiological factors in humans as well as animals. IF affects intestinal immunity through new interactions between macrophages and group 3 innate lymphoid cells (ILC3), increasing ILC3 secretion of IL-22 [92].

IF Improves Immune Cell Functions Immune cells are very sensitive to any psychological or nutritional changes since immune cells express on their surfaces certain receptors that bind to neurotransmitters and hormones secreted by the nervous system and the endocrine system, respectively. It has been proven at the level of humans and experimental animals that any psychological disorder, including anxiety, leads to a significant increase in the secretion of these molecules, which, in turn, leads to a negative effect on the functions of immune cells. Because the fasting person is in a state of mental clarity, the levels of these molecules are in the best condition compared to the non-fasting periods. As such, fasting has been considered a psychological treatment for all disorders of the nervous system and endocrine glands [104]. Additionally, immune cells are severely negatively affected by saturated and trans fatty acids, which are stored in many places in the body, the most important of which are the liver, abdomen, stomach, and intestines. Fasting leads to the decomposition of these fats in a process called autolysis as a source of energy [18].

Previous studies have proven a significant increase in the number of functions of phagocytic cells that are known to attack microbes and kill them. This may also explain the reduction in the symptoms of atherosclerosis in fasting people because phagocytic cells have an unusual ability to swallow fats deposited in the blood vessels that cause atherosclerosis. What is very interesting is that fasting significantly increases the numbers and functions of immune T cells, which play a major role in improving the specialized functions of the immune system against tumors and various microbes [105].

Some studies were conducted on fasting during the month of Ramadan on healthy and sick adults, the most important of which was the study that we conducted in the year 2009 and which was published in the *Journal of Nutrition Research* in the year 2012, where the effect of IF during the month of Ramadan was tested on 50 males and females healthy adults. The results of the study showed the absence of any negative change due to fasting during the month of Ramadan in any of the immune variables among the investigated subjects [106]. The results of this study were reinforced by another study on 120 healthy volunteers using several functional indicators of the immune system. This study concluded that fasting during the month of Ramadan has no harmful effect on the efficiency and functions of the immune system in healthy adults. In a third, similar study on 21 healthy people, the results showed the absence of any negative effect of fasting during the month of Ramadan on white blood cells and neutrophils, which are responsible for protecting the body from infections, especially bacterial ones [107].

In a recent review article, 45 peer-reviewed scientific studies on the effect of fasting during the month of Ramadan on the body's immunity were reviewed. This review concluded that fasting has no negative impact on immune indicators in healthy individuals and that it is not associated with an increased risk of infection or immune disorders. The study also showed that the immune changes that accompany fasting during the month of Ramadan are minor and temporary. This review also reported the absence of any negative effect of fasting during the month of Ramadan on immune indicators in patients with respiratory bronchitis [108].

One of the most important studies related to fasting and immunity is one that was conducted on the effect of fasting during the month of Ramadan on the mechanisms of preventing oxidation and resisting inflammation. It is scientifically proven that increases in these factors weaken immunity and increase the risk of bacterial infection. Our research team collected and analyzed data from 12 scientific studies (including 311 fasting adults) that addressed the effect of Ramadan fasting on oxidative factors and inflammation. The results of the analysis showed a significant decrease in several oxidation and inflammation indicators at the end of the month of Ramadan, which enhances the role of fasting in activating immunity and increasing its efficiency in resisting infection and refutes the claim that fasting may increase the chances of infection [109].

In our recent research on the effect of fasting during the month of Ramadan on the expression of several genes regulating the processes of preventing oxidation and inflammation in approximately 60 healthy adults, the results of the study showed the ability of Ramadan fasting to increase the expression of these genes, namely mitochondrial transcription factor A (TFAM), superoxide dismutase 2 (SOD2), and nuclear factor erythroid 2–related factor 2 (NRF2), at levels as high as 90.5%, 54.1%, and 411.5%, respectively, compared to their levels before Ramadan. These are extremely important results in proving the ability of fasting to prevent the state of oxidative stress and inflammation that is responsible for weakening the immune system and reducing its efficiency in resisting infections [110].

In a preclinical study, IF was also found to increase the efficiency of the immune system in resisting the pathogenic bacteria [*Salmonella typhimurium*], which causes typhoid fever. Fasting was also found to prevent and reduce diseases associated with aging and the state of immune senescence [111]. The results of one study showed that animals were subjected to IF for thirty consecutive days and were injected with toxic inflammatory compounds (lipopolysaccharides (LPS)). The results of the study showed a beneficial effect on animals subjected to fasting against inflammatory factors stimulated by the toxic substance LPS. It also demonstrated the ability of IF for thirty days to protect brain cells from the damage and memory impairment that this toxic substance can cause [112].

Another animal study showed the ability of IF to suppress negative changes and reduce the rise in inflammatory indicators in an animal model of multiple sclerosis (MS), a type of autoimmune disease in which the immune system attacks the patient's own body. The results also showed the fasting's ability to change the bacterial content of the intestine. Fasting is believed to have a role in causing autoimmune diseases such as the sclerosis above, as it improves the bacterial content of the intestine and reduces inflammatory factors that trigger the disease itself [113]. This indicates a possible positive effect of IF on patients with MS and other autoimmune diseases [113].

The results of another murine study showed that IF has a role in improving the immune response in experimental animals by increasing the secretion of interferon-gamma (IFN-γ), which increases the body's resistance to infections. It protects brain cells in the hippocampus from damage and aging. It represents a protective factor against the risk of neurological spasms, stroke, and neurodegenerative diseases such as Alzheimer's disease, dementia, tremors, and other neuro-aging diseases [114]. In a simulation of fasting during the month of Ramadan, animals were injected with the toxic substance carbon tetrachloride (CCl4) and subjected to IF for 12 hours a day for 30 days. The results of the study showed the ability of fasting to improve immunity and metabolism and reduce the toxic effects of oxidative stress on animals that were subjected to fasting, as compared to other animals that were not subjected to fasting [115]. In the same model that simulates Ramadan fasting in experimental animals, IF for 12 hours a day over 30 days showed the ability of fasting to improve immune indicators and enhance the flow of neurotransmitters in animals that were subjected to IF [116].

Clinical studies confirmed the abovementioned preclinical observations. In one study, blood samples of 30 fasting volunteers were used to test the effect of fasting during the month of Ramadan on the body's ability to resist pathogenic bacterial infection that causes pulmonary tuberculosis, which is caused by *Mycobacterium tuberculosis bacteria*. The study showed the ability of fasting to reduce the chances of infection with this pathogenic bacterium and increase the body's resistance to it by increasing the number of macrophages. The study also demonstrated the ability of fasting to increase the secretion of IFN-γ, which can stimulate immune mechanisms resistant to bacterial and viral infections. Studies of fasting and immunity were not limited to healthy people but rather extended to studying the effect of fasting during the month of Ramadan on Muslim patients suffering from acquired immunodeficiency syndrome (AIDS), who are infected with the human immunodeficiency virus (HIV). The results of the study on these Muslim patients showed the absence of any negative effect on their immunity [117]. The effect of time-restricted feeding (TRF), which is a pattern like Ramadan fasting, was investigated on 40 volunteers, both old and young. The results of the study showed the ability of this pattern of fasting to reduce the state of inflammation by reducing the number of inflammatory cells, including NK (NKCD16$^+$ and KCD56$^+$) cells, whose temporary decrease in the body is linked to a reduction in the severity of inflammation. Recently, we have reviewed these preclinical and clinical studies [109].

Fasting and Reduction of Inflammation IF can significantly affect the regulation of inflammation and modulation of immune cell differentiation. Various fasting regimes have been shown to enhance health, alleviate chronic immunological problems, and enhance age-related factors. Inflammation is the immune system's natural response to defending the body from dangerous stimuli such as viruses, injuries, and toxins. However, persistent inflammation has been related to several health issues, including heart disease, diabetes, and cancer. Incorporating IF into your lifestyle can help repair and renew cells, reduce inflammation, improve general health, and potentially lengthen your life. IF has been shown to have anti-inflammatory effects on the body. Some studies have suggested that IF may help protect against age-related diseases like Alzheimer's disease and Parkinson's disease, although more research is needed to understand these effects fully [37].

IL-6 is a pro-inflammatory cytokine released by connective tissues and inflammatory cells that eventually enter the bloodstream and liver. Several studies have indicated that abdominal or visceral adipose tissue produces approximately 30% of IL-6, particularly from macrophages and other innate immune cells that assault these fat cells. High amounts of IL-6 protein are produced during inflammation and are therefore utilized as a marker of inflammation, such as hepatitis. There is currently a considerable body of evidence suggesting that high levels of this protein are a strong risk factor for cardiovascular disease. One of the ways IF reduces inflammation is by lowering the levels of pro-inflammatory markers in the blood [118].

Fasting has been found to result in significant reductions in the level of IL-6 and TNF-α that persist for at least 20 days beyond the fasting period, leading to a considerable reduction in inflammation. The decrease in the secretion of IL-6 by IF has also been found to be associated with a decrease in C- reactive protein (CRP) and homocysteine. These substances play a major role in driving inflammation by interacting with various body proteins, especially in the context of fat accumulation. This interaction leads to protein degradation and causes damage to multiple organs, including inflammation of blood vessels. Because these substances play a major role in increasing inflammation, the effect of fasting on these substances explains the reduction in inflammation, especially in vascular and heart diseases [118].

IF also stimulates the creation of anti-inflammatory chemicals, including adiponectin, a hormone that regulates glucose levels and fatty acid breakdown in the body. Low adiponectin levels have been linked to insulin resistance and inflammation. Increasing adiponectin levels by IF reduces inflammation and improves insulin sensitivity [119]. In addition to its direct effects on inflammation, IF can also help improve gut health, which plays a key role in regulating inflammation in the body. Fasting has been shown to promote the growth of beneficial gut bacteria while reducing the growth of harmful bacteria. A healthy gut microbiome is essential for reducing inflammation and maintaining overall health [100].

Homocysteine is an amino acid that is broken down by vitamins B12 and B6 to form other compounds. High homocysteine levels may indicate a vitamin deficit. Without therapy, excessive homocysteine raises the risk of dementia, heart disease, and stroke. Fasting also influences the level of homocysteine. Several studies have shown an increase in folate and B12, which have the opposite effect on inflammation and improve the functions of the immune system. When there are low levels of folate and B12, the amino acid methionine is converted to cysteine after the formation of homocysteine. However, in the presence of high levels of folate/B12, as happens during fasting, the formation of cystine is not accompanied by the formation of homocysteine [120].

IF and Modulation of miRNA

Many studies demonstrate that dietary habits can modulate endogenous microRNA (miRNA) levels and subsequently regulate the expression of their related genes [121]. It is noteworthy that these genes may be oncogenes, tumor suppressor genes, or cancer-related proteins. Further, many studies reveal the pivotal role of miRNAs in carcinogenesis or cancer proliferation. Yet the interplay between IF, as a method of diet restriction; miRNAs; and their health implications during cancer is still unclear. Hence, IF, as a part of healthy dietary habits, may potentially influence cancer regulation through miRNA implication.

Typically, miRNAs are considered small noncoding molecules that play a significant role in posttranscriptional gene expression [122]. The endogenous miRNA sequences are approximately 22 nucleotides in length. The biogenesis events of miRNA start with RNA polymerase II (Pol II) transcription of the miRNA gene into a large pri-miRNA in the nucleus, which is cleaved into a hairpin structure called pre-miRNA70 nucleotides by a complex composed of the RNase III enzyme

DROSHA and the DiGeorge syndrome critical region gene 8 (DGCR8) protein, which binds to double-stranded RNA [123]. After that, the pre-miRNAs are carried outside the nucleus to the cytoplasm by Exportin 5 and cleaved into small double-stranded miRNAs, 18–24 nucleotides in length, by the RNase III enzyme Dicer, which is associated with TAR RNA–binding protein (TRBP). On the other hand, Dicer also initiates the formation of the RNA-induced silencing complex (RISC). The duplex is then unwound by helicase to generate mature miRNA that is finally incorporated into RISC and guided to target-specific mRNA. The Argonaut (Ago) family of proteins is a major component and protector of RISC to prevent degradation. Finally, this mature version of miRNA is directed to the 3′ UTR of the mRNAs through base pairing, leading to the repression of mRNAs' translation of target genes [124].

Potentially, miRNA–mRNA interactions showed that each mature miRNA can target the expression of multiple mRNAs, and several miRNAs can modulate one mRNA. Since miRNA circulates intracellularly, it is also expressed extracellularly through carriers called exosomes, so it serves as a pivotal communicator in cell-to-cell interactions [125]. miRNA plays many essential biological roles in cell proliferation, differentiation, and apoptosis. Recently, microRNAs have been considered metabolic modulators that conserve metabolic hemostasis. The initial miRNA linked to metabolic control, miR-122, is expressed early in the liver and has been shown to influence lipid metabolism, specifically hepatic cholesterol. It has also been implicated in the maintenance of liver cell differentiation [126].

The main lipid biosynthesis signaling is regulated by endoplasmic reticulum–bound sterol regulatory element–binding proteins (SREBPs). The SREBP family consists of SREBP-1a, SREBP-1c, and SREBP-2 transcription proteins that are encoded by Srebp-1 and Srebp-2 genes. Additionally, SREBP-1c controls the transcription of genes involved in fatty acid metabolism, such as fatty acid synthase (FASN) [127]. Furthermore, SREBP-2 controls the transcription of cholesterol-related genes, such as 3-hydroxy-3-methylglutaryl CoA reductase (HMGCR), which mainly catalyzes cholesterol biosynthesis rates, and the low-density lipoprotein receptor (LDLr), which imports cholesterol from the blood [128]. Any upregulation in SREBP activity leads to the accumulation of cholesterol and fatty acids [129]. In this way, the cross-link between miRNAs and metabolism was examined.

Interestingly, miR-33a, within the intronic sequences of the SREBP genes transcribed by host gene SREBP-2, resulted in increased cellular cholesterol levels by the limitation of cholesterol export through the downregulation of ABC transporters, ABCA1 and ABCG1. On the other hand, miR-33b is regulated by the SREBP1 gene and targets genes involved in fatty acid oxidation and insulin signaling [130]. miR-33a specifically targets genes that regulate β-oxidation of fatty acid and insulin through the inhibition of AMP kinase subunit-α (AMPKα) and insulin receptor substrate 2 (IRS2) genes [131]. miR-33b markedly downregulates the activity of a mitochondrial enzyme CPT1 that mediates the transport of long fatty acids across the membrane by binding them to carnitine, and it is the rate-limiting enzyme that regulates fatty acid oxidation [132].

Obviously, miR-33a and b have a significant role in controlling cholesterol and lipid metabolism by modulating their host genes and the SREBP transcription factors [132]. Moreover, miR-103 and miR-107 are considered key regulators of hepatic lipid homeostasis, such as regulating insulin and glucose homeostasis. Depending on the biology of miRNAs in lipid metabolism and insulin signaling modulation, therapeutic miRNAs have promising frontiers in controlling cardiovascular diseases, atherosclerosis, type 2 diabetes, obesity, and fatty liver conditions [133].

Many clinical trials and studies have emerged to identify the consequences of diet on human miRNAs and their correlation with health conditions. Diet is the main source of energy and nutrients, and it also contains bioactive nutrients that can modulate the biological impact on health status. Diet compounds such as vitamins, polyphenols, and fatty acids, as well as exogenous diet-derived miRNAs, regulate metabolism according to mechanisms involving the modulation of endogenous miRNAs [134]. Exogenous miRNAs present in foods can also be absorbed through the gastrointestinal tract during the digestive process and subsequently integrated with host gene expression [135].

Recent studies showed plant-derived miRNAs in human milk exosomes as ath-miR-166a, pab-miR-951, PTC-miR-472a, and bid-miR-168. Another study confirmed the presence of significant levels of exogenous plant miRNAs, ath-miR-156a, ath-miR-166a, and osa-miR-168a, in human serum [121]. As shown in Fig. 11.1, these studies suggest the potential interplay of diet-derived miRNAs to reach human plasma from the gastrointestinal tract and subsequently regulate the expression of human target genes [136]. Endogenous miRNAs were expressed differentially during a time-restricted regimen. The downregulated miRNA targets suggested an increased expression of transcripts, such as PTEN, TSC1, and ULK1, which are involved in the inhibition of cell growth pathways and activate the pathways of cell survival to promote healthy aging and longevity [137].

Certain miRNAs that are upregulated during fasting, such as miR-146a, exert anti-inflammatory effects by suppressing the production of pro-inflammatory cytokines. Additionally, miR-132 enhances cognitive function and neuroprotection [138]. Another miRNA is miR-124, which promotes neuronal differentiation and function, while miR-126 promotes angiogenesis and vascular health [139]. Furthermore, miR-21 is involved in oxidative stress response, promoting cellular repair, as mentioned previously; miR-34a is a tumor suppressor, which inhibits cancer cell proliferation; and miR-499 enhances cardiac resilience and function (Table 11.1) [140]. Taken together, this upregulation of miRNAs during IF provides many health benefits, such as improved insulin sensitivity by miR-7 upregulation, enhanced stress response, and improved metabolism [141]. On the other hand, the downregulated miRNAs during fasting include miR-122, which reduces lipid synthesis and enhances lipid metabolism [142]. miR-33a/33b, which enhances cholesterol efflux and fatty acid oxidation by downregulating these miRNAs [143].

miR-33a and miR-33b regulate cholesterol efflux and fatty acid oxidation by downregulating key genes involved in these pathways; thus, inhibiting these miRNAs can enhance cholesterol efflux and promote fatty acid oxidation [144]. Furthermore, miR-208 protects against heart disease by modulating the miRNA involved in cardiac hypertrophy, and miR-1 protects against heart disease by modulating this miRNA involved in cardiac fibrosis (Table 11.1) [145]. A previous study

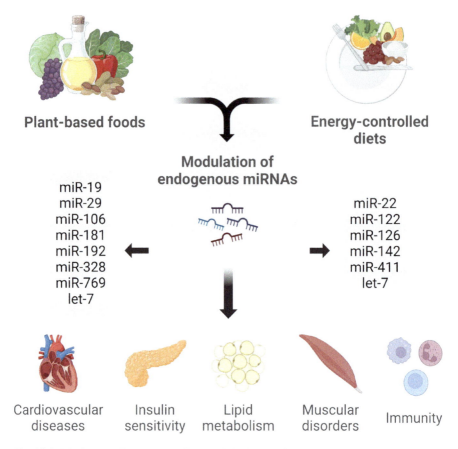

Fig. 11.1 The impact of exogenous miRNAs derived from diet on circulatory endogenous miR-NAs [145]

implicates the influence of a CR diet in the inhibition of a set of 18 circulating miR-NAs that increased in the aging process in the serum of young and old mice. This set of age-modulated miRNAs is predicted to regulate genes involved in metabolic disorders that are directly relevant to the manifestations of aging. There is growing evidence supporting a relationship between these miRNAs and the effects of calorie restriction (CR), which include downregulating apoptosis and promoting neuronal survival, thereby contributing to improved healthspan and resistance to age-related neurodegeneration. A single study confirmed that CR prevented the age-dependent overexpression of miR-181a-1, miR-30e, and miR-34a, along with the reciprocal increase of their target Bcl-2 gene in mouse brain tissues [74, 146]. Another study showed that the expression of serum miR-500-3p and miR-770-3p specifically increased with aging, whereas their levels declined with the CR diet. CR-modulated circulatory miR-500-3p and miR-770-3p could be used as informative aging-related biomarkers, which need more investigation to clarify this data on humans [147].

Table 11.1 Alternative miRNA expression levels during various aspects of IF regarding health benefits

Fasting duration	Upregulated miRNAs	Downregulated miRNAs	Health benefits
Early-fasting [8–16 h]	miR-146a miR-132	miR-122 miR-33a miR-33b	Upregulation outcomes: Anti-inflammatory effects Immune modulation Neuroprotection inhibits brain inflammation Downregulation outcomes: Improvement in liver function Enhancement of lipid metabolism
Mid-fasting [16–24 h]	miR-21 miR-34a miR-499	miR-155 miR-208 miR-1	Upregulation outcomes: Improvement of heart function, anticancer role Regulating cell cycles, apoptosis, and antiaging Regeneration of injured cardiac muscle Inhibition of autoimmune disorders Improvement of cardiac hypertrophy Improvement of muscle regeneration, performance
Extended fasting [24+ hours]	miR-124 miR-126	miR-122 miR-33a	Upregulation outcomes: Inhibition of neurodegenerative diseases, Alzheimer's disease Promotion of vascular health and wound healing Downregulation outcomes: Enhancement of liver antiviral response
Alternate-day fasting and 6-hour eating window	miR-7 miR-221 miR-222	miR-181a miR-181b miR-210	Upregulation outcomes: Metabolic switching from glucose to fat Enhancing cellular stress resistance Improving insulin sensitivity Downregulation outcomes: Improving tissue oxygenation Improving vascular health
5:2-hour IF	–	miR-148a	Downregulation outcomes: Decreasing the lipid metabolism of LDL Enhancing insulin sensitivity Tumor suppression
Short-term calorie restriction [CR] in mice	–	miR-500-3p miR-770-3p	Downregulation outcomes: Control age-related inflammatory diseases Biomarkers for age-related pathophysiological conditions

Interestingly, the levels of seven microRNAs [miR-19b-3p, miR-22-3p, miR-122-5p, miR-126-3p, miR-142-3p, miR-143-3p, and miR-145-5p] were significantly altered following long-term fasting [10-day fasting intervention], which engages homeostatic mechanisms associated with specific microRNAs to improve metabolic signaling regardless of health status. Importantly, the levels of these miRNAs have been previously found to be deregulated and linked to inflammation [148].

Recent studies have highlighted the potential role of miRNA in glucose regulation while fasting in pregnancy. They revealed that specific plasmatic miRNAs measured in the first trimester are robustly associated with fasting glucose levels in the late second trimester of pregnancy. Identified miRNAs during fasting glycemia could contribute to regulating fasting glucose levels. Interestingly, five of the 18 miRNAs associated with fasting glucose were implicated in the extracellular matrix–receptor interaction pathway. More specifically, the targets of these five miRNAs, *COL5A2* [hsa-miR-516b-5p], *LAMB1* [hsa-miR-512-3p], and *COL6A2* [hsa-miR-516a-5p], were *COL1A1* [hsa-miR-518a-5p] as well as *COL1A2* and *FN1* [hsa-miR-145-3p] genes. These data suggested that miRNAs could serve as early biomarkers for predicting gestational diabetes mellitus [GDM] and offer potential targets for early intervention [148].

IF and Cancer

Cancer cells have heightened metabolic demands, requiring ample sources of essential nutrients, such as sugars and amino acids, to support their accelerated expansion and replication. Despite the presence of oxygen and functional mitochondria, cancer cells preferentially utilize anaerobic glycolysis a metabolic strategy widely recognized as the Warburg effect—to produce ATP for energy rather than mitochondrial oxidative phosphorylation. This metabolic preference is a hallmark of cancer cells and supports their aggressive growth and survival [149].

Fasting was found to help prevent tumor incidence by assisting the body in removing damaged and weak cells that do not have nutrients to help them grow and are, therefore, more susceptible to self-decomposition. In this regard, early studies, notably by Moreschi, highlighted the benefits of fasting and calorie restriction on animal tumor development, resulting in significant reductions in both metabolic and endocrine factors implicated in cancer vulnerability, enhancing the resilience of tissues and organs to metabolic stresses, potentially mitigating the development of chronic diseases [150].

During fasting, the body automatically breaks down the fats accumulated in the liver into fatty acids, which are used to create energy for the body by converting them into glucose [5]. This process helps clear toxins and fat-derived waste products from the liver, preventing their accumulation, which otherwise can impair liver function. Continuing this process of emptying the liver and cleaning it regularly [12 hours of washing and 12 hours of rest] leads to a significant improvement in the liver function, which, in turn, leads to improving other body functions, especially the immune system, which can kill microbes and tumors. Of note is that this process of breaking down fats also takes place in tumor cells if they are present in the body. Because tumor cells grow much faster than normal cells, more than ten times, the tumor shrinks during fasting due to the lack of sufficient quantities of nutritional components for it [5].

IF affects tumor cell metabolism, inhibiting growth and improving immune cell function, suggesting its potential in tumor immunotherapy. It may also enhance cancer prevention and treatment by improving the effectiveness and tolerance of anticancer drugs. Additionally, IF can enhance the quality of life for cancer patients through a variety of adaptive biological processes.

Calorie restriction (CR) induces a series of metabolic changes that result in lower blood glucose levels, diminished growth factor signaling, reduced inflammation and angiogenesis, and enhanced protection against oxidative stress [151]. Implementing a CR regimen results in notable reductions in systemic glucose levels and insulin-like growth factors, pivotal for tumor proliferation through the activation of critical pathways such as Ras/MAPK and PI3K/AKT. Furthermore, CR stimulates AMP-activated protein kinase (AMPK) activation, thereby fostering heightened apoptosis. Moreover, fasting has demonstrated the ability to induce an anti-Warburg effect, fostering apoptosis in cancer cells cultured in vitro [152]. The way IF suppresses the growth of tumor cells can be outlined through its molecular mechanism as follows. IF initiates CR, leading to metabolic reprogramming, characterized by a systemic reduction in various nutrient and hormone levels in the bloodstream, primarily glucose, thereby lowering insulin levels in the blood, resulting in decreased expression of IGF-1. Consequently, the decrease in IGF-1 plasma level results in the downregulation of key molecular pathways, particularly those mediated by IGF-1R, AKT, and mTOR [153]. Reduced signaling through the mTOR pathway alerts the cell to limited resources, prompting metabolic adjustments to ensure survival [153]. These adjustments involve decreasing metabolic demands and shifting cell metabolism toward alternative energy sources; for instance, elevated glucagon levels promote the accelerated breakdown of liver glycogen stores into glucose and the hydrolysis of triglycerides into glycerol and free fatty acids. Consequently, over time, fasting elicits advantageous effects on the hepatocytes, fat tissue, the brain, and muscles via a range of biochemical mechanisms [98].

Ketones, which are produced in hepatocytes from fatty acids, glycerol, and protein amino acids, serve as the fuel for gluconeogenesis in the ketogenic condition. This process helps maintain glucose levels at approximately 70 mg/dL, primarily utilized by the brain. Ketone bodies inhibit histone deacetylases, potentially decelerating tumor progression [98]. During IF, fibroblast growth factor 21 (FGF21) is significantly regulated, which is essential in lowering IGF-1 levels because it inhibits hepatic phosphorylated STAT5. Additionally, circulating IGF-1 is bound by elevated amounts of insulin-like growth factor–binding protein 1 (IGFBP1), which prevents IGF-1 from interacting with the proper surface cell receptor. This process diminishes the biological impact of IGF-1 during IF. All these outcomes are recognized to influence cancer development, leading to antitumor effects, reduced production of free radicals, and enhanced bodily resilience to stress [98].

During IF, AMPK becomes active. Nicotinamide adenine dinucleotide (NAD+), a crucial coenzyme, is essential for the function of sirtuins, which include SIRT1

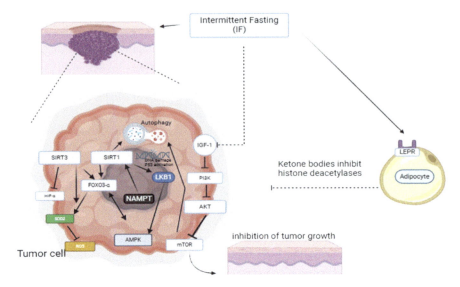

Fig. 11.2 IF inhibits tumor growth by suppressing the IGF-1/AKT and mTOR pathways and activating AMPK, SIRT1, and SIRT3. AMPK and sirtuins enhance each other, boosting FOXO3a and SOD to reduce ROS and regulate HIF-1α. IF also upregulates the leptin receptor [LEPR], further inhibiting tumor growth. De Groot et al. performed a study with 131 patients diagnosed with stage II/III HER2-negative breast cancer, all of whom were receiving neoadjuvant chemotherapy. Participants followed a fasting-mimicking diet [FMD] for three days before and during their chemotherapy sessions. The study observed no significant differences in grade 3 or 4 toxicity between the fasting group and those receiving standard care. However, the FMD group showed a higher prevalence of Miller–Payne 4/5 pathological responses. Additionally, patients who strictly followed the FMD had a higher percentage of Miller–Payne 4/5 scores. This indicates that factors other than change in weight may contribute to the consequences of fasting. These factors may include changes in glucose, insulin, and IGF-1 levels, as evidenced by studies in mice and rats

and SIRT3 (Fig. 11.2). These proteins, part of the NAD + -dependent deacetylase family, play pivotal roles in cellular regulation and stress responses, consequently impeding tumor cell growth. Notably, there is a mutual dependence between AMPK and SIRTs in the metabolic adaptation associated with IF. AMPK can elevate SIRT1 activity through the enzyme nicotinamide phosphoribosyl transferase (NAMPT), and SIRT1 can, in turn, enhance AMPK activity via liver kinase B1 (LKB1). Furthermore, the protein FOXO3a controls the expression of genes related to the replication of cells, growth, and longevity. SIRT1/SIRT3 and AMPK can increase the transcriptional activity of FOXO3a. In addition, SIRT3 reduces the production of hypoxia-inducible factor-1α (HIF-1α), which is frequently involved in tumor growth under low oxygen conditions, and increases the levels of superoxide dismutase 2 [SOD2], an enzyme that neutralizes reactive oxygen species (ROS) [154]. Moreover, the leptin receptor (LEPR) and its subsequent signaling protein, PR/SET domain 1 (PRDM1), are essential for a variety of cellular activities. IF can increase the expression of LEPR and PRDM1, further inhibiting tumor growth [154].

Elevated levels of IGF-1 have been linked to cancers of the colon, prostate, and breast, as they contribute to reduced apoptosis, enhanced cell proliferation, and increased genetic instability. In a study conducted by Bianchi in 2015 involving Balb/c CT26 colon cancer models, mice underwent a 48-hour fasting period followed by treatment with oxaliplatin, a chemotherapy drug. The study found that fasting enhanced the effects of oxaliplatin on the cancer cells. Specifically, fasting led to a decrease in aerobic glycolysis and glutaminolysis while promoting oxidative phosphorylation, a process that generates energy in cells. This shift in cellular metabolism induced by fasting contributed to increased oxygen consumption, which is referred to as the anti-Warburg effect. Overall, fasting appeared to make cancerous cells more sensitive to the effects of oxaliplatin by altering their metabolic processes, potentially enhancing the efficacy of the chemotherapy treatment [155].

Zorn et al. conducted a study involving patients with gynecological cancer at various stages, with 30 individuals undergoing neoadjuvant chemotherapy, consisting of a minimum of four cycles with the same treatment regimen. Participants fasted for 96 hours during half of their chemotherapy cycles, while following a regular diet for the other cycles. The study revealed that fasting was associated with elevated levels of ketone bodies and reduced insulin and IGF-1 levels in the blood. Patients reported decreased incidences of stomatitis, headaches, and weakness, as well as a lower general toxicity index and fewer chemotherapeutic drug delays during fasting periods. However, there were no observed enhancements in patient-reported quality of life, chemotherapy-induced neuropathy, or weariness [156].

In hematologic malignancies, IF was found to slow the progression of acute lymphoblastic leukemia [157]. Mice that underwent fasting had a considerably lower percentage of leukemic green fluorescent protein (GFP)-positive cells in their peripheral blood than control mice seven weeks after transplantation. However, IF did not have a similar effect on the incidence of acute myeloid leukemia in mice models with these tumors. Additionally, alternate day fasting (ADF) for four months significantly reduced lymphoma incidence by 33% in OF1 mice, suggesting that ADF may have potential as a preventive strategy against certain types of cancer. Interestingly, despite the fasting mice consuming almost double the daily amount as control mice on their feast days, no significant distinction in body weight was observed between the fasting group and the control group [157].

In an investigation conducted by Badar et al., 11 patients with non-Hodgkin lymphoma and acute myeloid leukemia received chemotherapy during Ramadan. The study showed that patients undergoing chemotherapy during Ramadan experienced safe and well-tolerated treatment without significant adverse effects. This suggests that fasting did not lead to negative outcomes on the patient's ability to undergo chemotherapy, indicating that it can be practiced without significant concerns regarding its impact on chemotherapy outcomes or patient well-being [98].

The quality of the tumor microenvironment is one of the main driving forces for the good or poor prognosis of tumor. Cold tumors (few immunostimulatory cells with high immunoregulatory cells) indicate poor prognosis, while hot tumors (high number of immunostimulatory cells and fewer regulatory cells) indicate good prognosis [158]. As such, tumor-associated macrophages (TAMs) are one of the most prevalent immune cell types in the tumor microenvironment. TAMs can polarize into M2-like macrophages, which stimulate immunosuppression and the growth of cancer, or M1-like macrophages, which prevent cancer from progressing. Depending on the location and stage of the tumor's growth, the ratio and quantity of these two macrophage subtypes might change [159]. To be more precise, M2-like macrophages prefer to live in hypoxic regions of the tumor, while M1-like macrophages are usually located close to tumor blood arteries, where oxygen levels are greater. As tumors grow and become more hypoxic, there is an increase in the number of M2-like macrophages, which is associated with poor patient prognosis [160].

Compared to conventional M2 macrophages, M2-like tumor-associated macrophages (TAMs) have a different metabolism in the hypoxic tumor microenvironment. Rather than depending on FAO and OXPHOS, M2-like TAM uses glycolysis to produce energy. The transcription factor HIF-1α and the results of the expression of pro-angiogenic and pro-metastatic cytokines mediate this. Thus, inhibiting the ability of TAM to utilize glycolysis may provide a potential antitumor strategy. A recent study showed that the main consumer of glucose in the tumor microenvironment is TAM, not the tumor [161]. Additionally, lactic acid derived from tumor cells might be associated with the promotion of M2 polarization. Preclinical and initial clinical data indicated that fasting or FMD reduces glucose and lactic acid levels [102]. These studies suggest that fasting may significantly affect the polarization of TAM, which contributes to the antitumor effect of fasting [162].

Reduction of total monocytes, M-myeloid-derived suppressor cells (MDSCs), and PMN-MDSCs, including the PMN-MDSC subset expressing LOX1. The boost of classical monocytes expresses HLA-DR (CMo DR+), intermediate monocytes [IMo], dendritic cells, and $CD16^+$ dendritic cells. Reduction of Tregs and $CD8^+$ regulatory T cells. Increase in cytotoxic T lymphocytes, activated $CD8^+$ T cells, NK cells, memory T cells, and NK cell subsets. An increase in the CD8/CD68 and CD8A/CD68 ratios is associated with better prognosis in cancer patients. Enrichment of immune signatures associated with favorable prognosis and better response to therapies in cancer patients. Activation of several antitumor immune programs at the tumor level, including a switch toward a favorable/cytotoxic Th1/M1-like phenotype [163].

Modulation of immune transcriptomic signatures with prognostic/predictive relevance, such as the IFNγ activating signature (IFNG.GS). Upregulation of immune-related genes associated with T cell activation and cytotoxicity, such as CTLA4 and LGALS9. Recruitment of activated and cytotoxic T cells occurs through the CCR5 and CX3CR1 chemokine receptor pathways, facilitating their migration to sites of inflammation or tumor tissues. These changes indicate that the FMD has a significant impact on reshaping the immune system in cancer patients, reducing biomarkers associated with immune suppression, and promoting the infiltration of activated and cytotoxic immune cell populations in tumors [164].

IF selectively inhibited the splenic accumulation of $CD205^+$ G-MDSCs in a murine breast cancer model. IF treatment was comparable to docetaxel in suppressing tumor growth. Fasting decreased the accumulation of $CD205^+$ G-MDSCs in the spleen by inhibiting cell trafficking and inducing apoptosis. The downregulation of CXCR4 correlated with a reduction in $CD205^+$ G-MDSC trafficking from the bone marrow to the spleen under IF treatment. Glucose deficiency and 2-deoxy-D-glucose (2DG) treatment induced massive death of splenic CD205$^+$ G-MDSCs, mimicking the effects of IF in suppressing their accumulation. IF inhibited cell trafficking through the downregulation of CXCR4 and induced apoptosis by altering glucose metabolism, thereby enhancing antitumor immunity [165].

The findings suggest that IF has suppressive effects on a specific subset of MDSCs known as CD205$^+$ G-MDSCs in murine breast cancer models. This suppression is achieved by inhibiting cell trafficking and inducing apoptosis by altering glucose metabolism. The study also showed that IF enhanced antitumor immunity by reducing the accumulation of tumor-induced splenic CD205$^+$ G-MDSCs [101]. These findings have implications for cancer immunotherapy. They suggest that IF could potentially enhance the efficacy of cancer immunotherapy by suppressing the development of MDSCs, thereby improving antitumor immunity.

11.9   Conclusion

Fasting can be beneficial for health by reducing risk factors connected to serious health conditions, including cancer. Although the mechanisms behind these beneficial effects of IF are not clear yet, the mechanisms can include enhancing ketone body production, autophagy, DNA repair, anti-stress abilities, and antioxidant defense. In tumor cells, these events result in the inhibition of the IGF-1/AKT and mTORC1 pathways and increase AMPK, which is dependent on the Sirtuin-1 (SIRT1) and SIRT3 pathways, thus hindering tumor cell growth. Furthermore, in cancer cells, IF alters autophagy, which is a conserved lysosomal degradation pathway for the intracellular recycling of macromolecules and clearance of damaged organelles and misfolded proteins to ensure cellular homeostasis. IF can also increase cancer sensitivity to chemotherapy and radiotherapy and reduce the side effects of traditional anticancer treatments. Furthermore, IF could influence gene expression regulation through miRNA implication. Besides, IF can enhance the quality and quantity of the immune cells by enhancing the functions of NK and dendritic cells, increasing cytokine production, and improving antitumor immune responses. Given these beneficial effects of IF, fasting could be considered as an adjuvant therapy for cancer treatment, including immunotherapy.

Acknowledgments S. Alwasel and W. Al-Dahmash would like to thank the Researchers Supporting Program [RSP-2021/59] at King Saud University, Riyadh, Saudi Arabia, for their support.

References

1. Zouhal H, Bagheri R, Triki R, Saeidi A, Wong A, Hackney AC, et al. Effects of Ramadan intermittent fasting on gut hormones and body composition in males with obesity. Int J Environ Res Public Health. 2020;17(15)

2. Hofer SJ, Carmona-Gutierrez D, Mueller MI, Madeo F. The ups and downs of caloric restriction and fasting: from molecular effects to clinical application. EMBO Mol Med. 2022;14(1):e14418.
3. Elortegui Pascual P, Rolands MR, Eldridge AL, Kassis A, Mainardi F, Le KA, et al. A meta-analysis comparing the effectiveness of alternate day fasting, the 5:2 diet, and time-restricted eating for weight loss. Obesity (Silver Spring). 2023;31(Suppl 1):9–21.
4. Paukkonen I, Torronen EN, Lok J, Schwab U, El-Nezami H. The impact of intermittent fasting on gut microbiota: a systematic review of human studies. Front Nutr. 2024;11:1342787.
5. Anton SD, Lee SA, Donahoo WT, McLaren C, Manini T, Leeuwenburgh C, et al. The effects of time restricted feeding on overweight, older adults: a pilot study. Nutrients. 2019;11(7)
6. Rozanski G, Pheby D, Newton JL, Murovska M, Zalewski P, Slomko J. Effect of different types of intermittent fasting on biochemical and anthropometric parameters among patients with metabolic-associated fatty liver disease (MAFLD)-a systematic review. Nutrients. 2021;14(1)
7. Harvie M, Howell A. Potential benefits and harms of intermittent energy restriction and intermittent fasting amongst obese, overweight and normal weight subjects-a narrative review of human and animal evidence. Behav Sci (Basel). 2017;7(1)
8. Anic K, Schmidt MW, Furtado L, Weidenbach L, Battista MJ, Schmidt M, et al. Intermittent fasting-short- and Long-term quality of life, fatigue, and safety in healthy volunteers: a prospective, clinical trial. Nutrients. 2022;14(19)
9. Nowosad K, Sujka M. Effect of various types of intermittent fasting (IF) on weight loss and improvement of diabetic parameters in human. Curr Nutr Rep. 2021;10(2):146–54.
10. Farhana A, Rehman A. Metabolic Consequences of Weight Reduction. In: StatPearls. Treasure Island (FL) ineligible companies. Disclosure: Anis Rehman declares no relevant financial relationships with ineligible companies; 2025.
11. Furman D, Campisi J, Verdin E, Carrera-Bastos P, Targ S, Franceschi C, et al. Chronic inflammation in the etiology of disease across the life span. Nat Med. 2019;25(12):1822–32.
12. Lange MG, Coffey AA, Coleman PC, Barber TM, Van Rens T, Oyebode O, et al. Metabolic changes with intermittent fasting. J Hum Nutr Diet. 2024;37(1):256–69.
13. Davis AE, Smyers ME, Beltz L, Mehta DM, Britton SL, Koch LG, et al. Differential weight loss with intermittent fasting or daily calorie restriction in low- and high-fitness phenotypes. Exp Physiol. 2021;106(8):1731–42.
14. Richard AJ, White U, Elks CM, Stephens JM. Adipose tissue: physiology to metabolic dysfunction. In: Feingold KR, Anawalt B, Blackman MR, Boyce A, Chrousos G, Corpas E, et al., editors. Endotext. South Dartmouth (MA); 2000.
15. Lessan N, Ali T. Energy metabolism and intermittent fasting: the Ramadan perspective. Nutrients. 2019;11(5)
16. Zhu S, Surampudi P, Rosharavan B, Chondronikola M. Intermittent fasting as a nutrition approach against obesity and metabolic disease. Curr Opin Clin Nutr Metab Care. 2020;23(6):387–94.
17. Zhang Y, Liu L, Hou X, Zhang Z, Zhou X, Gao W. Role of autophagy mediated by AMPK/DDiT4/mTOR Axis in HT22 cells under oxygen and glucose deprivation/Reoxygenation. ACS Omega. 2023;8(10):9221–9.
18. Stockman MC, Thomas D, Burke J, Apovian CM. Intermittent fasting: is the wait worth the weight? Curr Obes Rep. 2018;7(2):172–85.
19. Vasim I, Majeed CN, DeBoer MD. Intermittent fasting and metabolic health. Nutrients. 2022;14:3.
20. Song DK, Kim YW. Beneficial effects of intermittent fasting: a narrative review. J Yeungnam Med Sci. 2023;40(1):4–11.
21. Macedo RCO, Santos HO, Tinsley GM, Reischak-Oliveira A. Low-carbohydrate diets: effects on metabolism and exercise – a comprehensive literature review. Clin Nutr ESPEN. 2020;40:17–26.

22. Santos HO, Lavie CJ. Weight loss and its influence on high-density lipoprotein cholesterol (HDL-C) concentrations: a noble clinical hesitation. Clin Nutr ESPEN. 2021;42:90–2.
23. Stekovic S, Hofer SJ, Tripolt N, Aon MA, Royer P, Pein L, et al. Alternate day fasting improves physiological and molecular markers of aging in healthy, non-obese humans. Cell Metab. 2019;30(3):462–76 e6.
24. Hoddy KK, Marlatt KL, Cetinkaya H, Ravussin E. Intermittent fasting and metabolic health: from religious fast to time-restricted feeding. Obesity (Silver Spring). 2020;28(Suppl 1):S29–37.
25. Park S, Yoo KM, Hyun JS, Kang S. Intermittent fasting reduces body fat but exacerbates hepatic insulin resistance in young rats regardless of high protein and fat diets. J Nutr Biochem. 2017;40:14–22.
26. Begum M, Choubey M, Tirumalasetty MB, Arbee S, Mohib MM, Wahiduzzaman M, et al. Adiponectin: a promising target for the treatment of diabetes and its complications. Life (Basel). 2023;13(11)
27. Yao K, Su H, Cui K, Gao Y, Xu D, Wang Q, et al. Effectiveness of an intermittent fasting diet versus regular diet on fat loss in overweight and obese middle-aged and elderly people without metabolic disease: a systematic review and meta-analysis of randomized controlled trials. J Nutr Health Aging. 2024;28(3):100165.
28. Yao J, Wu D, Qiu Y. Adipose tissue macrophage in obesity-associated metabolic diseases. Front Immunol. 2022;13:977485.
29. Mattson MP, Longo VD, Harvie M. Impact of intermittent fasting on health and disease processes. Ageing Res Rev. 2017;39:46–58.
30. Chijiokwu EA, Nwangwa EK, Oyovwi MO, Naiho AO, Emojevwe V, Ohwin EP, et al. Intermittent fasting and exercise therapy abates STZ-induced diabetotoxicity in rats through modulation of adipocytokines hormone, oxidative glucose metabolic, and glycolytic pathway. Physiol Rep. 2022;10(20):e15279.
31. Elesawy BH, Raafat BM, Muqbali AA, Abbas AM, Sakr HF. The impact of intermittent fasting on brain-derived neurotrophic factor, Neurotrophin 3, and rat behavior in a rat model of type 2 diabetes mellitus. Brain Sci. 2021;11(2)
32. Kant AK, Graubard BI. Association of self-reported sleep duration with eating behaviors of American adults: NHANES 2005-2010. Am J Clin Nutr. 2014;100(3):938–47.
33. Joaquim L, Faria A, Loureiro H, Matafome P. Benefits, mechanisms, and risks of intermittent fasting in metabolic syndrome and type 2 diabetes. J Physiol Biochem. 2022;78(2):295–305.
34. Naous E, Achkar A, Mitri J. Intermittent fasting and its effects on weight, Glycemia, lipids, and blood pressure: a narrative review. Nutrients. 2023;15(16)
35. Ensminger DC, Salvador-Pascual A, Arango BG, Allen KN, Vazquez-Medina JP. Fasting ameliorates oxidative stress: a review of physiological strategies across life history events in wild vertebrates. Comp Biochem Physiol A Mol Integr Physiol. 2021;256:110929.
36. Amorim JA, Coppotelli G, Rolo AP, Palmeira CM, Ross JM, Sinclair DA. Mitochondrial and metabolic dysfunction in aging and age-related diseases. Nat Rev Endocrinol. 2022;18(4):243–58.
37. Longo VD, Di Tano M, Mattson MP, Guidi N. Intermittent and periodic fasting, longevity and disease. Nat Aging. 2021;1(1):47–59.
38. Savencu CE, Linta A, Farcas G, Bina AM, Cretu OM, Malita DC, et al. Impact of dietary restriction regimens on mitochondria, heart, and endothelial function: a brief overview. Front Physiol. 2021;12:768383.
39. Kazmirczak F, Hartweck LM, Vogel NT, Mendelson JB, Park AK, Raveendran RM, et al. Intermittent fasting activates AMP-kinase to restructure right ventricular lipid metabolism and microtubules. JACC Basic Transl Sci. 2023;8(3):239–54.
40. Liu Z, Dai X, Zhang H, Shi R, Hui Y, Jin X, et al. Gut microbiota mediates intermittent-fasting alleviation of diabetes-induced cognitive impairment. Nat Commun. 2020;11(1):855.

41. Kyriazis ID, Vassi E, Alvanou M, Angelakis C, Skaperda Z, Tekos F, et al. The impact of diet upon mitochondrial physiology (review). Int J Mol Med. 2022;50(5)
42. Mani K, Javaheri A, Diwan A. Lysosomes mediate benefits of intermittent fasting in Cardiometabolic disease: the janitor is the undercover boss. Compr Physiol. 2018;8(4):1639–67.
43. Minchew CL, Didenko VV. Dual detection of Nucleolytic and proteolytic markers of lysosomal cell death: DNase II-type breaks and Cathepsin D. Methods Mol Biol. 2017;1554:229–36.
44. Trivedi PC, Bartlett JJ, Pulinilkunnil T. Lysosomal biology and function: modern view of cellular debris bin. Cells. 2020;9(5)
45. Settembre C, Fraldi A, Medina DL, Ballabio A. Signals from the lysosome: a control center for cellular clearance and energy metabolism. Nat Rev Mol Cell Biol. 2013;14(5):283–96.
46. Fang Y, Qian J, Xu L, Wei W, Bu W, Zhang S, et al. Short-term intensive fasting enhances the immune function of red blood cells in humans. Immun Ageing. 2023;20(1):44.
47. Finkbeiner S. The autophagy lysosomal pathway and neurodegeneration. Cold Spring Harb Perspect Biol. 2020;12(3).
48. Kim BH, Joo Y, Kim MS, Choe HK, Tong Q, Kwon O. Effects of intermittent fasting on the circulating levels and circadian rhythms of hormones. Endocrinol Metab (Seoul). 2021;36(4):745–56.
49. Ozkul C, Yalinay M, Karakan T. Structural changes in gut microbiome after Ramadan fasting: a pilot study. Benef Microbes. 2020;11(3):227–33.
50. van den Burg EL, van Peet PG, Schoonakker MP, van de Haar DE, Numans ME, Pijl H. Metabolic impact of intermittent energy restriction and periodic fasting in patients with type 2 diabetes: a systematic review. Nutr Rev. 2023;81(10):1329–50.
51. Martinez-Garza U, Torres-Oteros D, Yarritu-Gallego A, Marrero PF, Haro D, Relat J. Fibroblast growth factor 21 and the adaptive response to nutritional challenges. Int J Mol Sci. 2019;20(19)
52. Chen L, Wang K, Long A, Jia L, Zhang Y, Deng H, et al. Fasting-induced hormonal regulation of lysosomal function. Cell Res. 2017;27(6):748–63.
53. Barbosa MC, Grosso RA, Fader CM. Hallmarks of aging: an Autophagic perspective. Front Endocrinol (Lausanne). 2018;9:790.
54. Ortega MA, Fraile-Martinez O, de Leon-Oliva D, Boaru DL, Lopez-Gonzalez L, Garcia-Montero C, et al. Autophagy in its (proper) context: molecular basis, biological relevance, pharmacological modulation, and lifestyle medicine. Int J Biol Sci. 2024;20(7):2532–54.
55. Yang H, Li C, Che M, Li Y, Feng R, Sun C. Gut microbiota mediates the anti-obesity effect of intermittent fasting by inhibiting intestinal lipid absorption. J Nutr Biochem. 2023;116:109318.
56. Allen EA, Baehrecke EH. Autophagy in animal development. Cell Death Differ. 2020;27(3):903–18.
57. Levine B, Klionsky DJ. Autophagy wins the 2016 Nobel prize in physiology or medicine: breakthroughs in baker's yeast fuel advances in biomedical research. Proc Natl Acad Sci USA. 2017;114(2):201–5.
58. Ichimiya T, Yamakawa T, Hirano T, Yokoyama Y, Hayashi Y, Hirayama D, et al. Autophagy and autophagy-related diseases: a review. Int J Mol Sci. 2020;21(23)
59. Lei Y, Klionsky DJ. The emerging roles of autophagy in human diseases. Biomedicines. 2021;9(11)
60. Mehrabani S, Bagheriya M, Askari G, Read MI, Sahebkar A. The effect of fasting or calorie restriction on mitophagy induction: a literature review. J Cachexia Sarcopenia Muscle. 2020;11(6):1447–58.
61. Shabkhizan R, Haiaty S, Moslehian MS, Bazmani A, Sadeghsoltani F, Saghaei Bagheri H, et al. The beneficial and adverse effects of Autophagic response to caloric restriction and fasting. Adv Nutr. 2023;14(5):1211–25.

62. Bou Malhab LJ, Madkour MI, Abdelrahim DN, Eldohaji L, Saber-Ayad M, Eid N, et al. Dawn-to-dusk intermittent fasting is associated with overexpression of autophagy genes: a prospective study on overweight and obese cohort. Clinical Nutrition ESPEN. 2024.
63. Karl JP, Hatch AM, Arcidiacono SM, Pearce SC, Pantoja-Feliciano IG, Doherty LA, et al. Effects of psychological, environmental, and physical stressors on the gut microbiota. Front Microbiol. 2018;9:2013.
64. Singh S, Sharma P, Sarma DK, Kumawat M, Tiwari R, Verma V, et al. Implication of obesity and gut microbiome Dysbiosis in the etiology of colorectal cancer. Cancers (Basel). 2023;15(6)
65. Milani C, Duranti S, Bottacini F, Casey E, Turroni F, Mahony J, et al. The first microbial colonizers of the human gut: composition, activities, and health implications of the infant gut microbiota. Microbiol Mol Biol Rev. 2017;81(4)
66. Mayer EA, Nance K, Chen S. The gut-brain Axis. Annu Rev Med. 2022;73:439–53.
67. Rinninella E, Tohumcu E, Raoul P, Fiorani M, Cintoni M, Mele MC, et al. The role of diet in shaping human gut microbiota. Best Pract Res Clin Gastroenterol. 2023;62–63:101828.
68. Wu J, Man D, Shi D, Wu W, Wang S, Wang K, et al. Intermittent fasting alleviates risk markers in a murine model of ulcerative colitis by modulating the gut microbiome and metabolome. Nutrients. 2022;14(24)
69. Su J, Wang Y, Zhang X, Ma M, Xie Z, Pan Q, et al. Remodeling of the gut microbiome during Ramadan-associated intermittent fasting. Am J Clin Nutr. 2021;113(5):1332–42.
70. Herz D, Karl S, Weiss J, Zimmermann P, Haupt S, Zimmer RT, et al. Effects of different types of intermittent fasting interventions on metabolic health in healthy individuals (EDIF): a randomised trial with a controlled-run in phase. Nutrients. 2024;16(8)
71. Zeb F, Wu X, Chen L, Fatima S, Haq IU, Chen A, et al. Effect of time-restricted feeding on metabolic risk and circadian rhythm associated with gut microbiome in healthy males. Br J Nutr. 2020;123(11):1216–26.
72. Popa AD, Nita O, Gherasim A, Enache AI, Caba L, Mihalache L, et al. A scoping review of the relationship between intermittent fasting and the human gut microbiota: current knowledge and future directions. Nutrients. 2023;15(9)
73. Ma RX, Hu JQ, Fu W, Zhong J, Cao C, Wang CC, et al. Intermittent fasting protects against food allergy in a murine model via regulating gut microbiota. Front Immunol. 2023;14:1167562.
74. Khan MN, Khan SI, Rana MI, Ayyaz A, Khan MY, Imran M. Intermittent fasting positively modulates human gut microbial diversity and ameliorates blood lipid profile. Front Microbiol. 2022;13:922727.
75. Shi H, Zhang B, Abo-Hamzy T, Nelson JW, Ambati CSR, Petrosino JF, et al. Restructuring the gut microbiota by intermittent fasting lowers blood pressure. Circ Res. 2021;128(9):1240–54.
76. Cadena-Ullauri S, Guevara-Ramirez P, Ruiz-Pozo VA, Tamayo-Trujillo R, Paz-Cruz E, Zambrano-Villacres R, et al. The effect of intermittent fasting on microbiota as a therapeutic approach in obesity. Front Nutr. 2024;11:1393292.
77. Wegman MP, Guo MH, Bennion DM, Shankar MN, Chrzanowski SM, Goldberg LA, et al. Practicality of intermittent fasting in humans and its effect on oxidative stress and genes related to aging and metabolism. Rejuvenation Res. 2015;18(2):162–72.
78. Brocchi A, Rebelos E, Dardano A, Mantuano M, Daniele G. Effects of intermittent fasting on brain metabolism. Nutrients. 2022;14(6)
79. Eroglu MN, Rodriguez-Longobardo C, Ramirez-Adrados A, Colina-Coca C, Burgos-Postigo S, Lopez-Torres O, et al. The effects of 24-h fasting on exercise performance and metabolic parameters in a pilot study of female CrossFit athletes. Nutrients. 2023;15(22)
80. Tang D, Tang Q, Huang W, Zhang Y, Tian Y, Fu X. Fasting: from physiology to pathology. Adv Sci (Weinh). 2023;10(9):e2204487.
81. Hwangbo DS, Lee HY, Abozaid LS, Min KJ. Mechanisms of lifespan regulation by calorie restriction and intermittent fasting in model organisms. Nutrients. 2020;12(4)

82. Qian J, Fang Y, Yuan N, Gao X, Lv Y, Zhao C, et al. Innate immune remodeling by short-term intensive fasting. Aging Cell. 2021;20(11):e13507.
83. Kanashiro A, Hiroki CH, da Fonseca DM, Birbrair A, Ferreira RG, Bassi GS, et al. The role of neutrophils in neuro-immune modulation. Pharmacol Res. 2020;151:104580.
84. Ju YJ, Lee KM, Kim G, Kye YC, Kim HW, Chu H, et al. Change of dendritic cell subsets involved in protection against listeria monocytogenes infection in short-term-fasted mice. Immune Netw. 2022;22(2):e16.
85. Perera Molligoda Arachchige AS. Human NK cells: from development to effector functions. Innate Immun. 2021;27(3):212–29.
86. Dang VT, Tanabe K, Tanaka Y, Tokumoto N, Misumi T, Saeki Y, et al. Fasting enhances TRAIL-mediated liver natural killer cell activity via HSP70 upregulation. PLoS One. 2014;9(10):e110748.
87. Delconte RB, Owyong M, Santosa EK, Srpan K, Sheppard S, McGuire TJ, et al. Fasting reshapes tissue-specific niches to improve NK cell-mediated anti-tumor immunity. Immunity. 2024;57(8):1923–38 e7.
88. Pan Y, Cao S, Tang J, Arroyo JP, Terker AS, Wang Y, et al. Cyclooxygenase-2 in adipose tissue macrophages limits adipose tissue dysfunction in obese mice. J Clin Invest. 2022;132(9)
89. Trott DW, Henson GD, Ho MHT, Allison SA, Lesniewski LA, Donato AJ. Age-related arterial immune cell infiltration in mice is attenuated by caloric restriction or voluntary exercise. Exp Gerontol. 2018;109:99–107.
90. Jordan S, Tung N, Casanova-Acebes M, Chang C, Cantoni C, Zhang D, et al. Dietary intake regulates the circulating inflammatory monocyte Pool. Cell. 2019;178(5):1102–14 e17.
91. DeMaio A, Mehrotra S, Sambamurti K, Husain S. The role of the adaptive immune system and T cell dysfunction in neurodegenerative diseases. J Neuroinflammation. 2022;19(1):251.
92. Chen H, Sun L, Feng L, Han X, Zhang Y, Zhai W, et al. Intermittent fasting promotes type 3 innate lymphoid cells secreting IL-22 contributing to the beigeing of white adipose tissue. elife. 2024;12:12.
93. Zhu X, Zhu J. CD4 T helper cell subsets and related human immunological disorders. Int J Mol Sci. 2020;21(21)
94. Xie Q, Ding J, Chen Y. Role of CD8(+) T lymphocyte cells: interplay with stromal cells in tumor microenvironment. Acta Pharm Sin B. 2021;11(6):1365–78.
95. Sun L, Su Y, Jiao A, Wang X, Zhang B. T cells in health and disease. Signal Transduct Target Ther. 2023;8(1):235.
96. Munteanu C, Schwartz B. The relationship between nutrition and the immune system. Front Nutr. 2022;9:1082500.
97. Bordon Y. Fast tracking immunity. Nat Rev Immunol. 2019;19(10):598.
98. Han K, Singh K, Rodman MJ, Hassanzadeh S, Wu K, Nguyen A, et al. Fasting-induced FOXO4 blunts human CD4(+) T helper cell responsiveness. Nat Metab. 2021;3(3):318–26.
99. Udumula MP, Singh H, Faraz R, Poisson L, Tiwari N, Dimitrova I, et al. Intermittent Fasting induced ketogenesis inhibits mouse epithelial ovarian tumors by promoting anti-tumor T cell response. bioRxiv. 2023.
100. Maifeld A, Bartolomaeus H, Lober U, Avery EG, Steckhan N, Marko L, et al. Fasting alters the gut microbiome, reducing blood pressure and body weight in metabolic syndrome patients. Nat Commun. 2021;12(1):1970.
101. Fu C, Lu Y, Zhang Y, Yu M, Ma S, Lyu S. Intermittent fasting suppressed splenic CD205+ G-MDSC accumulation in a murine breast cancer model by attenuating cell trafficking and inducing apoptosis. Food Sci Nutr. 2021;9(10):5517–26.
102. Nencioni A, Caffa I, Cortellino S, Longo VD. Fasting and cancer: molecular mechanisms and clinical application. Nat Rev Cancer. 2018;18(11):707–19.
103. Cheng CW, Adams GB, Perin L, Wei M, Zhou X, Lam BS, et al. Prolonged fasting reduces IGF-1/PKA to promote hematopoietic-stem-cell-based regeneration and reverse immunosuppression. Cell Stem Cell. 2014;14(6):810–23.
104. Stec K, Pilis K, Pilis W, Dolibog P, Letkiewicz S, Glebocka A. Effects of fasting on the physiological and psychological responses in middle-aged men. Nutrients. 2023;15(15)

105. Di Biase S, Lee C, Brandhorst S, Manes B, Buono R, Cheng CW, et al. Fasting-mimicking diet reduces HO-1 to promote T cell-mediated tumor cytotoxicity. Cancer Cell. 2016;30(1):136–46.
106. Faris MA, Kacimi S, Al-Kurd RA, Fararjeh MA, Bustanji YK, Mohammad MK, et al. Intermittent fasting during Ramadan attenuates proinflammatory cytokines and immune cells in healthy subjects. Nutr Res. 2012;32(12):947–55.
107. Adawi M, Watad A, Brown S, Aazza K, Aazza H, Zouhir M, et al. Ramadan fasting exerts immunomodulatory effects: insights from a systematic review. Front Immunol. 2017;8:1144.
108. Rouhani MH, Azadbakht L. Is Ramadan fasting related to health outcomes? A review on the related evidence. J Res Med Sci. 2014;19(10):987–92.
109. Faris MAE, Madkour MI, Obaideen AK, Dalah EZ, Hasan HA, Radwan H, et al. Effect of Ramadan diurnal fasting on visceral adiposity and serum adipokines in overweight and obese individuals. Diabetes Res Clin Pract. 2019;153:166–75.
110. Madkour MI, El-Serafi AT, Jahrami HA, Sherif NM, Hassan RE, Awadallah S, et al. Ramadan diurnal intermittent fasting modulates SOD2, TFAM, Nrf2, and sirtuins (SIRT1, SIRT3) gene expressions in subjects with overweight and obesity. Diabetes Res Clin Pract. 2019;155:107801.
111. Gasmi M, Sellami M, Denham J, Padulo J, Kuvacic G, Selmi W, et al. Time-restricted feeding influences immune responses without compromising muscle performance in older men. Nutrition. 2018;51-52:29–37.
112. Vasconcelos AR, Yshii LM, Viel TA, Buck HS, Mattson MP, Scavone C, et al. Intermittent fasting attenuates lipopolysaccharide-induced neuroinflammation and memory impairment. J Neuroinflammation. 2014;11:85.
113. Kafami L, Raza M, Razavi A, Mirshafiey A, Movahedian M, Khorramizadeh MR. Intermittent feeding attenuates clinical course of experimental autoimmune encephalomyelitis in C57BL/6 mice. Avicenna J Med Biotechnol. 2010;2(1):47–52.
114. Lee J, Kim SJ, Son TG, Chan SL, Mattson MP. Interferon-gamma is up-regulated in the hippocampus in response to intermittent fasting and protects hippocampal neurons against excitotoxicity. J Neurosci Res. 2006;83(8):1552–7.
115. Sadek K, Saleh E. Fasting ameliorates metabolism, immunity, and oxidative stress in carbon tetrachloride-intoxicated rats. Hum Exp Toxicol. 2014;33(12):1277–83.
116. Faris MAE, Salem ML, Jahrami HA, Madkour MI, BaHammam AS. Ramadan intermittent fasting and immunity: an important topic in the era of COVID-19. Ann Thorac Med. 2020;15(3):125–33.
117. Yakasai AM, Muhammad H, Babashani M, Jumare J, Abdulmumini M, Habib AG. Once-daily antiretroviral therapy among treatment-experienced Muslim patients fasting for the month of Ramadan. Trop Dr. 2011;41(4):233–5.
118. Mulas A, Cienfuegos S, Ezpeleta M, Lin S, Pavlou V, Varady KA. Effect of intermittent fasting on circulating inflammatory markers in obesity: a review of human trials. Front Nutr. 2023;10:1146924.
119. Yanai H, Yoshida H. Beneficial effects of adiponectin on glucose and lipid metabolism and atherosclerotic progression: mechanisms and perspectives. Int J Mol Sci. 2019;20(5)
120. Koklesova L, Mazurakova A, Samec M, Biringer K, Samuel SM, Busselberg D, et al. Homocysteine metabolism as the target for predictive medical approach, disease prevention, prognosis, and treatments tailored to the person. EPMA J. 2021;12(4):477–505.
121. Zhang L, Hou D, Chen X, Li D, Zhu L, Zhang Y, et al. Exogenous plant MIR168a specifically targets mammalian LDLRAP1: evidence of cross-kingdom regulation by microRNA. Cell Res. 2012;22(1):107–26.
122. Saliminejad K, Khorram Khorshid HR, Soleymani Fard S, Ghaffari SH. An overview of microRNAs: biology, functions, therapeutics, and analysis methods. J Cell Physiol. 2019;234(5):5451–65.
123. Macias S, Cordiner RA, Caceres JF. Cellular functions of the microprocessor. Biochem Soc Trans. 2013;41(4):838–43.

124. Cai Y, Yu X, Hu S, Yu J. A brief review on the mechanisms of miRNA regulation. Genomics Proteomics Bioinformatics. 2009;7(4):147–54.
125. Ruiz GP, Camara H, Fazolini NPB, Mori MA. Extracellular miRNAs in redox signaling: health, disease and potential therapies. Free Radic Biol Med. 2021;173:170–87.
126. Antoni R, Johnston KL, Collins AL, Robertson MD. Effects of intermittent fasting on glucose and lipid metabolism. Proc Nutr Soc. 2017;76(3):361–8.
127. Horton JD, Goldstein JL, Brown MS. SREBPs: activators of the complete program of cholesterol and fatty acid synthesis in the liver. J Clin Invest. 2002;109(9):1125–31.
128. Zelcer N, Tontonoz P. Liver X receptors as integrators of metabolic and inflammatory signaling. J Clin Invest. 2006;116(3):607–14.
129. Phillips MC. Molecular mechanisms of cellular cholesterol efflux. J Biol Chem. 2014;289(35):24020–9.
130. Rayner KJ, Suarez Y, Davalos A, Parathath S, Fitzgerald ML, Tamehiro N, et al. MiR-33 contributes to the regulation of cholesterol homeostasis. Science. 2010;328(5985):1570–3.
131. Goedeke L, Vales-Lara FM, Fenstermaker M, Cirera-Salinas D, Chamorro-Jorganes A, Ramirez CM, et al. A regulatory role for microRNA 33* in controlling lipid metabolism gene expression. Mol Cell Biol. 2013;33(11):2339–52.
132. Davalos A, Goedeke L, Smibert P, Ramirez CM, Warrier NP, Andreo U, et al. miR-33a/b contribute to the regulation of fatty acid metabolism and insulin signaling. Proc Natl Acad Sci USA. 2011;108(22):9232–7.
133. Rottiers V, Naar AM. MicroRNAs in metabolism and metabolic disorders. Nat Rev Mol Cell Biol. 2012;13(4):239–50.
134. Cena H, Calder PC. Defining a healthy diet: evidence for the role of contemporary dietary patterns in health and disease. Nutrients. 2020;12(2)
135. Otsuka K, Yamamoto Y, Matsuoka R, Ochiya T. Maintaining good miRNAs in the body keeps the doctor away?: perspectives on the relationship between food-derived natural products and microRNAs in relation to exosomes/extracellular vesicles. Mol Nutr Food Res. 2018;62(1)
136. Humphreys KJ, Conlon MA, Young GP, Topping DL, Hu Y, Winter JM, et al. Dietary manipulation of oncogenic microRNA expression in human rectal mucosa: a randomized trial. Cancer Prev Res (Phila). 2014;7(8):786–95.
137. Saini SK, Singh A, Saini M, Gonzalez-Freire M, Leeuwenburgh C, Anton SD. Time-restricted eating regimen differentially affects circulatory miRNA expression in older overweight adults. Nutrients. 2022;14(9)
138. Wang L, Wang HC, Chen C, Zeng J, Wang Q, Zheng L, et al. Differential expression of plasma miR-146a in sepsis patients compared with non-sepsis-SIRS patients. Exp Ther Med. 2013;5(4):1101–4.
139. Zhang H, Liu R, Deng T, Wang X, Lang H, Qu Y, et al. The microRNA-124-iGluR2/3 pathway regulates glucagon release from alpha cells. Oncotarget. 2016;7(17):24734–43.
140. Zia A, Farkhondeh T, Sahebdel F, Pourbagher-Shahri AM, Samarghandian S. Key miRNAs in modulating aging and longevity: a focus on signaling pathways and cellular targets. Curr Mol Pharmacol. 2022;15(5):736–62.
141. Withers SB, Dewhurst T, Hammond C, Topham CH. MiRNAs as novel Adipokines: obesity-related circulating MiRNAs influence Chemosensitivity in cancer patients. Noncoding. RNA. 2020;6(1)
142. Esau C, Davis S, Murray SF, Yu XX, Pandey SK, Pear M, et al. miR-122 regulation of lipid metabolism revealed by in vivo antisense targeting. Cell Metab. 2006;3(2):87–98.
143. Horie T, Ono K, Horiguchi M, Nishi H, Nakamura T, Nagao K, et al. MicroRNA-33 encoded by an intron of sterol regulatory element-binding protein 2 (Srebp2) regulates HDL in vivo. Proc Natl Acad Sci USA. 2010;107(40):17321–6.
144. Johnson C, Ct D, Virtue A, Gao T, Wu S, Hernandez M, et al. Increased expression of Resistin in MicroRNA-155-deficient White adipose tissues may be a possible driver of metabolically healthy obesity transition to classical obesity. Front Physiol. 2018;9:1297.
145. DeLucas M, Sanchez J, Palou A, Serra F. The impact of diet on miRNA regulation and its implications for health: a systematic review. Nutrients. 2024;16(6)

146. Khanna A, Muthusamy S, Liang R, Sarojini H, Wang E. Gain of survival signaling by down-regulation of three key miRNAs in brain of calorie-restricted mice. Aging (Albany NY). 2011;3(3):223–36.
147. Lee EK, Jeong HO, Bang EJ, Kim CH, Mun JY, Noh S, et al. The involvement of serum exo-somal miR-500-3p and miR-770-3p in aging: modulation by calorie restriction. Oncotarget. 2018;9(5):5578–87.
148. Ravanidis S, Grundler F, de Toledo FW, Dimitriou E, Tekos F, Skaperda Z, et al. Fasting-mediated metabolic and toxicity reprogramming impacts circulating microRNA levels in humans. Food Chem Toxicol. 2021;152:112187.
149. Antunes F, Erustes AG, Costa AJ, Nascimento AC, Bincoletto C, Ureshino RP, et al. Autophagy and intermittent fasting: the connection for cancer therapy? Clinics (Sao Paulo). 2018;73(suppl 1):e814s.
150. Nogueira S, Barbosa J, Faria J, Sa SI, Cardoso A, Soares R, et al. Unhealthy diets induce distinct and regional effects on intestinal inflammatory Signalling pathways and Long-lasting metabolic dysfunction in rats. Int J Mol Sci. 2022;23(18)
151. Tiwari S, Sapkota N, Han Z. Effect of fasting on cancer: a narrative review of scientific evi-dence. Cancer Sci. 2022;113(10):3291–302.
152. Kolluru GK, Bir SC, Kevil CG. Endothelial dysfunction and diabetes: effects on angiogen-esis, vascular remodeling, and wound healing. Int J Vasc Med. 2012;2012:918267.
153. de Gruil N, Pijl H, van der Burg SH, Kroep JR. Short-term fasting synergizes with solid can-cer therapy by boosting antitumor immunity. Cancers (Basel). 2022;14(6)
154. Zhao X, Yang J, Huang R, Guo M, Zhou Y, Xu L. The role and its mechanism of intermittent fasting in tumors: friend or foe? Cancer Biol Med. 2021;18(1):63–73.
155. Bianchi G, Martella R, Ravera S, Marini C, Capitanio S, Orengo A, et al. Fasting induces anti-Warburg effect that increases respiration but reduces ATP-synthesis to promote apoptosis in colon cancer models. Oncotarget. 2015;6(14):11806–19.
156. Kikomeko J, Schutte T, van Velzen MJM, Seefat R, van Laarhoven HWM. Short-term fasting and fasting mimicking diets combined with chemotherapy: a narrative review. Ther Adv Med Oncol. 2023;15:17588359231161418.
157. Clifton KK, Ma CX, Fontana L, Peterson LL. Intermittent fasting in the prevention and treat-ment of cancer. CA Cancer J Clin. 2021;71(6):527–46.
158. Xie HY, Shao ZM, Li DQ. Tumor microenvironment: driving forces and potential therapeutic targets for breast cancer metastasis. Chin J Cancer. 2017;36(1):36.
159. Jayasingam SD, Citartan M, Thang TH, Mat Zin AA, Ang KC, Ch'ng ES. Evaluating the polarization of tumor-associated macrophages into M1 and M2 phenotypes in human cancer tissue: technicalities and challenges in routine clinical practice. Front Oncol. 2019;9:1512.
160. Lewis C, Murdoch C. Macrophage responses to hypoxia: implications for tumor progression and anti-cancer therapies. Am J Pathol. 2005;167(3):627–35.
161. Missiaen R, Lesner NP, Simon MC. HIF: a master regulator of nutrient availability and meta-bolic cross-talk in the tumor microenvironment. EMBO J. 2023;42(6):e112067.
162. Chelakkot C, Chelakkot VS, Shin Y, Song K. Modulating glycolysis to improve cancer ther-apy. Int J Mol Sci. 2023;24(3)
163. Zhang J, Li S, Liu F, Yang K. Role of CD68 in tumor immunity and prognosis prediction in pan-cancer. Sci Rep. 2022;12(1):7844.
164. Cortellino S, Longo VD. Metabolites and immune response in tumor microenvironments. Cancers (Basel). 2023;15(15)
165. Pajak B, Siwiak E, Soltyka M, Priebe A, Zielinski R, Fokt I, et al. 2-Deoxy-d-glucose and its analogs: from diagnostic to therapeutic agents. Int J Mol Sci. 2019;21(1)

Part IV
Special Populations

Chapter 12
Diabetes and Ramadan Fasting: Opportunities and Challenges

Mohammaed M Hassanein

Abstract Ramadan fasting presents unique challenges for Muslim individuals with diabetes, necessitating a comprehensive understanding and preparation by healthcare professionals (HCPs). Epidemiological studies reveal that a significant majority of diabetic Muslims partake in fasting; however, variations in fasting behaviors emerge across regions. Pre-Ramadan evaluations are crucial to assess the risks associated with fasting, considering factors such as age, diabetes type, and comorbidities. Risk stratification frameworks assist HCPs in categorizing individuals into low-, moderate-, and high-risk groups, guiding tailored medical advice. Structured pre-Ramadan education programs have demonstrated efficacy in enhancing glycemic control and reducing hypoglycemic incidents. Furthermore, the need for individualized insulin management and dietary adaptations during Ramadan is highlighted, particularly for vulnerable populations, including the elderly, pregnant women, and those with chronic conditions. Ultimately, an inclusive approach combining medical and religious guidance is essential for fostering safe fasting practices among diabetic patients during Ramadan.

Keywords Ramadan fasting · Diabetes management · Risk stratification · Healthcare professionals · Pre-Ramadan evaluation

12.1 Introduction

The vast majority of Muslim people with diabetes observe Ramadan fasting. Given that Islam is the second most popular religion in the world [1], healthcare professionals (HCPs) need to comprehend the potential challenges associated with Ramadan fasting. Recent epidemiological studies, such as the DAR 2020 Global Survey, showed that over 83% of participants chose to fast, and 94.8% fasted for

M. M Hassanein (✉)
Department of Endocrinology, Mohamed Bin Rashid University Dubai, Dubai, United Arab Emirates

≥15 days, with the average number of days fasting during Ramadan being 27 and 6 days, respectively [2]. The decision to fast during Ramadan varied widely among different countries, ranging from the lowest in Morocco (42.6%) to the highest in KSA and Bangladesh, 97.1% and 98.1%, respectively, highlighting significant regional differences among Muslim-majority countries [2]. Other important factors, such as age and comorbidities, should not be overlooked, as the same study found that, for instance, a significantly higher proportion of those ≥65 years did not fast—28.8% vs. 12.7% of those <65 years [2]. For some patients, the month of Ramadan can bring about an increase in their rates of hypo- and hyperglycemia due to changes in eating and sleeping habits, and numerous studies have shown an increase in the risk of dehydration and diabetic ketoacidosis when fasting [3]. It is important to point out that most people fast without apparent risk; in fact, some studies found that there were brief improvements in blood pressure, weight, and metabolic indicators without any appreciable impact on renal function [4]. Healthcare professionals should also be aware of other special considerations, such as the voluntary 1- to 2-day fasts per week that many Muslims practice throughout the year and the effect of prolonged fasting (more than 18 hours a day) in regions far from the equator during Ramadan.

12.2 Pre-Ramadan Evaluation for Safe Fasting

Ideally, several weeks prior to Ramadan, a comprehensive assessment regarding the safety of fasting is required. This assessment should cover the following:

- Evaluation of the individual risk of fasting.
- Guide healthy dieting and fluid consumption; fasting is not considered.
- Guide timing and intensity of physical activity during fasting hours.
- Optimizing blood glucose monitoring.
- Reinforcement of signs of hypo- and hyperglycemia.
- Advice on when to break the fast.
- Proper adjustment of medication for Ramadan.

12.3 Risk Stratification of Individuals with Diabetes for Fasting During Ramadan

When advising people with diabetes who wish to fast during Ramadan, risk stratification is a crucial first step. All ensuing advice and choices should be made with the anticipated risk level in mind. The most recent IDF-DAR recommendations introduced a revolutionary grading system for each risk element based on the best clinical judgment and available data in the literature, with the goal of empowering clinicians from multiple disciplines [3]. It is critical to keep in mind that risk stratification is an ongoing process that is subject to change. Indeed, it could empower people with diabetes who wish to improve on some of the risk elements pre-Ramadan quickly, which could eventually improve their risk level.

During the pre-Ramadan evaluation, each risk element should be examined, and points should be added to provide the total risk level for the individual (Table 12.1). The risk categories are:

Table 12.1 Elements for risk calculation and suggested risk score for people with diabetes mellitus (DM) who seek to fast during Ramadan

Risk element	Risk score	Risk element	Risk score
1. Diabetes type		8. MVD complications/comorbidities	
Type 1 diabetes	1	Unstable MVD	6.5
Type 2 diabetes	0	Stable MVD	2
		No MVD	0
2. Duration of diabetes (years)		9. Renal complications/comorbidities	
A duration of ≥10	1	eGFR <30 mL/min	6.5
A duration of <10	0	eGFR 30–45 mL/min	4
		eGFR 45–60 mL/min	2
		eGFR >60 mL/min	0
3. Presence of hypoglycemia		10. Pregnancy*	
Hypoglycemia unawareness	6.5	Pregnant not within targets*	6.5
Recent severe hypoglycemia	5.5	Pregnant within targets*	3.5
Multiple weekly hypoglycemia	3.5	Not pregnant	0
Hypoglycemia less than one time per week	1		
No hypoglycemia	0		
4. Level of glycemic control		11. Frailty and cognitive function	
HbA1c levels >9% (11.7 mmol/L)	2	Impaired cognitive function or frailty	6.5
HbA1c levels 7.5–9% (9.4–11.7 mmol/L)	1	> 70 years old with no home support	3.5
HbA1c levels <7.5% (9.4 mmol/L)	0	No frailty or loss in cognitive function	0
5. Type of treatment		12. Physical labor	
Multiple daily mixed insulin injections	3	Highly intense physical labor	4
Basal-bolus/insulin pump	2.5	Moderately intense physical labor	2

(continued)

Table 12.1 (continued)

Risk element	Risk score	Risk element	Risk score
Once daily, mixed insulin	2	No physical labor	0
Basal insulin	1.5		
Glibenclamide	1		
Medications include Gliclazide MR, Glimepiride, or Repaglinide	0.5		
Other therapies, not including SU or insulin	0		
6. Self-monitoring of blood glucose (SMBG)		13. Previous Ramadan experience	
Indicated but not conducted	2	Overall negative experience	1
Indicated but conducted sub-optimally	1	No negative or positive experience	0
Conducted as indicated	0		
7. Acute complications		14. Fasting hours (location)	
DKA/HONC in the last 3 months	3	≥ 16 h	1
DKA/HONC in the last 6 months	2	< 16 h	0
KA/HONC in the last 12 months	1		
No DKA or HONC	0		

Abbreviations: *DKA* Diabetic ketoacidosis, *HONC* Hyperglycemic hyperosmolar nonketotic coma, *eGFR* Estimated glomerular filtration rate, *MVD* Macrovascular disease

[a]Pregnant and breastfeeding women have the right not to fast, regardless of whether they have diabetes

- High risk, when it is probably not safe to fast
- Moderate risk, where the safety of fasting is unknown
- Low risk, when fasting is most likely safe

Table 12.2 summarizes the medical and religious recommendations that the highest Egyptian religious regulatory authority has approved. However, religious rulings vary considerably between countries and regions, so further regional discussions are required when presenting advice based on such recommendations.

HCPs need to discuss the level of risks associated with fasting during Ramadan with people with diabetes. This would help them understand and accept the risk level. Those who insist on fasting in spite of their risk category need to adhere to the necessary advice and guidelines to minimize potential risks.

Table 12.2 Medical and religious risk score recommendations

Risk score/ level	Medical recommendations	Religious recommendations
Low risk 0–3 points	**Fasting is safe**	1. Fasting is obligatory
	1. Medical evaluation	2. Advice not to fast is not allowed unless the patient is unable to fast due to the physical burden of fasting or needing to take medication or food or drink during the fasting hours
	2. Medication adjustment	
	3. Strict monitoring	
Moderate risk 3.5–6 points	**Fasting safety is uncertain**	1. Fasting is preferred, but patients may choose not to fast if they are concerned about their health after consulting the doctor and taking into account the full medical circumstances and the patient's own previous experiences
	1. Medical evaluation	2. If the patient does fast, they must follow medical recommendations, including regular blood glucose monitoring
	2. Medication adjustment	
	3. Strict monitoring	
High risk > 6 points	**Fasting is probably unsafe**	Advise against fasting

12.4 Pre-Ramadan Structured Education

Numerous research studies on pre-Ramadan organized education have shown that participation in such programs can enhance glycemic control and/or lower rates of hypoglycemia [5]. The aspects of pre-Ramadan education are as follows:

1. **Dietary and Lifestyle Changes and Guidance During Ramadan**

   During Ramadan, most people will see a change in their eating habits, regardless of their fasting status, as many view it as a time for celebration. However, people with diabetes must adjust their meals to maintain good glycemic control. The DAR International Alliance created the Ramadan Nutrition Plan (RNP), a web-based/mobile program designed to assist healthcare professionals and people with diabetes with medical nutrition therapy throughout Ramadan (www.daralliance.org).

   While mild-to-moderate physical activity is encouraged during fasting hours, strenuous activity should be avoided during these hours to prevent hypoglycemia and dehydration, particularly during hot summer days [6].

2. **Self-Monitoring of Blood Glucose**

   The cornerstone in identifying/preventing hypo- and hyperglycemia incidents is frequent monitoring of blood glucose. The frequency and timing of monitoring will vary according to the individual's needs. The blood glucose monitoring guide for people with diabetes fasting during Ramadan should include the following times during the week for better assessment:

- Pre-dawn meal (*Suhoor*)
- Morning
- Midday
- Midafternoon
- Pre-sunset meal (*iftar*)
- Two hours after *iftar*
- Any time there are symptoms of hypo-/hyperglycemia or feelings of being unwell

People with diabetes should also be assured that taking a blood glucose test does not break the fast.

3. **Management of Individuals with Diabetes When Fasting During Ramadan**

12.4.1   Type 1 Diabetes Mellitus (T1DM) [7]

Despite the consensus among religious authorities that people with chronic conditions such as diabetes are exempt from fasting, many individuals with T1DM will pursue participation in Ramadan fasting even against the advice of their healthcare professionals in some circumstances [8]. The IDF-DAR guidelines caution against allowing fasting for some persons with T1DM, particularly those at high risk [9]. There is minimal information on the safety of fasting in individuals with type 1 diabetes; hence, a tailored approach is recommended [10].

12.4.2   Insulin Regimens and Blood Glucose Monitoring Among Adolescents with T1DM

Four different types of insulin therapy are commonly employed in managing DM in adolescents: Basal-bolus regimens, continuous subcutaneous insulin infusion (CSII) with or without sensors, conventional twice-daily NPH/regular short-acting (human) insulin, and premixed insulins.

The recommendations for adolescents not on CSII therapy are:

- Adolescents with T1DM benefit from a basal-bolus regimen rather than traditional twice-daily regimens, as demonstrated in Flowchart 1.
- Premixed insulin regimens lack flexibility for fasting due to strict nutritional requirements.
- Perform SMBG routinely when fasting and when feeling sick. When available, continuous glucose monitoring (CGM) or flash glucose monitoring (FGM) are preferable tools for monitoring blood glucose levels.

Basal insulin	
Good glycemic control (HBA1C < 7.5%)	Poor glycemic control (HBA1C > 7.5%)
Reduce dose by 20–30%. Take it at iftar, late evening, or pre-Ramadan bedtime	Keep the same dose and follow up. Take it at iftar, late evening, or before Ramadan bedtime

Prandial insulin	
Patients on ICR/ISF correction	Patients on fixed doses
To continue the same for iftar and Suhoor	No change at iftar, but the Suhoor dose by 20–30%
Notes on prandial insulin: For better postprandial control, it is advised to take the bolus 20 mins prior to iftar to account for high-fat and/or high-protein meals High blood glucose values may require extra correction doses based on insulin sensitivity ratio and target blood glucose Correction doses must not be given more frequently than every 3 h to avoid insulin stacking and hypoglycemia	An individualized approach is essential for treatment adjustment according to the patient's SMBG or CGM data

Adolescents with T1DM are prime candidates for CSII/insulin pump therapy when appropriate. Insulin pumps can lower the incidence of glucose excursions and hypoglycemia while fasting [11]. Additional investigation is needed to properly examine the effectiveness of these treatments during RF and provide more detailed recommendations. The current recommended use is shown in Box 12.1.

Box 12.1: Recommendations for Insulin Pump Therapy Usage among Adolescents with Type 1 Diabetes Mellitus (T1DM) Who Are Fasting During Ramadan
Basal insulin:

- Reduce basal insulin by 20–35% in the last 4–5 h before iftar.
- Increase dose by 10–30% after iftar up to midnight.

Bolus insulin:

- Prandial insulin bolus is calculated based on usual ICR and insulin sensitivity factor.

Notes on bolus insulin:

- Bolus doses of insulin can be delivered in three different patterns:

    *Immediately known as standard bolus
    *Slowly over a certain period (extended or square bolus)
    *A combination of the two, a combo or dual-wave bolus

(continued)

Box 12.1 (continued)

- Meals higher in fat content may need an extended or combo bolus as the rise in glucose following the meal.
- It is recommended to use bolus calculators in determining carbohydrate and correction dosing to avoid

(ICR: insulin to carbohydrate ratio).

12.4.3 Insulin Regimens and Blood Glucose Monitoring Among Adults with T1DM

Limited research has been conducted on Ramadan fasting in adults with type 1 diabetes. Table 12.3 suggests adjustments to insulin regimens that should be tailored to individual needs.

Table 12.3 Recommendations for insulin dose adjustments based on type of regimen

Type of insulin regimen	Adjustment for fasting during Ramadan	Methods of monitoring during Ramadan
CSII/insulin pump	*Basal rate adjustment:* 20–40% decrease for the last 3–4 h of fast 10–30% increase for the first few hours after iftar bolus doses Same principles as prior to Ramadan	CGM
MDI (basal-bolus) with analog insulin	*Basal insulin:* 30–40% reduction in dose and to be taken at iftar rapid analog insulin Dose at Suhoor to be reduced by 30–50% Prelunch dose to be skipped The dose around iftar to be adjusted based on the 2-h post-iftar glucose reading	7-point glucose monitoring
MDI (basal-bolus) with conventional insulin	*NPH insulin:* The usual pre-Ramadan morning dose to be taken in the evening during Ramadan 50% of the pre-Ramadan dose to be taken at Suhoor *regular insulin:* Dose at evening meal remains unchanged Suhoor dose to be 50% of the pre-Ramadan evening dose Afternoon dose to be skipped	7-point blood glucose monitoring or 2–3 staggered readings throughout the day
Premixed (analog or conventional)	Shift the usual pre-Ramadan morning dose to iftar 50% of the pre-Ramadan evening dose at Suhoor	At least 2–3 daily readings and whenever any hypoglycemic symptoms develop

CGM continuous glucose monitoring, *CSII* continuous subcutaneous insulin infusion, *MDI* multiple daily injections

12.4.4 Type 2 Diabetes Mellitus

Certain drugs may increase the risk of hypoglycemia during Ramadan, necessitating adjustments to the dose, timing, and frequency of use. This also applies to those taking several antidiabetic treatments simultaneously. Among the drugs that present a low risk of hypoglycemia and so require no dose modification during Ramadan are metformin, dipeptidyl peptidase-4 (DPP-4) inhibitors, acarbose, thiazolidinediones (TZDs), sodium-glucose cotransporter-2 (SGLT-2) inhibitors, and glucagon-like peptide-1 receptor agonists (GLP-1 RAs). There is a slightly higher risk of hypoglycemia during Ramadan with modern sulfonylureas (glimepiride, gliclazide, and gliclazide MR) that warrants dose adjustment in those susceptible [12]. Recent studies have confirmed the safety of SGLT-2 inhibitors, but certain recommendations should be followed when using this class of drugs:

A lower pre-Ramadan dose is advised if indicated for cardiovascular or renal protection. It is best administered 2 weeks to a month before the holy month. No dosage modification is required during Ramadan, but coadministration of other antidiabetic medications necessitates monitoring the risk of hypoglycemia. Proper hydration should be maintained during nonfasting hours. In view of the potential GIT side effects, the initiation or intensification of glucagon-like peptide-1 receptor agonists (GLP-1 RAs) during the last 2–4 weeks before Ramadan is not recommended. Table 12.4 summarizes the suggested use of antidiabetic drugs during Ramadan.

12.4.5 Insulin Treatment for T2DM

Ramadan fasting increases the risk of hypoglycemia associated with insulin; the particular type of insulin also plays a role in this risk. Tables 12.5 and 12.6 summarize the adjustments needed to insulin timing, dosage, and frequency to minimize hypoglycemic risk.

12.4.5.1 Special Populations

12.4.6 Elderly Individuals with Diabetes

Despite being considered high risk for fasting during Ramadan, many older adults with diabetes have enjoyed fasting for many years. Comorbidities such as dementia, repeated falls, amputation, and vision impairment all increase their risk of fasting.

Older adults with diabetes are more likely to experience complications than younger adults [13]. Identifying preexisting comorbidities during the pre-Ramadan screening is crucial for proper risk stratification. One serious concern in older people is the development of hypoglycemia and hyperglycemia. Hypoglycemia is particularly dangerous

Table 12.4 Recommended dose and regimen modifications for noninsulin-based antidiabetic medications during Ramadan fasting

Antidiabetic medications	Regimen/dose modifications	Level of evidence supporting recommendation and grading from IDF-DAR writing group (Tables 12.5 and 12.6)
Metformin	*Once daily:* No dose modifications Take at iftar *Twice daily:* No dose modifications Take at iftar or Suhoor *Three times daily:* Morning dose is taken before Suhoor Combine the afternoon dose with the iftar dose. *Prolonged release:* No dose modifications Take at iftar	Level 4 and grade D
Acarbose	No dose modifications	Level 4 and grade D
TZDs	No dose modifications, but doses can be taken with iftar or Suhoor	Pioglitazone—level 2 grade B Other TZDs grade D
Short-acting insulin secretagogues	Three-meal dosing can be redistributed to two doses according to meal sizes	Repaglinide—level 2 grade B Gliclazide, gliclazide MR, and glimepiride—level 3 grade C
GLP-1 RAs	No dose modifications after appropriate dose titrations have been achieved	Exenatide, liraglutide, lixisenatide—level 2 grade B Other GLP-1 RAs—grade D
DPP-4 inhibitors	No dose modifications	Vildagliptin, sitagliptin—level 1A/B grade A Other DPP-4 inhibitors grade D
SUs	Use newer drugs, e.g., gliclazide, gliclazide MR, glimepiride *Once daily:* Reductions in well-controlled individuals Take at iftar *Twice daily:* Reductions of Suhoor in well-controlled individuals	Level 3 and grade C
SGLT-2 inhibitors	No dose modifications Extra fluids to maintain hydration	Dapagliflozin, canagliflozin—Level 3 grade C Other SGLT-2 inhibitors grade D

DPP-4 dipeptidyl peptidase-4, *GLP-1 RAs* glucagon-like peptide-1 receptor agonists, *SGLT-2* sodium-glucose cotransporter-2, *SUs* sulfonylureas, *TZDs* thiazolidinediones

Table 12.5 Dose adjustments for long- or short-acting insulins and premixed insulins

Changes to premixed insulin dosing during Ramadan		
Once-daily dosing	Twice-daily dosing	Three-times-daily dosing
Take the normal dose at iftar	Take the normal dose at iftar	Omit afternoon dose Adjust iftar and Suhoor doses
	Reduce Suhoor dose by 20–50%	Carry out dose titration every 3 days

Table 12.6 Dose titrations for long- and short-acting insulins and premixed insulins based on blood glucose levels

Fasting/pre-iftar/pre-Suhoor blood glucose	Pre-iftar	Pre-iftar[a]/post-Suhoor[b]
	Basal insulin/premixed	Short-acting insulin
<70 mg/dL (3.9 mmol/L) or symptoms	Reduce by 4 units	Reduce by 4 units
<90 mg/dL (5.0 mmol/L)	Reduce by 2 units	Reduce by 2 units
90–126 mg/dL (5.0–7.0 mmol/L)	No change required	No change required
>126 mg/dL (7.0 mmol/L)	Increase by 2 units	Increase by 2 units
>200 mg/dL (16.7 mmol/L)	Increase by 4 units	Increase by 4 units

Source: Adapted from Hassanein et al. (2014)
[a]Reduce the insulin dose taken before Suhoor
[b]Reduce the insulin dose taken before iftar

since it leads to neuroglycopenic manifestations in the form of dizziness, delirium, and confusion and results in hypoglycemia unawareness. Countering these risks is best carried out by frequent SMBG and medication adjustments, among other recommendations adapted from the IDF-DAR guidelines (Box 12.2).

> **Box 12.2: Specific Guidance for the Elderly Population**
> *Medications and regimens:*
>
> - Have an assessment and discussion prior to Ramadan to modify and adjust medications to reduce the risk of hypoglycemia.
>
> *SMBG:*
>
> - Increase the frequency of SMBG and consider using a CGM.
>
> *Diet:*
>
> - There needs to be an emphasis on staying properly hydrated and ensuring adequate nutrients. *Physical activity:*
> - Physical activity levels should be curtailed but not halted during fasting hours.

(continued)

Box 12.2 (continued)

Social considerations and community support:

- Adequate support mechanisms should be in place to ensure that elderly individuals with diabetes wishing to fast receive support from family members, friends, carers, or community members. This should provide greater levels of safety and confidence.

Risks of complications and awareness:

- The effects of fasting in people with comorbidities such as dementia, impaired renal function, CVD, and others should be seriously considered and discussed prior to conducting Ramadan fasting.

CGM continuous glucose monitoring, *CVD* cardiovascular disease, *SMBG* self-monitoring of blood glucose.

12.4.7 Fasting During Ramadan and Congestive Heart Failure, Acute Coronary Syndrome, or Stroke

Several studies on the correlation between fasting and congestive heart failure (CHF) or acute coronary syndrome (ACS) failed to establish any difference in outcomes before and after Ramadan. Few studies have even pointed to fewer ACS occurrences during Ramadan. Still, more randomized controlled trials are needed to confirm the safety of fasting in this cohort of patients.

Multiple studies have shown conflicting findings on the link between Ramadan fasting (RF) and stroke. Some studies found no increase in the risk of ischemic or hemorrhagic strokes, while others found that fasting during Ramadan may increase that risk ($p = 0.03$) [14]. According to DAR guidelines, patients with diabetes who have unstable macrovascular problems should remain classified as high risk and discouraged from fasting until further research presents more evidence. Table 12.7 provides recommendations for people with macrovascular disease who are willing to fast.

12.4.8 Impact of Fasting During Ramadan for People with Diabetes and Chronic Kidney Disease

The evidence on the impact of fasting on renal function is conflicting, with few studies showing deterioration and others showing no discernible effect by the end of the fast. The same argument can be made about patients undergoing dialysis, where evidence is lacking and hard to interpret since most available data comes from high-income countries where facilities and medical services differ significantly from the

Table 12.7 Macrovascular complications and safety of fasting during Ramadan

Macrovascular complications	Recommendations
Congestive heart failure (CHF) Acute coronary syndrome (ACS) Stroke	Receive a thorough risk assessment from their diabetes specialist, cardiologist, and/or neurologist well in advance of Ramadan
	Receive pre-Ramadan education and understand how to conduct safe fasting with diabetes properly
	Obtain individualized advice based on their current health status and treatment regimens
	Practice safe fasting as discussed in these guidelines wherever applicable
	Make appropriate adjustments to therapies in accordance with their symptoms. For example, diuretics, antihypertensives, antidiabetic medication, and insulin regimens will need adjusting to give the greatest chance of achieving safe fasting during Ramadan
	Make a concerted effort to stay hydrated and get an adequate amount of sleep and nutrition prior to conducting fasting

Table 12.8 Recommendation for patients with chronic kidney disease

Chronic kidney disease	Recommendation
Renal impairment Dialysis Renal transplant	All individuals with diabetes (both T1DM and T2DM) and chronic kidney disease (CKD) or with any other renal issues should discuss their intentions to fast during Ramadan with diabetes and renal specialists at least 3 months prior to Ramadan and attend Ramadan-focused education
	Individuals with diabetes (both T1DM and T2DM) and CKD of stages 3–5 or on dialysis should be considered high risk, and fasting ought to be discouraged
	Those who are considered high risk and still choose to fast must:
	*Be carefully monitored and have weekly reviews during Ramadan
	*Make a concerted effort to stay hydrated outside of fasting periods
	*Monitor electrolyte and creatinine levels at various points during Ramadan to ensure safe fasting is being conducted and whether it should continue
	*Avoid foods with high potassium or phosphorous content

rest of the Islamic world. Fasting during Ramadan is generally safe for patients who have undergone kidney transplants, but more studies are needed to bolster current evidence.

For now, the risk for fasting remains high in cases of unstable renal impairment, and should those patients choose to fast despite the medical advice against it, certain recommendations to be considered are listed in Table 12.8.

12.4.8.1   Pregnant Women

Islamic teachings have exempted all pregnant women from fasting. With limited data on fasting with preexisting diabetes during pregnancy and its effects on the newborn, it is recommended that pregnant women with diabetes not fast until further research is available.

For pregnant women who still insist on observing fasting against religious and medical advice, the following measures should be taken:

Pre-Ramadan assessment with individualized expert nutritional and diabetes education.
Frequent monitoring of blood glucose to detect the presence of hyper- and/or hypoglycemia.
SMBG needs to be done throughout the day, including during fasting hours, before and after meals, and while feeling poorly.

Insulin is the drug of choice for managing diabetes during pregnancy, but a specific regimen has yet to be established [15]. The IDF-DAR guidelines advocate aligning insulin doses and blood glucose monitoring regimens in pregnancy with individuals with type 1 diabetes (Table 12.3).

12.5   Conclusion

Armed with the knowledge and understanding of every risk involved with Ramadan fasting, both healthcare professionals and people with diabetes can make the right decision about fasting. A crucial first step is a pre-Ramadan assessment that guides the HCP toward an individualized, tailored Ramadan-focused education program on changes in treatment and nutrition to avoid both acute and chronic complications [16]. The role of religious figures and other prominent community members in raising awareness and overcoming barriers that can impede the implementation of guidelines cannot be overstated. An inclusive strategy of modern methods using social media and telemedicine should ensure safer fasting for all people with diabetes.

All tables and figures in this chapter have been adapted from the IDF-DAR Diabetes and Ramadan: Practical Guidelines 2021 [3].

References

1. Hackett C, Connor P, Stonawski M, Skirbekk V, Potančoková M, Abel G. The future of world religions: population growth projections, 2010–2050. Washington: Pew Research Center; 2015.
2. Hassanein M, Hussein Z, Shaltout I, Seman WJW, Tong CV, Noor NM, et al. The DAR 2020 global survey: Ramadan fasting during COVID 19 pandemic and the impact of older age on fasting among adults with type 2 diabetes. Diabetes Res Clin Pract. 2021;173:108674.
3. Hassanein M, Afandi B, Yakoob Ahmedani M, et al. Diabetes and Ramadan: practical guidelines 2021. Diabetes Res Clin Pract. 2022 Mar;185:109185. https://doi.org/10.1016/j.diabres.2021.109185.
4. Lessan N, Saadane I, Alkaf B, Hambly C, Buckley AJ, Finer N, et al. The effects of Ramadan fasting on activity and energy expenditure. Am J Clin Nutr. 2018;107(1):54–61.

5. Zainudin SB, Abu Bakar KNB, Abdullah SB, Hussain AB. The diabetes education and medication adjustment in Ramadan (DEAR) program prepares for self-management during fasting with telehealth support from pre-Ramadan to post-Ramadan. Ther Adv Endocrinol Metabol. 2018;9(8):231–40.
6. BaHammam A, Alrajeh M, Albabtain M, Bahammam S, Sharif M. Circadian pattern of sleep, energy expenditure, and body temperature of young, healthy men during the intermittent fasting of Ramadan. Appetite. 2010;54(2):426–9.
7. Al Awadi FF, Echtay A, Al Arouj M, Sabir Ali S, Shehadeh N, Al-Shaikh A, et al. Patterns of diabetes care among people with type 1 diabetes during Ramadan: an international prospective study (DAR-MENA T1DM). Adv Ther. 2020;37(4):1550–63.
8. Hassanein M, Alamoudi RM, Kallash MA, Aljohani NJ, Alfadhli EM, Tony LE, et al. Ramadan fasting in people with type 1 diabetes during COVID-19 pandemic: the DaR global survey. Diabetes Res Clin Pract. 2021;172:108626.
9. Afandi B, Kaplan W, Al Kuwaiti F, Al Dahmani K, Nagelkerke N. Ramadan challenges: fasting against medical advice. J Nutr Fasting Health. 2017;5(3):133–7.
10. Kaplan W, Afandi B. Blood glucose fluctuation during Ramadan fasting in adolescents with type 1 diabetes: findings of continuous glucose monitoring. Diabetes Care. 2015;38(10):e162–3.
11. barbary NS. Effectiveness of the low-glucose suspend feature of insulin pump during fasting during Ramadan in type 1 diabetes mellitus. Diabetes Metab Res Rev. 2016;32(6):623–33.
12. Hassanein M, Al Sifri S, Shaikh S, Abbas Raza S, Akram J, Pranoto A, et al. A real-world study in patients with type 2 diabetes mellitus treated with gliclazide modified-release during fasting: DIA-RAMADAN. Diabetes Res Clin Pract. 2020;163:108154.
13. Hassanein M, et al. An update on the current characteristics and status of care for Muslims with type 2 diabetes fasting during Ramadan: the DAR global survey 202. Curr Med Res Opin. 2024;40(9):1515–23. https://doi.org/10.1080/03007995.2024.2385057.
14. Assy MH, Awd M, Elshabrawy AM, Gharieb M. Effect of Ramadan fasting on the incidence of cerebrovascular stroke in Egyptian patients with type 2 diabetes mellitus. Diabetes Res Clin Pract. 2019;151:299–304.
15. Afandi BO, Hassanein MM, Majd LM, Nagelkerke NJD. Impact of Ramadan fasting on glucose levels in women with gestational diabetes mellitus treated with diet alone or diet plus metformin: a continuous glucose monitoring study. BMJ Open Diabetes Res Care. 2017;5(1):e000470.
16. Afandi B, Beshyah SA, Hassanein MM, Jabbar A, Khalil AB. The individualization of care for people with diabetes during Ramadan fasting: a narrative review. Ibnosina J Med Biomed Sci. 2020;12(2):98.

Chapter 13
Pregnancy and Ramadan Fasting: Implications for Maternal and Fetal Health

Leen Al Kassab, Lobna Raya, and Sarrah Shahawy

Abstract Pregnant Muslims may be religiously exempt from fasting during the month of Ramadan if there is any concern for undue hardship or maternal or fetal harm. The current data on the effect of Ramadan fasting (RF) on maternal health outcomes show insufficient evidence of an association with hypertension and pre-eclampsia. There is conflicting data regarding the negative vs. protective association of RF on developing gestational diabetes mellitus (GDM) and glycemic control. Some evidence exists regarding changes in different hormone concentrations, lipid profiles, and ketonuria. There is no association with changes in uterine artery pulsatility indices. Some data suggest an association with signs and symptoms of maternal fatigue and dehydration, equivalent to lower mean maternal weight gain. There is conflicting data on mode of delivery. Data suggest a potential decrease in placental weight and possible effect on macronutrients of breast milk. The current data on the impact of RF on fetal health outcomes show some associations with impact on antenatal fetal testing indices, including nonstress tests (NSTs), lower amniotic fluid levels, and lower biophysical profile (BPP) scores. There is an increase or no difference in intrauterine growth indices in fasters. Little to no clinically significant effect on neonatal birthweight or preterm delivery has been found. There are possible adverse long-term effects on offspring of fasting mothers, but more data are required. The variation in defining "Ramadan fasting" in pregnancy and in study size and design breed many potential confounders and negatively impact the quality of the

L. Al Kassab (✉)
Department of Obstetrics & Gynecology, Harvard Medical School, Mass General Brigham, Boston, MA, USA
e-mail: lalkassab@mgb.org

L. Raya
Department of Obstetrics and Gynecology, Beth Israel Deaconess Medical Center, Boston, MA, USA

S. Shahawy
Department of Obstetrics and Gynecology, Harvard Medical School, Beth Israel Deaconess Medical Center, Boston, MA, USA

© The Author(s), under exclusive license to Springer Nature Singapore Pte Ltd. 2025
M. E. Faris et al. (eds.), *Health and Medical Aspects of Ramadan Intermittent Fasting*, https://doi.org/10.1007/978-981-96-6783-3_13

217

existing evidence. More research is needed to better understand the true effect of fasting during Ramadan on certain outcomes. Obstetric providers need to demonstrate cultural and religious awareness and confidently counsel their patients on the nuances of the literature while making individualized recommendations.

Keywords Ramadan fasting · Muslim · Maternal fetal outcomes · Pregnancy · Obstetrics

13.1   Introduction

The month of Ramadan has, on average, a 75% chance of falling during any Muslim woman's nine-month pregnancy (nine/twelve months). Many Islamic scholarly interpretations indicate that pregnant women may be religiously exempt from Ramadan fasting (RF), especially if there is any concern for *undue hardship* or *maternal or fetal harm* [1]. Several studies conducted primarily in Muslim-majority countries show that most Muslim women still choose to fast during pregnancy at a rate of 70% to 85% [2–4] despite this possible religious exemption.

   Studies and reviews, including systematic reviews on the effects of RF during pregnancy measured by different outcomes, have illustrated various conflicting results [5]. It is important to understand these data and utilize them to better guide pregnant Muslim patients' prenatal care, as this decision of whether to fast during Ramadan will come up for at least 75% of this population. Below is our summary of the existing literature on the impact of RF on maternal and fetal health outcomes.

13.2   Maternal Health

13.2.1   Preeclampsia

Few studies have examined the relationship between RF during pregnancy and the development of preeclampsia, a disease unique to pregnancy involving high blood pressure and proteinuria as a result of multifactorial pathophysiology, including abnormal placentation and resultant tissue hypoxia causing endothelial damage [6]. Current opinion on the pathogenesis of preeclampsia also explains a predictive role for oxidative stress parameters, defined as an imbalance between the cellular production of reactive oxygen species and the ability of antioxidants to prevent oxidative damage [6]. Ozturk et al.'s [7] prospective control study examined this outcome by looking at oxidative stress indices in fasting maternal serum samples and found no significant association between RF and maternal oxidative stress regarding total oxidant status or oxidative stress index. There was a significantly higher total antioxidant status in those who fasted for more than 10 days than in non-fasters [7]. The authors concluded that, given this suggested pathophysiology, there was no association between RF and the development of preeclampsia.

Similarly, Safari et al. [2] found no relationship between RF during pregnancy and preeclampsia. Existing studies thus suggest no significant association between RF and the development of preeclampsia. Glazier et al. [8] ran a meta-analysis of 22 observational and randomized-controlled trial studies that were English-only and published before April 2018. Overall, this encompassed 31,374 pregnancies that were exposed to intermittent RF in all pregnancy stages. They did not report sufficient data to carry out a meta-analysis for the association between RF and hypertension [8].

13.2.2   Gestational Diabetes

The relationship between RF during pregnancy and the development of gestational diabetes mellitus (GDM) has been explored in multiple studies. One case-control study determined an increase in the rate of GDM between fasting and non-fasting patients (17% vs. 14%), although these findings were not statistically significant [9]. A study in the United Arab Emirates (UAE) showed that 150 low-risk patients with similar body mass index (BMI) and age, and gestational age between 20 and 36 weeks had no significant change in fasting blood glucose level but showed a mean blood glucose level one hour after breaking the 14-hour summer fast was higher in the RF group vs. one hour after the main meal in non-fasters [10]. Another study ($n = 324$) by Mirghani and Hamud [11] showed an increase in GDM and induction of labor rates (for post-term or GDM) in patients fasting a mean of 9.4 hours at a mean gestational age of 34.6 weeks; however, the study did not correct for BMI and weight gain. The same study identified a higher risk of developing GDM in fasting patients than in those who were not fasting (20.2% vs. 7.1%, respectively; $P < 0.001$). However, this study did not collect data on participants' prepregnancy BMI, physical activity, diet changes, or weight gain, which other studies suggest may be confounding variables.

Contrary to these findings, in one case-control study ($n = 301$) in which prepregnancy BMIs were controlled for, participants who *did not* fast were 1.51 times more likely to develop GDM (prevalence of 8.3%) compared to their RF counterparts (prevalence of 2.6%) (OR, 1.51; 95% CI, 0.06–0.74; $P = 0.01$) [2]. Furthermore, one retrospective study ($n = 37$) focusing on the glycemic control of people with diabetes on insulin who chose to fast found that glycemic control was improved among participants during RF [12].

A separate study ($n = 345$) found that patients who already had GDM who chose to fast did not experience any difference in macrosomia, mean birthweight, or maternal outcomes [13]. However, RF was associated with a higher rate of neonatal hyperbilirubinemia in that group but a lower rate of neonatal hypoglycemia [13]. Additionally, another study ($n = 32$) found increased rates of maternal hypoglycemia in patients with GDM who chose to fast [14]. With many limitations, some studies suggest an association between RF and the development of GDM and 1-hour glucose levels. In contrast, others suggest a protective effect of RF on the development of GDM and improved glycemic control. Glazier et al.'s meta-analysis [8] did not report sufficient data to carry out a meta-analysis of GDM as an outcome.

13.2.3 Biochemical Changes

Many studies have shown a wide range of maternal biochemical changes during pregnancy with RF. An analysis of fasting pregnant women ($n = 30$) at 7–35 weeks gestation, with variable maternal age and BMI, measured follicle-stimulating hormone (FSH), luteinizing hormone, estrogen, progesterone, and leptin and found variations in these levels throughout the first, second, and fourth weeks of Ramadan and in the second week post-Ramadan [15]. Hypo-leptinemia (seen in the second week of Ramadan and the second week post-Ramadan) may be correlated with adverse effects on maternal health and intrauterine growth restriction. Interpretation of these results is limited by the levels of FSH and estrogen fluctuations depending on gestational age, which varied in this study [15].

A Turkish study found that fasters' maternal serum cortisol was significantly higher on day 20 of Ramadan compared to one week prior [16]. It also found a higher nonsignificant increase in total cholesterol and triglyceride levels, a nonsignificant decrease in LDL and VLDL, a slight increase in HDL levels, and a significant decrease in the LDL/HDL ratio in fasters. Another study in women who fasted for more than 10 consecutive days found lower levels of VLDL and triglycerides and a higher incidence of 1+ ketonuria than non-fasters [17]. A study in Lebanon [18] also found that fasting women had a higher rate of ketosis and ketonuria. In contrast, another study ($n = 36$ fasters and $n = 29$ non-fasters) found that RF was not associated with ketonemia or ketonuria [19]. One study found that RF was associated with an increase in the frequency of asymptomatic bacteriuria as the intake of fluids decreased [20]. It is unclear whether the changes outlined above in hormone concentration, lipid profiles, and ketonuria are significant associations and if they affect pregnancy outcomes.

13.2.4 Uterine Arterial Blood Flow

Some studies have evaluated the impact of RF on uterine arterial blood flow, peak systolic velocity, end-diastolic velocity, systolic/diastolic ratio, uterine artery pulsatility index, and resistance index (measured on Doppler flow velocimetry). These indices are measures of uteroplacental perfusion; a higher index would imply impaired placental perfusion, which can be associated with increased risk for maternal and fetal harm, including preeclampsia, fetal growth restriction, placental abruption, and neonatal stillbirth [21]. One cross-sectional observational study ($n = 106$) showed a similar mean (95% CI) of all the above indices between participants fasting at 20–24 weeks gestational age and the non-fasting control group, indicating no statistically significant difference between fasting and non-fasting participants [22]. Another study ($n = 52$) also found no statistically significant difference in uterine and umbilical artery Doppler indices in those who fasted during Ramadan in their second and third trimesters compared to those who did not fast [23]. Uterine artery pulsatility indices are similar in fasting and non-fasting groups, and inherently, there may be no significant association between RF and uteroplacental perfusion.

13.2.5 Maternal Weight Gain and Fatigue

A few studies have suggested a statistically significant lower mean weight gain (<1 lb) in pregnant patients who chose to fast Ramadan compared to those who did not [2, 18]. Poor weight gain was also seen in a study in which weight and BMI remained unchanged during the pregnancy of fasting women [15] and another that showed a lower mean increase in maternal weight [2]. Other studies have found no significant difference in maternal weight gain between fasting and non-fasting groups [7, 16]. One study examining the lifestyle changes during Ramadan of patients with gestational and pregestational diabetes in pregnancy found a higher tendency among patients to eat sugar and fatty foods while also decreasing physical exercise and the quality and quantity of sleep [24]. Various studies have indicated that RF is associated with symptoms like fatigue and dehydration due to occurrences of vomiting, diarrhea, and dizziness [18], increased weakness [25], and decreased maternal energy [26]. Mean weight gain likely ranges from equivalent to lower in fasters as compared to non-fasters. RF may also be associated with fatigue. Glazier et al. [8] did not include additional primary or secondary outcomes concerning maternal symptoms in their meta-analysis.

13.2.6 Mode of Delivery

Although various studies have been conducted to investigate whether RF impacts the mode of delivery, most of these studies did not indicate statistically significant findings [2, 9, 17, 27]. One study ($n = 402$) by Awwad et al. [18] found that the cesarean preterm delivery rate was lower in patients who did fast compared to patients who did not fast (28.4% vs. 39.3%; $P = 0.027$). On the other hand, one study ($n = 324$) by Mirghani and Hamud [11] identified a higher rate of cesarean delivery (12% vs. 4.5% for fetal distress in 35% vs. 14%) and induction of labor for post-term or GDM (15.5% vs. 5.8%) among patients who did fast. The data on the association between RF and the mode of delivery are mixed, likely with no significant effect, though some studies conflict, suggesting both lower and higher cesarean section rates.

13.2.7   Placental Weight

A robust systematic review and meta-analysis found that placental weight was significantly lower in maternal fasters compared to non-fasters [7], which was dominated by one large study [28]. However, this study defined Ramadan exposure from birth records and the overlap with the month of Ramadan, with unrecorded RF status. The same author in Saudi Arabia found that mean placental weight and ratio in babies exposed to Ramadan in the second or third trimester were lower than those not exposed in utero (14.4% vs. 14.9% in boys, 14.8% vs.15.1% in girls) [29]. Actual maternal RF status was also unknown in this study. However, no association with neonatal birthweight was found in either group, suggesting that despite the described reduced size, placentas can maintain an adequate level of activity. There may be a decrease in placental weight in fasters, though the significance of this finding is unclear.

13.2.8   Breastfeeding

Various studies have been carried out regarding Muslim women's perspectives on breastfeeding while fasting during Ramadan. Some studies noted that participants viewed it favorably [30], while others cited concerns, including whether breast milk supply decreases while fasting [31–33] and symptoms of thirst, hunger, and general weakness [34]. Studies have tested whether RF could affect the macronutrients produced in breast milk. One study in Sudan ($n = 24$) compared 100 mL breast milk samples taken while fasting during and two weeks after Ramadan. It was found that lactose, sodium, potassium, calcium, phosphate, and protein quantities dropped ($p = 0.01$) in fasters compared to non-fasters [35]. Similarly, another study found a significant decrease in the amount of magnesium, potassium, and zinc produced in the breast milk of fasting participants [36].

Conversely, one study examining whether RF could impact the macronutrients of lactating women ($n = 21$ fasters, 27 non-fasters) of similar education, age, and BMI backgrounds found no substantial change upon examining the protein, lipid, carbohydrate, and energy levels of the breast milk of both fasting and non-fasting participants [37]. Similarly, a UAE study ($n = 26$) found no significant difference in the amount of lactose, protein, triglycerides, cholesterol, fat, total solids, and nonfat solids in breast milk collected while fasting vs. two weeks after the end of Ramadan [38].

A separate study compared growth parameters of exclusively breastfed infants between one and six months of age whose mothers fasted during Ramadan while breastfeeding ($n = 20$) vs. those who did not fast ($n = 35$) [39]. The study found no statistical significance in mean weight, mean height, and mean head circumference between the two groups of children.

Different studies suggest RF may or may not be associated with changes in the macronutrients of breast milk. Studies have noted that participants did not usually share their RF status with physicians, and physicians did not ask [31, 32]. Yate and Soliman recommend that healthcare professionals, especially lactation consultants, offer support and open dialogue with Muslim breastfeeding women to help them navigate the decision-making process regarding fasting during Ramadan, considering both clinical and cultural/religious values [40].

13.3 Fetal Health

13.3.1 Antenatal Parameters and Fetal Testing

Several studies examined the relationship between RF and intrauterine indices and fetal monitoring, which evaluate fetal well-being during pregnancy. Four "medium-quality" studies were carried out, and no notable effects on reactivity of nonstress test (NST), amniotic fluid index (AFI), biophysical profile (BPP), and Doppler indices of the umbilical and middle cerebral arteries were determined [16]. Three other studies found RF may be associated with a decrease in AFI due to maternal dehydration in fasting participants [22, 41, 42].

One cross-sectional observational study, which included RF participants who were more than 30 weeks pregnant, found no change in mean umbilical artery pulsatility index, vertical amniotic pool depth, or fetal bladder volume [43]. BPP measures heart rate, amniotic fluid level, breathing movement, body movement, and muscle tone with two points each for a score out of 10, or 8, as a marker for fetal well-being. This study noted an increase in 6/8 BPP scores in fasting participants compared to their non-fasting counterparts (37% vs. 13.6%, $P = 0.001$), possibly due to a decrease in fetal breathing movements, with lower maternal and fetal glucose levels [43, 44].

A separate cross-sectional observational study noted that fetal heart rate indices did not differ between fasting and non-fasting participants aside from a lower frequency of large accelerations (1.1 vs. 3.6 in the fasting vs. non-fasting group, $P = 0.001$) [44]. Overall, there was no resulting difference in the number of reactive tracings in the fasting group. Oosterwijk et al. [45] conducted a systematic review that included 43 studies published before March 2020. They divided these into three categories, "low," "medium," and "high-quality," and ranked them by study design and size, exposure, outcome, and adjustments. They determined no relationship between RF and most fetal growth indices and antenatal testing metrics. In contrast, a few "medium-quality" studies did find a relationship between RF and a decrease in AFI and antenatal fetal test scores (BPP and NST). The impact of these on ultimate pregnancy outcomes is unclear.

13.3.2 Intrauterine Fetal Growth Indices

A prospective case-control study in Turkey of 106 women in their second and third trimesters during a summertime Ramadan showed the fasting group had a significant increase in fetal head circumference, biparietal diameter (BPD), and femur length (FL) [22]. No difference was seen in abdominal circumference (AC) or fetal weight gain [22]. In contrast, another study ($n = 52$) found there was no statistically significant difference in BPD or FL in addition to AC, fetal weight, and AFI [23] in those who fasted during Ramadan in their second and third trimesters compared to those who did not fast. Conflicting data suggest an increase or no difference in intrauterine growth indices in fasters; a decrease was not observed.

13.3.3 Preterm Birth

A retrospective study of births by Arabic-speaking women in Canada ($n = 78,109$) found a relationship between RF and preterm birth (PTB), where second-trimester fasting was associated with a 1.33 to 1.53 times risk of PTB (delivery at 28–31 weeks) in comparison to not fasting, with risk increasing as participants progressed throughout the second trimester [46]. However, no association was determined between RF and extreme PTB (delivery at 22–27 weeks) or late PTB (delivery at 32–36 weeks), regardless of the trimester of pregnancy. Although understanding of PTB pathophysiology is still growing, authors suggest that one possible explanation for an increase in PTB may be due to a *stress response* triggered by less placental and uterine blood flow, as well as suboptimal metabolic eating patterns [46]. One important limitation of this study was that the "Arabic language" was used as a surrogate for ethnicity and religion in women whose pregnancy time overlapped with one day of Ramadan [1]. As a result, the number of Muslim patients who fasted during pregnancy was not accurately accounted for, making associations found between RF and PTB difficult to interpret. In another study in Saudi Arabia ($n = 967$) [47], in which RF status was also not recorded, newborn girls had a 0.4-week shorter gestation period in mothers in their second trimester during Ramadan than newborn girls who were not in utero in the second trimester during Ramadan.

Awwad et al. [18] found that BMI was the only factor associated with PTB, regardless of fasting trimester and duration. No relationship was determined between RF and PTB in other large-scale reviews, with the majority of studies not finding any correlation [2, 13, 17, 18, 48–50]. Additionally, Glazier et al.'s [8] review ($n = 5600$ pregnancies) did not determine any significant effect of RF on the rate of PTB (OR, 0.99; 95% CI, 0.72–1.37). Likewise, Oosterwijk et al. [45] determined no significant difference in the occurrence of PTB between "medium" and "high-quality" studies examining fasting and non-fasting participants.

13.3.4 Neonatal Birth Weight

In Glazier et al.'s [8] meta-analysis that included 21 studies on the effects of RF on neonatal birthweight, 19,030 of 31,441 pregnancies were not affected by fasting (standard mean difference, 0.03; 95% confidence interval [CI], 0.00–0.05), and no significant influence was found on the proportion of low-birthweight babies (odds ratio [OR], 1.05; 95% CI, 0.87–1.26). Additionally, the meta-analysis showed no single trimester significantly affecting birthweight, and no differences were found between pregnancies in the first, second, or third trimester. Similarly, the results of 13 "medium" and "high-quality" studies found no significant effect on birthweight [7, 11, 17, 26, 28, 45, 48–50] regardless of gestational age [51] in adjusted and non-adjusted analysis for covariables [49]. Oosterwijk et al.'s systematic review [45] did not report any studies that found a statistically significant relationship between neonatal birthweight and the number of fasted days by patients [26, 49, 52].

However, one "high-quality" study in Lebanon ($n = 402$) found that newborns with mothers who chose to fast did show a significantly lower mean birthweight compared to mothers who did not fast (3094 + −467 g vs. 3202 + −473 g, $P = 0.024$). There was no significant difference in neonates less than 2500 grams, the cap for low-birthweight babies. Caloric intake was not accounted for [18]. One study by Almond and Mazumder [53] also found a statistically significant decrease of 50 grams in neonatal birth weight. However, this study was not included in Glazier et al.'s [8] meta-analysis due to its use of Michigan natality data of Arab patients who may not have been Muslim or fasting during Ramadan. Another study ($n = 130$) showed that fasting more than two weeks during the first trimester was associated with a statistically significant decrease ($P = 0.05$) in neonatal birthweight (3226 g) compared to participants fasting two weeks or less (3439 g) or participants who chose not to fast (3421 g). This finding was hypothesized to be secondary to "accelerated starvation," which involves "more rapid and marked metabolic and endocrine alterations" and a potential maladaptive placental response [26, 53]. Yet, no statistically significant difference in neonatal birthweight was determined when fasting later in pregnancy [26]. A more recent systematic review and meta-analysis similarly found no association between RF and neonatal birthweight [54].

Variable findings also illustrate the impact of the duration of RF in terms of the number of hours and number of days, where two of these studies were conducted by the same research group [4, 26] and showed different results. In a study in the Netherlands, a 13- to15-hour summer fast was associated with lower birth weight when fasting for more than 15 days [26]. However, in a study in Indonesia, fasting for more than one day (mean 14 days) during the summer was not associated with a difference in birthweight [4]. This may demonstrate a contribution of differences in cultural and dietary habits, variations in the climate, duration, and the number of fasting days to measured outcomes. Taking the aforementioned data into consideration, though an association with lower birthweight is suggested in several studies, there is no clearly established, clinically significant relationship between RF and neonatal birthweight overall.

13.3.5 Long-Term Outcomes of Offspring

Concerns about long-term effects on offspring may arise when considering the impact of RF on pregnancy. A systematic review, which included 16 retrospective longitudinal studies, found that offspring with in-utero Ramadan exposure during conception or the first trimester may experience negative long-term health and eco-nomic outcomes [55]. Examples of these effects include higher mortality rates for children under 3 months and under 5 years of age, decreased height and BMI, an increase in the number of vision, hearing, and learning disabilities, lower test scores in mathematics, reading, and writing, and a lower probability of owning a home, although the authors acknowledge the evidence is limited [55]. The authors propose an etiology of the first-trimester fasting environment that mostly affects a "fetal pro-gramming theory" and has a lasting lifespan influence on health and well-being [56].

It is important to note that six out of 16 of these studies investigated children of Muslim parents without known Ramadan exposure, and nine investigated children of Ramadan-exposed Muslim mothers who experienced Ramadan during their preg-nancy with unknown fasting status. Only one study identified Ramadan exposure as the offspring of participants who fasted more than 27 days, which found no notable change in children's IQ scores [57]; the other studies included in the systemic review did not clearly identify Ramadan exposure as offspring born to fasting participants. Furthermore, Oosterwijk et al. [45] noted the poor quality of existing articles that examine the cognitive and long-term effects of RF during pregnancy on offspring, with no substantial evidence to support findings. Significant findings were only noted in "low-quality" studies, with "medium-quality" and "high-quality" studies finding few and none, respectively.

One "medium-quality" study by van Ewijk et al. [58] ($n = 12,900$ Muslims and 1220 non-Muslims) noted that adults exposed to Ramadan during gestation had a shorter height (8 mm) and lower BMI (~1 kg) when compared to adults not exposed to Ramadan ($P < 0.05$). While statistically significant, these findings may not be clini-cally important. A separate retrospective study ($n = 759,799$) assessing offspring between 2003 and 2020 from 103 demographic health surveys in 56 countries deter-mined no statistically significant relationship between RF during pregnancy and height or weight stunting in children under age five [59]. One study from Pakistan studying offspring born from 2003 to 2018 under 5 years of age and exposed to Ramadan deter-mined a substantial risk of stunted growth and lower BMI [60]. Results showed off-spring experiencing a 22% higher risk of stunted growth when exposed to Ramadan during the fourth month of pregnancy and a 20% higher risk of being underweight when exposed during the third month of pregnancy [60]. Another study in Tunisia [61] found intergenerational effects of RF; offspring whose mothers had been in utero dur-ing Ramadan were smaller and thinner and had smaller placentas than those whose mothers had not been in utero during Ramadan. These findings were also seen in off-spring who themselves were exposed to Ramadan in late gestation, independent of maternal intrauterine exposure and independent of the trimester of Ramadan exposure. However, this study similarly did not identify the mother's fasting status.

Another study conducted by van Ewijk [62] showed that offspring exposed to Ramadan during gestation ($n = 43,643$ from the Indonesian Family Life Survey) exhibited worse general health (standard deviation 6.1%) as rated by providers using various health metrics like anemia, chest pain, and wound healing time in exposed Muslims. This finding was particularly evident in the offspring of mothers greater than 45 years of age (18.5%; $P < 0.01$) and offspring exposed to Ramadan during the second trimester.

Again, these studies do not clearly define "Ramadan exposure" as having specifically fasted during Ramadan. Various studies claim that Ramadan exposure may indeed have long-term effects on children [55, 58, 62], while other studies do not [59]. Oosterwijk et al. [45] deem the quality of the data inadequate. It is difficult to definitively extrapolate or conclude long-term effects on offspring, especially due to misclassification bias, since offspring not exposed to RF (just to Ramadan generally) may be conflated with offspring that were exposed to RF in many of these studies. Additionally, there is a need for more "high-quality" data on cognitive outcomes to further understand the long-term effects of RF on children. Despite these limitations, the evidence currently available suggests long-term effects on offspring may exist if one chooses to fast during pregnancy.

13.4 Limitations

The available data on the impact of RF on maternal and fetal health have many limitations with regard to study size and design. There is a wide range of definitions of "Ramadan fasting," from fasting periods to utilizing patient ethnicity, language, or geography as profiling substitutes to identify intersections between pregnancy and the month of Ramadan, leading to misclassification and confounding with "Ramadan exposure" rather than RF [29, 46]. Practically, roughly 75% of all children born to Muslim mothers are potentially exposed to RF [53]. This exposure may mean active fasting or participating in common practices of the month. In studies in which RF status was recorded, there is inconsistency in the duration of fasting in terms of the number of days: many studies did not report this, while others defined fasting as >1 day and others as >27 days. Studies also varied in the length of the daily fast in hours: the variation in geographic regions and seasons results in a wide range of possible fasting hours, from anywhere between 9 to 22 hours. Gestational age during the fast is not always recorded, and the outcomes reported are not specifically correlated with fasting in a specific trimester. In very few studies is the nutritional intake, with the variation in consumption of different types and quantities of food in Ramadan, controlled for or recorded, and it is often based on recall in questionnaires when recorded. Investigators did not always account for differences in participant age, parity, socioeconomic status, prepregnancy BMI, and sleep patterns (given possible longer nocturnal wake periods for prayer or other exercises during Ramadan). There was a large variation in the number of participants, from the multiple of thousands in studies based on databases, where RF status is usually unknown, to multiples of tens to low one hundreds in the more informative studies.

13.5 Conclusion

The existing literature shows mixed evidence on the associations between RF during pregnancy and maternal and fetal outcomes, but it has many limitations. The limitations in existing data highlight the need for further research, especially for studies that uniformly define "Ramadan exposure" as true RF, control for the duration of time fasted in hours and days, and stratify by trimester of fasting on all outcomes discussed above. Further research is also needed to elucidate the effects on less-studied outcomes, such as GDM, hypertension, stillbirth, neonatal death, and admission to the neonatal intensive care unit.

Given these limitations, it is important to be able to interpret these data and utilize them to provide individualized recommendations to patients who seek input from their perinatal care provider on whether RF contributes to undue hardship or maternal or fetal harm. Shahawy et al. [1] provide a counseling framework for perinatal care providers to engage with their patients in shared decision-making, including a patient infographic.

References

1. Shahawy S, Al Kassab L, Rattani A. Ramadan fasting and pregnancy: an evidence-based guide for the obstetrician. Am J Obstet Gynecol. 2023;228(6):689–95.
2. Safari K, Piro TJ, Ahmad HM. Perspectives and pregnancy outcomes of maternal Ramadan fasting in the second trimester of pregnancy. BMC Pregnancy Childbirth. 2019;19(1):128.
3. Seiermann AU, Al-Mufti H, Waid JL, Wendt AS, Sobhan S, Gabrysch S. Women's fasting habits and dietary diversity during Ramadan in rural Bangladesh. Matern Child Nutr. 2021;17(3):e13135.
4. van Bilsen LA, Savitri AI, Amelia D, Baharuddin M, Grobbee DE, Uiterwaal CSPM. Predictors of Ramadan fasting during pregnancy. J Epidemiol Global Health. 2016;6(4):267–75.
5. Faris MAIE, Al-Holy MA. Implications of Ramadan intermittent fasting on maternal and fetal health and nutritional status: a review. Mediterr J Nutr Metab. 2014;7(2):107–18.
6. Bisson C, Dautel S, Patel E, Suresh S, Dauer P, Rana S. Preeclampsia pathophysiology and adverse outcomes during pregnancy and postpartum. Front Med (Lausanne). 2023;10:1144170.
7. Ozturk E, Balat O, Ugur MG, Yazıcıoglu C, Pence S, Erel Ö, et al. Effect of Ramadan fasting on maternal oxidative stress during the second trimester: a preliminary study. J Obstet Gynaecol Res. 2011;37(7):729–33.
8. Glazier JD, Hayes DJL, Hussain S, D'Souza SW, Whitcombe J, Heazell AEP, et al. The effect of Ramadan fasting during pregnancy on perinatal outcomes: a systematic review and meta-analysis. BMC Pregnancy Childbirth. 2018;18(1):421.
9. Hossain N, Samuel M, Mughal S, Shafique K. Ramadan fasting: perception and maternal outcomes during pregnancy. Pak J Med Sci. 2021;37(5):1262–7.
10. Baynouna Al Ketbi LM, Niglekerke NJ, Zein Al Deen SM, Mirghani H. Diet restriction in Ramadan and the effect of fasting on glucose levels in pregnancy. BMC Res Notes. 2014;7(1):392.
11. Mirghani HM, Hamud OA. The effect of maternal diet restriction on pregnancy outcome. Am J Perinatol. 2006;23(01):021–4.
12. Ismail NAM, Olaide Raji H, Abd Wahab N, Mustafa N, Kamaruddin NA, Abdul JM. Glycemic control among pregnant diabetic women on insulin who fasted during Ramadan. Iran J Med Sci. 2011;36(4):254–9.
13. AlMogbel TA, Ross G, Wu T, Molyneaux L, Constantino MI, McGill M, et al. Ramadan and gestational diabetes: maternal and neonatal outcomes. Acta Diabetol. 2022;59(1):21–30.
14. Afandi BO, Hassanein MM, Majd LM, Nagelkerke NJD. Impact of Ramadan fasting on glucose levels in women with gestational diabetes mellitus treated with diet alone or diet plus metformin: a continuous glucose monitoring study. BMJ Open Diabetes Res Care. 2017;5(1):e000470.

15. Khoshdel A, Kheiri S, Hashemi-Dehkordi E, Nasiri J, Shabanian-Borujeni S, Saedi E. The effect of Ramadan fasting on LH, FSH, estrogen, progesterone, and leptin in pregnant women. J Obstet Gynaecol. 2014;34(7):634–8.
16. Dikensoy E, Balat O, Cebesoy B, Ozkur A, Cicek H, Can G. The effect of Ramadan fasting on maternal serum lipids, cortisol levels, and fetal development. Arch Gynecol Obstet. 2008;279(2):119.
17. Hızlı D, Yılmaz SS, Onaran Y, Kafalı H, Danışman N, Mollamahmutoğlu L. Impact of maternal fasting during Ramadan on fetal Doppler parameters, maternal lipid levels and neonatal outcomes. J Matern Fetal Neonatal Med. 2012;25(7):975–7.
18. Awwad J, Usta I, Succar J, Musallam K, Ghazeeri G, Nassar A. The effect of maternal fasting during Ramadan on preterm delivery: a prospective cohort study. BJOG. 2012;119(11):1379–86.
19. Dikensoy E, Balat O, Cebesoy B, Ozkur A, Cicek H, Can G. Effect of fasting during Ramadan on fetal development and maternal health. J Obstet Gynaecol Res. 2008;34(4):494–8.
20. Gur E, Turan G, Ince O, Karadeniz M, Tatar S, Kasap E, et al. Effect of Ramadan fasting on metabolic markers, dietary intake and abdominal fat distribution in pregnancy. Hippokratia. 2015;19(4):298–303.
21. Barati M, Shahbazian N, Ahmadi L, Masihi S. Diagnostic evaluation of uterine artery Doppler sonography for the prediction of adverse pregnancy outcomes. J Res Med Sci. 2014;19(6):515–9.
22. Sakar MN, Gultekin H, Demir B, Bakir VL, Balsak D, Vuruskan E, et al. Ramadan fasting and pregnancy: implications for fetal development in the summer season. J Perinat Med. 2015;43(3):319–23.
23. Moradi M. The effect of Ramadan fasting on fetal growth and Doppler indices of pregnancy. J Res Med Sci. 2011;16(2):165–9.
24. Leila B, Salma B, Haraj NE, El AS, Chadli A. Impact of Ramadan on the course of diabetic pregnancy. In: Endocrine Abstracts. Bioscientifica; 2023 [cited 2024 Mar 2]. Available from: https://www.endocrine-abstracts.org/ea/0090/ea0090ep335
25. Mubeen SM, Mansoor S, Hussain A, Qadir S. Perceptions and practices of fasting in Ramadan during pregnancy in Pakistan. Iran J Nurs Midwifery Res. 2012;17(7):467–71.
26. Savitri AI, Amelia D, Painter RC, Baharuddin M, Roseboom TJ, Grobbee DE, et al. Ramadan during pregnancy and birth weight of newborns. J Nutr Sci. 2018;7:e5.
27. Jamilian M, Hekmatpou D, Jamilian HR, Ardalan SH, Shamsi M. The effect of Ramadan fasting on outcome of pregnancy. J Sci Res. 2015;23(7):1270–5.
28. Alwasel SH, Abotalib Z, Aljarallah JS, Osmond C, Alkharaz SM, Alhazza IM, et al. Secular increase in placental weight in Saudi Arabia. Placenta. 2011;32(5):391–4.
29. Alwasel SH, Abotalib Z, Aljarallah JS, Osmond C, Alkharaz SM, Alhazza IM, et al. Changes in placental size during Ramadan. Placenta. 2010;31(7):607–10.
30. Al-Qahtani AM, Mohamed H, Ahmed AM. Knowledge, attitude, and practice of Saudi women in the Najran area towards breastfeeding during Ramadan. Sudan J Paediatr. 2020;20(1):42–8.
31. Ertem IO, Kaynak G, Kaynak C, Ulukol B, Gulnar SB. Attitudes and practices of breastfeeding mothers regarding fasting in Ramadan. Child Care Health Dev. 2001;27(6):545–54.
32. Özsoy S, Adana F, Uyar HH. Fasting behavior of breastfeeding mothers in Ramadan. HealthMED. 2014;8:102–7.
33. Gunduz S, Usak E, Karacan C. Does Ramadan fasting influence breastmilk? HealthMED. 2013;7:837–41.
34. Lakho NUSRAT, Saeed S, Mahmood A, Lakho S, Madhu Das C, Shaikh NB. Health beliefs and breastfeeding practices during Ramadan fasting. Pak J Med Health Sci. 2021;15(4):1371–3.
35. Salah ET, Malik NME, Hassan MS, Mohammed IA, Mohamed M, Mohamed MO, et al. How does the fasting of Ramadan affect breast Milk constituents? Sudan J Med Sci. 2016;11(1):17–22.
36. Rakicioğlu N, Samur G, Topçu A, Topçu AA. The effect of Ramadan on maternal nutrition and composition of breast milk. Pediatr Int. 2006;48(3):278–83.

37. Başıbüyük M, Karabayır N, Aktaç Ş, Kundakçı S, Büke Ö. Breast milk macronutrients in fasting vs. non-fasting lactating women. 2024.; Available from: https://avesis.marmara.edu.tr/yayin/52a2cfa8-f57b-44f2-84cc-7e61fdc968bd/breast-milk-macronutrients-in-fasting-vs-nonfasting-lactating-women
38. Bener A, Galadari S, Gillett M, Osman N, Al-Taneiji H, Al-Kuwaiti MHH, et al. Fasting during the holy month of Ramadan does not change the composition of breast milk. Nutr Res. 2001;21(6):859–64.
39. Haratipour H, Sohrabi MB, Ghasemi E, Karimi A, Zolfaghari P, Yahyaei E. Impact of maternal fasting during Ramadan on growth parameters of exclusively breastfed infants in Shahroud, 2012. J Nutr Fasting Health. 2013;1(2):66–9.
40. Yate Z, Abdelghani Soliman SM. Lactation assessment for Muslim breastfeeding women who fast during Ramadan: understanding an Islamic legal dispensation. J Hum Lact. 2022;38(3):525–30.
41. Seckin KD, Yeral MI, Karslı MF, Gultekin IB. Effect of maternal fasting for religious beliefs on fetal sonographic findings and neonatal outcomes. Int J Gynecol Obstet. 2014;126(2):123–5.
42. Karateke A, Kaplanoglu M, Avci F, Kurt RK, Baloglu A. The effect of Ramadan fasting on fetal development. Pak J Med Sci. 2015;31(6):1295–9.
43. Mirghani HM, Weerasinghe DSL, Ezimokhai M, Smith JR. The effect of maternal fasting on the fetal biophysical profile. Int J Gynecol Obstet. 2003;81(1):17–21.
44. Mirghani HM, Weerasinghe S, Al-Awar S, Abdulla L, Ezimokhai M. The effect of intermittent maternal fasting on computerized fetal heart tracing. J Perinatol. 2005;25(2):90–2.
45. Oosterwijk VNL, Molenaar JM, van Bilsen LA, Kiefte-de Jong JC. Ramadan fasting during pregnancy and health outcomes in offspring: a systematic review. Nutrients. 2021;13(10):3450.
46. Tith RM, Bilodeau-Bertrand M, Lee GE, Healy-Profitós J, Auger N. Fasting during Ramadan increases risk of very preterm birth among Arabic-speaking women. J Nutr. 2019;149(10):1826–32.
47. Alwasel SH, et al. Sex differences in birth size and intergenerational effects of intrauterine exposure to Ramadan in Saudi Arabia. Am J Hum Biol. 2011;23(5):651–4.
48. Abd-Allah Rezk M, Sayyed T, Abo-Elnasr M, Shawky M, Badr H. Impact of maternal fasting on fetal well-being parameters and fetal–neonatal outcome: a case-control study. J Matern Fetal Neonatal Med. 2016;29(17):2834–8.
49. Petherick ES, Tuffnell D, Wright J. Experiences and outcomes of maternal Ramadan fasting during pregnancy: results from a sub-cohort of the born in Bradford birth cohort study. BMC Pregnancy Childbirth. 2014;14(1):335.
50. Ziaee V, Kihanidoost Z, Younesian M, Akhavirad MB, Bateni F, Kazemianfar Z, et al. The effect of Ramadan fasting on outcome of pregnancy. Iran J Pediatr. 2010;20(2):181–6.
51. Cross JH, Eminson J, Wharton BA. Ramadan and birth weight at full term in Asian Muslim pregnant women in Birmingham. Arch Dis Child. 1990;65(10):1053–6.
52. Jürges H. Ramadan fasting, sex-ratio at birth, and birth weight: no effects on Muslim infants born in Germany. Econ Lett. 2015;137:13–6.
53. Almond D, Mazumder B. Health capital and the prenatal environment: the effect of maternal fasting during pregnancy. National Bureau of Economic Research; 2008 [cited 2022 Jan 8]. (Working Paper Series). Report No.: 14428. Available from: http://www.nber.org/papers/w14428
54. Chen YE, Loy SL, Chen LW. Chrononutrition during pregnancy and its association with maternal and offspring outcomes: a systematic review and meta-analysis of Ramadan and non-Ramadan studies. Nutrients. 2023;15(3):756.
55. Mahanani MR, Abderbwih E, Wendt AS, Deckert A, Antia K, Horstick O, et al. Long-term outcomes of in utero Ramadan exposure: a systematic literature review. Nutrients. 2021;13(12):4511.
56. Van Ewijk R, Pradella F. Ramadan during pregnancy and offspring health over the life course: a systematic review. Eur J Pub Health. 2023;33(Supplement_2):ckad160.1519.
57. Azizi S, et al. Intellectual development of children born of mothers who fasted in Ramadan during pregnancy. Int J Vitam Nutr Res. 2004;74(5):374–80.

58. van Ewijk RJG, Painter RC, Roseboom TJ. Associations of prenatal exposure to Ramadan with small stature and thinness in adulthood: results from a large Indonesian population-based study. Am J Epidemiol. 2013;177(8):729–36.
59. Chu H, Goli S, Rammohan A. *In utero* Ramadan exposure and child nutrition. J Dev Orig Health Dis. 2023;14(1):96–109.
60. Chaudhry TT, Mir A. The impact of prenatal exposure to Ramadan on child anthropomorphic outcomes in Pakistan. Matern Child Health J. 2021;25(7):1136–46.
61. Alwasel SH, et al. Intergenerational effects of in utero exposure to Ramadan in Tunisia. Am J Hum Biol. 2013;25(3):341–3.
62. van Ewijk R. Long-term health effects on the next generation of Ramadan fasting during pregnancy. J Health Econ. 2011;30(6):1246–60.

Chapter 14
Ramadan Fasting and Sports Performance

Mohamed Kerkeni, Manel Kerkeni, Omar Boukhris, and Hamdi Chtourou

Abstract In the last decade, there has been a significant focus on examining the effects of Ramadan fasting on Muslim athletes. Ramadan, one of the five pillars of Islam, mandates that nondisabled Muslims refrain from eating, drinking, engaging in sexual activity, and smoking from sunrise to sunset for 29–30 days each year. Restricting energy intake to nighttime, along with additional social and religious activities, can disrupt regular sleep and normal eating patterns for those who fast, which may negatively affect athletic performance. Scientific studies have shown conflicting findings regarding the impact of Ramadan observance on athletic performance. Systematic reviews with meta-analyses have found that Ramadan fasting has a negative effect on mean and peak power during afternoon anaerobic Wingate cycle exercises, as well as on morning sprint running performance. However, no associations have been observed with strength, jump height, fatigue index (FI), or aerobic performance. Despite the lack of adjustments to the sports calendar to accommodate religious requirements, Ramadan fasting presents a challenge for Muslim athletes who are required to

M. Kerkeni · M. Kerkeni
High Institute of Sport and Physical Education, University of Sfax, Sfax, Tunisia

Research laboratory, Education, Motricity, Sport and Health (EM2S), LR15JS01, High Institute of Sport and Physical Education, University of Sfax, Sfax, Tunisia

O. Boukhris
Sport, Performance, and Nutrition Research Group, School of Allied Health, Human Services, and Sport, La Trobe University, Melbourne, VIC, Australia

SIESTA Research Group, School of Allied Health, Human Services and Sport, La Trobe University, Melbourne, VIC, Australia

H. Chtourou (✉)
High Institute of Sport and Physical Education, University of Sfax, Sfax, Tunisia

Physical Activity, Sport, and Health, UR18JS01, National Observatory of Sport, Tunis, Tunisia
e-mail: hamdi.chtourou@isseps.usf.tn

compete or prepare for important events while fasting. They are unable to consume nutrients and fluids for recovery during daylight competitions or training sessions, which can negatively affect their hydration and nutritional status. Additionally, Muslim athletes observing Ramadan may face a competitive disadvantage depending on their sport, the time of day, and the environmental conditions during physical activities. This chapter examines the impact of Ramadan fasting on performance during exercise testing and explore the potential mechanisms behind the performance decline noted in some studies during this month.

Keywords Muslims · Athletes · Performance · Ramadan · Fasting · Sport

14.1 Introduction

Ramadan, the ninth month of the Islamic lunar calendar, is a period of spiritual reflection and self-discipline observed by Muslims worldwide. During this month, Muslims refrain from eating, drinking, and engaging in other activities from sunrise to sunset for about 29–30 days [1]. This practice, known as fasting, is one of the fundamental pillars of Islam. While Ramadan is a deeply spiritual experience, it can also pose unique challenges, particularly for athletes who are required to maintain peak physical performance. The duration of Ramadan fasting varies based on geographic location and time of year, ranging from approximately 10 h to over 18 h per day [2, 3]. This variability, coupled with the potential for dehydration and sleep disturbances, could significantly impact an athlete's physical capacity and athletic performance.

Numerous studies have been conducted in the last two decades to investigate the influence of Ramadan fasting on athletic performance. However, these studies have produced contrasting results. Consequently, an increasing number of systematic reviews, some including meta-analyses, have been conducted on this topic. These reviews provide a chance to integrate and summarize the collective findings from published studies on Ramadan fasting and athletic performance [4–6].

Some studies have indicated that the decline in physical performance observed during Ramadan may be caused by several factors [4, 5]. These factors include lower muscle glycogen stores, dehydration, and sleep disturbances [4, 5]. However, other studies have discovered that there is no significant correlation between fasting during Ramadan and performance in specific athletic disciplines. These studies indicated that implementing appropriate nutritional and hydration strategies, as well as adopting mental resilience, could help alleviate any possible detrimental effects [5].

Despite the absence of adjustments to the sports calendar to accommodate religious requirements, Muslim athletes face the challenge of participating in competitions or preparing for crucial events while fasting during Ramadan (e.g., Olympic Games 2012, 2016; World Cup 2014; Mediterranean Games 2018; World Cup 2018) [7, 8]. As a result, numerous studies have been undertaken to assess how

Ramadan fasting affects physical performance, identify factors contributing to any potential decline, and propose strategies for athletes to sustain their fitness and performance during this period.

Considering these factors, this chapter aims to provide a comprehensive review of the current literature on the impact of Ramadan fasting on physical performance.

14.2 Effect of Ramadan Observance on Sports Performance

Concerning the jumping performance during Ramadan observance, inconclusive results have been reported by seven studies [9–15] (Table 14.1). In this context, it has been shown that jumping performance (i.e., vertical jump [10, 14], squat jump [12], countermovement jump [12], and 5-jump performance [15]) did not change during Ramadan observance in comparison with control periods. However, three studies reported that Ramadan observance decreased performance in the squat jump [13], countermovement jump [11, 13], and 30-s repeated jump test [12]. Conversely, Bouhlel et al. [14] found higher post-RSA vertical jump performances at the end of Ramadan (ER) than before Ramadan (BR). Similarly, Zerguini et al. [9] showed better vertical jump performance at ER compared to after Ramadan (AR).

Concerning the agility performance during Ramadan observance (Table 14.2), no changes in agility performance (i.e., the 4-line test [10] and the 4×10 m agility test [11]) were observed between periods during and before Ramadan. However, Zerguini et al. [9] found that 4-line test results were higher both at ER and AR than at BR.

Concerning maximal voluntary contraction (MVIC) during Ramadan observance (Table 14.3), it has been reported that MVIC was lower during Ramadan observance compared to BR [13, 16, 20]. On the other hand, Aloui et al. [13] reported that MVIC recorded immediately and 5 min after the RSA test were unchanged during Ramadan observance. Likewise, Zarrouk et al. [18, 19] reported no significant effect of Ramadan on MVIC.

Regarding the sprint performance during Ramadan observance (Table 14.4), inconclusive results have been reported by five studies [9–12, 21]. Three studies revealed no changes in sprint performance between periods during and outside Ramadan [10–12]. However, it has been reported that speed in the 20 m sprint decreased at ER and AR compared to BR, time in the 5 m sprint decreased at AR compared to BR, time in the 10 m sprint decreased at AR compared to ER, and time in the 20 m sprint did not change between periods [9]. Similarly, Aziz et al. [21] reported that speed attained at 0–15, 45–60, 60–75, and 75–90 min was lower during Ramadan observance compared to BR, and speed attained at 15–30 and 30–45 min did not change between periods before and during Ramadan.

Concerning the Wingate test during Ramadan observance (Table 14.5), although Abedelmalek et al. [27], Chtourou et al. [25, 26], and Souissi et al. [23] found decreases in peak and mean power compared to BR, Abedelmalek et al. [24]

Table 14.1 Influence of Ramadan on jumping ability

Study	Sample size	Age	Sex	Activity (level of practice)	Training schedule	Fasting period	Assessment periods	Test outcomes	Effect
Zerguini et al. [9]	55	17 to 34	Male	Soccer (professional)	NM	~12–13 h	BR; ER; AR	Vertical jump (cm)	↓ at AR vs. ER
Kirkendall et al. [10]	Fasting (n = 21)	18 ± 1	Male	Soccer (professional)	Each session had a duration of 60 to 80 minutes	~12.5–13.5 h	BR; SWR; ER	Vertical jump (cm)	No change
	Non-fasting (n = 18)								No change
Meckel et al. [11]	19	15.1 ± 0.9	Male	Soccer (first division youth league)	Weekly training time decreased from an average of 6.4 h (before Ramadan) to 4.5 h during Ramadan	NM	BR; ER	Countermovement jump (cm)	↓ at ER vs. BR
Chaouachi et al. [12]	15	18 ± 1	Male	Judo (elite)	The training schedule consisted of 9 sessions per week, averaging 17 h total, with workouts lasting at least 2 h per day, 6 days a week	~12–13 h	BR; MR; ER; AR	Height and peak power during squat jump	No change
								Height and peak power during countermovement jump	No change
								30-s repeated jumps test	↓ at ER vs. BR

								Squat jump (cm)	↓ at ER vs. BR
Alouni et al. [13]	12	13.3 ± 0.4	Male	Soccer (NM)	NM	15 h	BR; ER	Countermovement jump (cm)	↓ at ER vs. BR
Bouhlel et al. [14]	10	18.8 ± 1	Male	Boxing (amateur)	5 × 1.5 h per week	15 h	BR; FWR; ER	Vertical jump before the RSA test	No change
								Vertical jump after RSA test	↑ at ER vs. BR
Hsouna et al. [15]	12	21.9 ± 2.4	Male	Running (moderately trained)	At least 3 h/week	16–17 h	BR; FR; ER; AR10; AR20	5-jump performance	No change

↓ = decrease, ↑ = increase, *NM* not mentioned, *RSA* repeated sprint ability, *AR* after Ramadan, *AR10* after 10 days of Ramadan, *AR20* after 20 days of Ramadan, *BR* before Ramadan, *ER* end of Ramadan, *FR* first 10 days of Ramadan, *FWR* first week of Ramadan, *MR* middle of Ramadan, *SWR* second week of Ramadan, *vs.* versus

Table 14.2 Influence of Ramadan observance on agility performance

Study	Sample size	Age	Sex	Activity (level of practice)	Training schedule	Fasting period	Assessment periods	Test outcomes	Effect
Zerguini et al. [9]	55	17 to 34	Male	Soccer (professional)	NM	~12–13 h	BR; ER; AR	Performance during the 4-line test (s)	↑ at ER and AR vs. BR
Kirkendall et al. [10]	Fasting (n = 21)	18 ± 1	Male	Soccer (professional)	Each session had a duration of 60 to 80 min	~12.5–13.5 h	BR; SWR; ER	Performance during the 4-line test (s)	No change
	Non-fasting (n = 18)								No change
Meckel et al. [11]	19	15.1 ± 0.9	Male	Soccer (first division youth league)	Weekly training time decreased from an average of 6.4 h (before Ramadan) to 4.5 h during Ramadan	NM	BR; ER	Performance in the 4 × 10 meter agility test (seconds)	No change

↓ = decrease, ↑ = increase, *BR* before Ramadan, *ER* end of Ramadan, *NM* not mentioned, *SWR* second week of Ramadan, *AR* after Ramadan, *vs.* versus

Table 14.3 Influence of Ramadan observance on maximal voluntary contraction

Study	Sample size	Age	Sex	Activity (level of practice)	Training schedule	Fasting period	Assessment periods	Test outcomes	Effect
Brisswalter et al. [16]	Fasting ($n = 9$)	23.6 ± 2.9	Male	Running (well trained)	Three weekly sessions include: Slow running (30 min) and intermittent running (30 s run-30 s rest) at maximal aerobic speed (100% MAS) Slow running (30 min) and two sets of 6 repetitions of 300 meters at 100% MAS Slow running (20 min) and four sets of 4-min intervals at specific competition running speed	NM	BR; ER	Maximal voluntary isometric contraction (MVIC)	↓ at ER vs. BR
	Non-fasting ($n = 9$)								No change
Aloui et al. [17]	12	20.1 ± 1.6	Male	Soccer (Tunisian amateur league)	Approximately 10 h of training per week	~16 h	BR; SWR; ER; AR	MVIC before RSA test (N)	↓ at SWR and ER vs. BR
								MVIC immediately after RSA test (N)	No change
								MVIC at 5 min after RSA test (N)	No change

(continued)

Table 14.3 (continued)

Study	Sample size	Age	Sex	Activity (level of practice)	Training schedule	Fasting period	Assessment periods	Test outcomes	Effect
Zarrouk et al. [18]	8	17.2 ± 0.5	Male	Karate (amateur)	5 × 2 h per week	14 h	BR; FWR; ER	Isometric maximal force of the knee extensors	No change
								Isometric muscle endurance of the knee extensors	No change
Zarrouk et al. [19]	8	17.2 ± 0.5	Male	Karate (amateur)	6 × 2 h per week	14 h	BR; FWR; ER	MVIC	No change
								Absolute endurance time at 75% MVC (Tlim) of elbow flexion	No change
Gueldich et al. [20]	10	22.06 ± 1.98	Male	NM	3 × 1.5 h per week	~16 h	BR; FWR; ER; AR	MVIC	↓ at FWR and at ER vs. BR

↓ = decrease, ↑ = increase, *RSA* repeated sprint ability, *AR* after Ramadan, *BR* before Ramadan, *ER* end of Ramadan, *FWR* first week of Ramadan, *MVIC* maximal voluntary isometric contraction, *SWR* second week of Ramadan, *vs.* versus, *NM* not mentioned

Table 14.4 Influence of Ramadan observance on sprint performance

Study	Sample size	Age	Sex	Activity (level of practice)	Training schedule	Fasting period	Assessment periods	Test outcomes	Effect
Zerguini et al. [9]	55	17 to 34	Male	Soccer (professional)	NM	~12–13 h	BR; ER; AR	Sprint speed in the 20-meter (m/s)	↓ at ER and at AR vs. BR
								Time for the 5-meter sprint (in seconds)	↓ at AR vs. BR
								Time for the 10-meter sprint (in seconds)	↓ at AR vs. ER
								Time in the 20 m sprint (seconds)	No change
Kirkendall et al. [10]	Fasting (n = 21)	18 ± 1	Male	Soccer (professional)	Each session had a duration of 60–80 min	~12.5–13.5 h	BR; SWR; ER	Time in the 10 m sprint (seconds)	No change
								Time for the 30-meter sprint (in seconds)	No change
								FI in the 10 m sprint (%)	No change
								FI in the 30 m sprint (%)	No change
	Non-fasting (n = 18)							Time for the 10-meter sprint (in seconds)	No change
								Time for the 30-meter sprint (in seconds)	No change
								FI in the 10 m sprint (%)	No change
								FI in the 30 m sprint (%)	No change
Meckel et al. [11]	19	15.1 ± 0.9	Male	Soccer (first division youth league)	Weekly training time decreased from an average of 6.4 h (before Ramadan) to 4.5 h during Ramadan	NM	BR; ER	Time in the 40 m sprint (seconds)	No change

(continued)

Table 14.4 (continued)

Study	Sample size	Age	Sex	Activity (level of practice)	Training schedule	Fasting period	Assessment periods	Test outcomes	Effect
Chaouachi et al. [12]	15	18 ± 1	Male	Judo (elite)	The training schedule consisted of 9 sessions per week, averaging 17 h total, with workouts lasting at least 2 h per day, 6 days a week	~12–13 h	BR; MR; ER; AR	Time for the 5-meter sprint (in seconds)	No change
								Time for the 10-meter sprint (in seconds)	No change
								Time for the 30-meter sprint (in seconds)	No change
Aziz et al. [21]	13	20.1 ± 0.9	Male	Soccer (amateur)	BR: 4 sessions per week + one league match at the end of the week; during Ramdan 2 or 3 sessions per week without a competitive match	~14 h	BR: During Ramadan	Speed attained at 0–15 min	↓during Ramadan vs. BR
								Speed attained at 15–30 min	No change
								The speed attained at 30–45 min	No change
								Speed attained at 45–60 min	↓during Ramadan vs. BR
								Speed attained at 60–75 min	↓during Ramadan vs. BR
								Speed attained at 75–90 min	↓during Ramadan vs. BR

↓ = decrease, ↑ = increase, *BR* before Ramadan, *ER* end of Ramadan, *FR* first 10 days of Ramadan, *MR* middle of Ramadan, *NM* not mentioned, *AR* after Ramadan, *SWR* second week of Ramadan, *vs.* versus

Table 14.5 Influence of Ramadan observance on Wingate test performance

Study	Sample size	Age	Sex	Activity (level of practice)	Training schedule	Fasting period	Assessment periods	Test outcomes	Effect
Karli et al. [22]	10	22.30 ± 1.25	Male	Athletes specializing in power sports: 7 sprinters, two wrestlers, and one thrower (elite level)	A minimum of four years dedicated to rigorous training, with athletes consistently engaging in sessions exceeding 2 h, 6 days per week	NM	BR; ER; AR	PP (w)	↑ at ER and AR vs. BR
								MP (W)	No change
								FI (%)	No change
Souissi et al. [23]	12	22.6 ± 1.3	Male	NM (physical education students)	NM	NM	BR; SWR; ER; AR	Pmax (W. Kg^{-1})	↓ at SWR and at ER vs. BR
								PP (W. Kg^{-1})	↓ at SWR and at ER vs. BR
								MP (W. Kg^{-1})	↓ at ER vs. BR
Abedelmalek et al. [24]	9	22.1 ± 0.2	Male	NM (physical education students)	NM	16 h	FWR; ER; AR	PP (W/kg)	No change
								MP (W/ kg)	No change
								FI (%)	No change

(continued)

Table 14.5 (continued)

Study	Sample size	Age	Sex	Activity (level of practice)	Training schedule	Fasting period	Assessment periods	Test outcomes	Effect
Chtourou et al. [25]	20	18 ± 1	Male	Soccer (Tunisian junior football team)	2 h a day, 4 days a week	15–16 h	BR; SWR; ER	PP (W·kg^{-1})	↓ at SWR and at ER vs. BR
								MP (W·kg^{-1})	↓ at SWR and at ER vs. BR
								FI (%)	↑ at SWR and at ER vs. BR
Chtourou et al. [26]	10	17.0 ± 0.5	Male	Soccer (Tunisian junior football team)	2 h a day, 4 days a week	15–16 h	BR; SWR; ER	PP (W·kg^{-1})	↓ at SWR and at ER vs. BR
								MP (W·kg^{-1})	↓ at SWR and at ER vs. BR
								FI (%)	↑ at SWR and at ER vs. BR
Abedelmalek et al. [27]	11	22.11 ± 0.2	Male	Soccer (NM)	3 times per week	15 h	BR; FWR; ER	PP (W/kg)	↓ at ER vs. BR and FWR
								MP (W/kg)	↓ at ER vs. BR and FWR
								IF (%)	No change

↓ = decrease, ↑ = increase, *BR* before Ramadan, *FI* fatigue index, *MP* mean power, *NM* not mentioned, *Pmax* maximal power, *PP* peak power, *ER* end of Ramadan, *AR* after Ramadan, *SWR* second week of Ramadan, *vs.* versus reported no significant changes in peak and mean power between periods during and outside Ramadan. Karli et al. [22] showed an increase in peak power at ER and AR compared to BR and no change in mean power. On the other hand, Chtourou et al. [25, 26] reported that the fatigue index (FI) during the Wingate test was higher during Ramadan observance compared to BR. However, Karli et al. [22] and Abedelmalek et al. [24, 27] showed that FI during the Wingate test did not change between periods during and outside Ramadan.

Nine studies have examined how observing Ramadan affects repeated sprint performance (Table 14.6). Concerning repeated cycling exercise, although Chtourou et al. [25] and Hammouda et al. [29] reported that total work was lower during Ramadan compared to BR, no changes in total work were observed in the study by Aloui et al. [17] between periods during and outside Ramadan. However, concerning FI, an increase during Ramadan compared to BR was observed in the study of Chtourou et al. [25], a decrease during Ramadan compared to BR was observed in the study of Aloui et al. [17], and no changes between periods of before and during Ramadan were observed in the study of Hammouda et al. [29]. Nevertheless, Bouhlel et al. [14] showed that 10×6 s repeated sprints on a cycle ergometer decreased during the first week of Ramadan compared to BR and recovered at the ER. Concerning repeated running exercise, Meckel et al. [11] reported that total distance (TD) time and performance decrement during 6×40 m sprints increased at ER compared to BR. However, Girard and Farooq [28] reported an increase in cumulated sprint time at ER compared to BR and no changes in initial sprint time and sprint decrement score between periods during and outside Ramadan. Concerning performance during the 5mSRT, although Boukhris et al. [3] did not show any significant effect of Ramadan fasting on the highest distance (HD), significant decreases in HD were observed in the studies of Hsouna et al. [30, 31] between ER and AR. Total distance (TD) during the 5mSRT was unchanged between periods before, during, and after Ramadan [3, 30, 31]. However, concerning fatigue index (FI), an increase at AR10 compared to BR was observed in the study of Boukhris et al. [3], an increase at AR10 compared to BR and the first 10 days of Ramadan was reported in the study of Hsouna et al. [30], and no changes between periods before, during and after Ramadan were reported in the study of Hsouna et al. [31] (Table 14.7).

Concerning endurance performance during Ramadan observance, it has been shown a significant effect (i.e., decrease compared to control periods) of Ramadan observance on total distance during a 12 min run [9], maximal aerobic velocity [32], distance covered in a 30-min run [33], total distance and maximal aerobic velocity (MAV) during the Yo-Yo intermittent recovery test [25, 29, 37, 38], and VO$_2$max determined from the multistage 20-m shuttle test [13]. In addition to that, there has been reported an increase during Ramadan compared to control periods of the time of the realization of 1000 m [34] and 3000 m [11] runs. However, according to Güvenç [36], the distance covered during the 20-meter multistage shuttle run test was higher at ER and the first week of Ramadan compared to BR and AR. The peak running time was higher at ER compared to the first week of Ramadan and also higher at AR compared to both the first week of Ramadan and BR. The peak running velocity was higher at the ER than it was during

Table 14.6 Influence of Ramadan observance on repeated sprint ability

Studies	Sample size	Age	Sex	Activity (level of practice)	Training schedule	Fasting period	Assessment periods	Test outcomes	Effect
Meckel et al. [11]	19	15.1 ± 0.9	Male	Soccer (first division youth league)	6.4 ± 0.2 h / week BR and 4.5 ± 0.1 h / week during Ramadan	NM	BR ER	Total distance during 6 × 40 m sprint (s)	↑ at ER vs. BR
								Performance decrement during 6 × 40 m sprint (%)	↑ at ER vs. BR
Chtourou et al. [25]	20	18 ± 1	Male	Soccer (Tunisian junior football team)	2 h a day, 4 days a week	16 h	BR SWR ER	Total work during RSE (W·kg⁻¹)	↓ at ER vs. BR
								Performance decrement during RSE (%)	↑ at ER and at SWR vs. BR
Girard and Farooq [28]	18	12.6 ± 1.5	Male	NM	NM		BR FWR ER AR2 AR4	Initial sprint time (s)	No change
								Cumulated sprint times (s)	↑ at ER vs. BR
								Sprint decrement score (%)	No change
Hammouda et al. [29]	10	17.3 ± 0.48	Male	Soccer (first division of the Tunisian national league)	2 h a day, 4 days a week	15–16 h	BR SWR ER	Total work during RSE (W·kg⁻¹)	↓ at ER vs. BR; ↓ at SWR vs. ER
								Performance decrement during RSE (%)	No change

Study	N	Sex	Sport/population	Training	Fasting duration	Conditions	Test/measure	Result
Aloui et al. [17]	12	Male	Soccer (Tunisian amateur league)	Approximately 10 h of training per week	~16 h	BR / SWR / ER / AR	Total work during RSA test (W·kg⁻¹)	No change
							Performance decrement during RSA test (%)	↓ at SWR and ER vs. BR
Bouhlel et al. [14]	10	Male	Boxing (amateur)	5 × 1.5 h per week	15 h	BR / FWR / ER	10 x 6 s repeated sprints on a cycle ergometer	↓ at FWR vs. BR and recovered at the ER
Boukhris et al. [3]	13	Male	Running (moderately trained)	At least 3 h/week	16–17 h	BR / FR / ER / AR10 / AR20	HD	No change
							TD	No change
							FI	↑ at AR10 vs. BR
Hsouna et al. [30]	12	Male	Running (moderately trained)	At least 3 h/week	16–17 h	BR / FR / ER / AR10 / AR20	HD	↓ at ER vs. AR10
							TD	No change
							FI	↑ at AR10 vs. BR and FR
Hsouna et al. [31]	14	Male	Running (moderately trained)	At least 3 h/week	16–17 h	BR / ER / AR	HD	↓ at ER vs. AR
							TD	No change
							FI	No change

↓ = decrease, ↑ = increase, RSA repeated sprint ability, AR after Ramadan, AR2 two weeks after Ramadan, AR4 four weeks after Ramadan, AR10 after 10 days of Ramadan, AR20 after 20 days of Ramadan, BR before Ramadan, ER end of Ramadan, FR first 10 days of Ramadan, FWR first week of Ramadan, HD higher distance, NM not mentioned, RSE repeated sprint exercise, SWR second week of Ramadan, TD total distance, vs. versus

Table 14.7 Influence of Ramadan observance on long-duration exercise

Studies	Sample size	Age	Sex	Activity (level of practice)	Training schedule	Fasting period	Assessment periods	Test outcomes	Effect
Zerguini et al. [9]	55	17 to 34	Male	Soccer (professional)	NM	~12–13 h	BR; ER; AR	Distance covered during a 12-minute run (in meters)	↓ at ER and AR vs. BR; ↓ at ER vs. AR
Kirkendall et al. [10]	Fasting (n = 21) Non-fasting (n = 18)	18 ± 1	Male	Soccer (professional)	Each session had a duration of 60 to 80 minutes	~12.5–13.5 h	BR; SWR; ER	Distance covered during the 20-meter multistage shuttle test (in meters)	No change No change
Meckel et al. [11]	19	15.1 ± 0.9	Male	Soccer (first division youth league)	Weekly training time decreased from an average of 6.4 h (before Ramadan) to 4.5 h during Ramadan	NM	BR; ER	Time of the realization of 3000 m run (s)	↑ at ER vs. BR
Chaouachi et al. [12]	15	18 ± 1	Male	Judo (elite)	The training schedule consisted of 9 sessions per week, averaging 17 h total, with workouts lasting at least 2 h per day, 6 days a week	~12–13 h	BR; MR; ER; AR	VO2max determined from the multistage fitness test	No change
Chennaoui et al. [32]	8	25 ± 1	Male	Middle-distance running (professional)	6 to 10 times per week for a minimum of 3 years	~13 h	BR; day 7 and 21 of Ramadan; AR	Maximal aerobic velocity (MAV)	↓ at day 7 and 21 of Ramadan vs. BR

Study	n	Age	Sex	Sport/activity	Training	Fasting duration	Conditions	Measure	Result
Aziz et al. [33]	10	27 ± 7	Male	Running (moderately trained)	2 to 4 times per week, covering between 15 and 25 kilometers per week, in the 3 months leading up to the start of the study	~13.5 h	BR; DR	Distance covered in a 30-minute run	↓ DR vs. BR
								Average speed during a 30-minute run	↓ during the 15th and 25th minute DR
Lotfi et al. [34]	11	20.45 ± 1.65	Male	NM	NM	~13–14 h	BR; FWR; TWR; AR	Time taken to cover a distance of 1000 meters (s)	↑ at FWR and at TWR vs. BR
Aziz et al. [35]	Fasting (n = 10)	18.0 ± 0.7	Male	Soccer (international level)	4 times/week	13.5 h	BR; AR	The 20-m multistage shuttle run test	No change
	Non-fasting (n = 8)	17.9 ± 0.7							No change
Chtourou et al. [25]	20	18 ± 1	Male	Soccer (Tunisian junior football team)	2 h a day, 4 days a week	16 h	BR; SWR; ER	Total distance covered during the Yo-Yo intermittent recovery test (in meters)	↓ at ER vs. BR
								MAV during the Yo-Yo intermittent recovery test (km·h^{-1})	↓ at ER vs. BR

(continued)

Table 14.7 (continued)

Studies	Sample size	Age	Sex	Activity (level of practice)	Training schedule	Fasting period	Assessment periods	Test outcomes	Effect
Güvenç [36]	16	17.4 ± 1.2	Male	Soccer (amateur soccer league)	3 times per week (2 h of each session)	NM	BR; FWR; ER; AR	Peak running distance during the 20-m multistage shuttle test (m)	↑ at ER and FWR vs. BR; ↑ AR and FWR vs. BR
								Peak running time during the 20-m multistage shuttle test (min)	↑ at ER vs. FR; ↑ at AR vs. FWR and BR
								Peak running velocity during the 20-m multistage shuttle test (km·h⁻¹)	↑ at ER vs. FWR; ↑ at AR vs. FWR and BR
								Running velocity at 4.0 mmol·l⁻¹ lactate concentration during the 20-m multistage shuttle test (km·h⁻¹)	↑ at ER vs. FWR; ↑ at AR vs. FWR and BR
Hammouda et al. [29]	10	17.3 ± 0.48	Male	Soccer (first division of the Tunisian national league)	2 h a day, 4 days a week	15–16 h	BR; SWR; ER	Total distance during the Yo-Yo intermittent recovery test (m)	↓ at SWR and at ER vs. BR

Aloui et al. [13]	12	13.3 ± 0.4	Male	Soccer (NM)	NM	15 h	BR; ER	VO2max determined from the multistage 20-m shuttle test (ml/min/kg)	↓ at ER vs. BR
Hammouda et al. [37]	15	17.3 ± 0.3	Male	Soccer (the first division of the Tunisian football league)	At least 4 times per week (2 h for each time)	15–16 h	BR; SWR; ER	Total distance during the Yo-Yo intermittent recovery test (m)	↓ at SWR and at ER vs. BR
Hammouda et al. [38]	12	17.52 ± 0.2	Male	Soccer (Tunisian f, first professional league)	At least 4 times per week (2 h for each time) + the weekend match	~16 h	BR; SWR; ER	Total distance during the Yo-Yo intermittent recovery test (m)	↓ at SWR and at ER vs. BR
Bouhlel et al. [39]	10	18.5 ± 0.5	Male	Karate (moderately trained)	5 × 2 h per week	NM	BR; FWR; ER	The maximum aerobic power	No change
								VO2max	No change

↓ = decrease, ↑ = increase, AR after Ramadan, BR before Ramadan, ER end of Ramadan, FWR first week of Ramadan, MR middle of Ramadan, NM not mentioned, SWR second week of Ramadan, DR during Ramadan, TWR third week of Ramadan, vs. versus the first week of Ramadan and AR. Running velocity at 4.0 mmol·L^{-1} lactate concentration was higher at ER in comparison to the first week of Ramadan and AR. However, there was no significant effect of Ramadan fasting on the distance covered during the 20-m multistage shuttle test [10, 35], VO$_2$max determined from the multistage fitness test [12], and the maximum aerobic power and VO$_2$max during a progressive cycle ergometer test to exhaustion [39].

14.3 Possible Mechanisms Behind Reduced Performance During Ramadan Fasting

Inconsistent findings across studies could be attributed to differences in age, training levels, exercise protocols, or sleep assessment techniques used with participants. For example, the duration of physical tests in the studies of Chaouachi et al. [12] and Hsouna et al. [15] may not be sufficient to induce muscular fatigue. Aziz et al. [40] proposed that the length of exercise might impact the effects of Ramadan fasting on performance, potentially contributing to the varied findings in the literature.

Moreover, the decrease in physical performance during Ramadan fasting can be linked to its impact on sleep quality [41]. The loss or fragmentation of sleep during Ramadan may be linked to nocturnal meals. Studies have shown that reduced physical and cognitive performance is associated with partial sleep deprivation [42–45]. Additionally, the duration of sleep for athletes during Ramadan observance does not align with the recommended sleep duration of 9–10 h per day [46, 47] or 8 h per day [48]. This sleep loss can also lead to increased daytime sleepiness, negatively impacting the performance of athletes [47].

Furthermore, decreases in mood states have been identified as contributing factors to reduced performance during Ramadan [49, 50]. As sleep quality and quantity are directly associated with mood states [50], it is not surprising to observe a negative effect on mood states during Ramadan when sleep is compromised.

Additionally, changes in dietary intake during Ramadan may affect physical performance. However, other studies have suggested that the decline in performance observed during Ramadan is not always related to changes in caloric consumption [7, 13, 15]. Furthermore, research has demonstrated that a brief period of energy restriction, even though it reduces muscle and liver glycogen stores, does not impact muscle strength and anaerobic power [23].

14.4 Conclusion

The impact of observing Ramadan on athletic performance is a topic that generates debate. Currently, the specific reasons behind the decline in performance during Ramadan are not well understood. While speculative, potential factors such as disruptions in sleep patterns and circadian rhythms, dehydration, changes in body composition, environmental conditions, modifications in training intensity and schedule, and fatigue may contribute to the adverse effects of Ramadan observance on athletic performance.

Athletes employ a variety of coping strategies to manage fasting while also training. However, while some athletes may find it relatively easy to balance fasting and athletic activities, others may struggle to maintain the necessary performance levels during this month. As a result, coaches and medical professionals must prioritize individualization in managing athletes during Ramadan. Future research is needed to explore the combination of various strategies to mitigate or minimize the negative effects of Ramadan fasting. This would involve including different elements such as frequency, intensity, timing, and types of training, as well as considering aspects of sleep, nutrition, rest, and even social behavioral approaches and personal lifestyle.

References

1. Trabelsi K, Ammar A, Boukhris O, Boujelbane MA, Clark C, Romdhani M, et al. Ramadan intermittent fasting and its association with health-related indices and exercise test performance in athletes and physically active individuals: an overview of systematic reviews. Br J Sports Med. 2024;58(3):136–43.
2. Trabelsi K, Ammar A, Boukhris O, Glenn M, et al. Effects of Ramadan observance on dietary intake and body composition of adolescent athletes: systematic review and meta-analysis. Nutrients. 2020;12(6):1574.
3. Boukhris O, Hsouna H, Chtourou L, Abdesalem R, BenSalem S, Tahri N, et al. Effect of Ramadan fasting on feelings, dietary intake, rating of perceived exertion and repeated high intensity short-term maximal performance. Chronobiol Int. 2019;36(1):1–10.
4. Chtourou H, Trabelsi K, Boukhris O, Ammar A, Shephard RJ, Bragazzi NL. Effects of Ramadan fasting on physical performances in soccer players: a systematic review. Tunis Med. 2019;97(10):1114–31.
5. Abaïdia AE, Daab W, Bouzid MA. Effects of Ramadan fasting on physical performance: a systematic review with meta-analysis. Sports Med Auckl NZ. 2020;50(5):1009–26.
6. DeLang MD, Salamh PA, Chtourou H, Saad HB, Chamari K. The effects of Ramadan intermittent fasting on football players and implications for domestic football leagues over the next decade: a systematic review. Sports Med Auckl NZ. 2022;52(3):585–600.
7. Boukhris O, Trabelsi K, Shephard RJ, Hsouna H, Abdessalem R, Chtourou L, et al. Sleep patterns, alertness, dietary intake, muscle soreness, fatigue, and mental stress recorded before, during and after Ramadan observance. Sports. 2019;7(5):118.
8. Trabelsi K, Masmoudi L, Ammar A, Boukhris O, Khacharem A, Jemal M, et al. The effects of Ramadan intermittent fasting on sleep-wake behaviour and daytime sleepiness in team sport referees. J Sports Sci. 2021;39(21):2411–7.
9. Zerguini Y, Kirkendall D, Junge A, Dvorak J. Impact of Ramadan on physical performance in professional soccer players. Br J Sports Med. 2007;41(6):398–400.
10. Kirkendall DT, Leiper JB, Bartagi Z, Dvorak J, Zerguini Y. The influence of Ramadan on physical performance measures in young Muslim footballers. J Sports Sci. 2008;26(sup3):S15–27.
11. Meckel Y, Ismaeel A, Eliakim A. The effect of the Ramadan fast on physical performance and dietary habits in adolescent soccer players. Eur J Appl Physiol. 2008;102(6):651–7.
12. Chaouachi A, Coutts AJ, Chamari K, Wong DP, Chaouachi M, Chtara M, et al. Effect of Ramadan intermittent fasting on aerobic and anaerobic performance and perception of fatigue in male elite judo athletes. J Strength Cond Res. 2009;23(9):2702–9.
13. Aloui A, Chtourou H, Hammouda O, Souissi H, Chaouachi A, Chamari K, et al. Effects of Ramadan on the diurnal variations of physical performance and perceived exertion in adolescent soccer players. Biol Rhythm Res. 2013a;44(6):869–75.

14. Bouhlel H, Bogdanis G, Hamila A, Miled A, Chelly MS, Denguezli M, et al. Effects of Ramadan observance on repeated cycle ergometer sprinting and associated inflammatory and oxidative stress responses in trained young men. J Fasting Health. 2016;4(1)
15. Hsouna H, Abdessalem R, Boukhris O, Trabelsi K, Chtourou L, Tahri N, et al. Short-term maximal performance, alertness, dietary intake, sleep pattern and mood states of physically active young men before, during and after Ramadan observance. Marocolo M, editor. PLoS One. 2019;14(6):e0217851.
16. Brisswalter J, Bouhlel E, Falola JM, Abbiss CR, Vallier JM, Hausswirth C. Effects of Ramadan intermittent fasting on middle-distance running performance in well-trained runners. Clin J Sport Med. 2011;21(5):422–7.
17. Aloui A, Chaouachi A, Chtourou H, Wong DP, Haddad M, Chamari K, et al. Effects of Ramadan on the diurnal variations of repeated-Sprint performance. Int J Sports Physiol Perform. 2013b;8(3):254–63.
18. Zarrouk N, Hug F, Hammouda O, Rebai H, Tabka Z, Dogui M, et al. Effect of Ramadan intermittent fasting on body composition and neuromuscular performance in young athletes: a pilot study. Biol Rhythm Res. 2013;44(5):697–709.
19. Zarrouk N, Hammouda O, Latiri I, Adala H, Bouhlel E, Rebai H, et al. Ramadan fasting does not adversely affect neuromuscular performances and reaction times in trained karate athletes. J Int Soc Sports Nutr. 2016;13:18.
20. Gueldich H, Zghal F, Borji R, Chtourou H, Sahli S, Rebai H. The effects of Ramadan intermittent fasting on the underlying mechanisms of force production capacity during maximal isometric voluntary contraction. Chronobiol Int. 2019;36(5):698–708.
21. Aziz AR, Che Muhamed AM, Ooi CH, Singh R, Chia MYH. Effects of Ramadan fasting on the physical activity profile of trained Muslim soccer players during a 90-minute match. Sci Med Footb. 2018;2(1):29–38.
22. Karli U, Guvenc A, Aslan A, Hazir T, Acikada C. Influence of Ramadan fasting on anaerobic performance and recovery following short time high intensity exercise. J Sports Sci Med. 2007;6(4):490–7.
23. Souissi N, Souissi H, Sahli S, Tabka Z, Dogui M, Ati J, et al. Effect of Ramadan on the diurnal variation in short-term high power output. Chronobiol Int. 2007;24(5):991–1007.
24. Abedelmalek S, Souissi N, Takayuki A, Hadouk S, Tabka Z. Effect of acute maximal exercise on circulating levels of Interleukin-12 during Ramadan fasting. Asian J Sports Med. 2011;2(3):154–60.
25. Chtourou H, Hammouda O, Souissi H, Chamari K, Chaouachi A, Souissi N. The effect of ramadan fasting on physical performances, mood state and perceived exertion in young footballers. Asian J Sports Med. 2011;2(3):177–85.
26. Chtourou H, Hammouda O, Chaouachi A, Chamari K, Souissi N. The effect of time-of-day and Ramadan fasting on anaerobic performances. Int J Sports Med. 2012;33(02):142–7.
27. Abedelmalek S, Denguezli M, Chtourou H, Souissi N, Tabka Z. Does Ramadan fasting affect acylated ghrelin and growth hormone concentrations during short-term maximal exercise in the afternoon? Biol Rhythm Res. 2015;46(5):691–701.
28. Girard O, Farooq A. Effects of Ramadan fasting on repeated sprint ability in young children. Sci Sports. 2012;27(4):237–40.
29. Hamouda O, Chtourou H, Farjallah MA, Davenne D, Souissi N. The effect of Ramadan fasting on the diurnal variations in aerobic and anaerobic performances in Tunisian youth soccer players. Biol Rhythm Res. 2012;43(2):177–90.
30. Hsouna H, Boukhris O, Trabelsi K, Abdessalem R, Ammar A, Irandoust K, et al. Effects of 25-min nap opportunity during Ramadan observance on the 5-m shuttle run performance and the perception of fatigue in physically active men. Int J Environ Res Public Health. 2020a;17(9):3135.
31. Hsouna H, Boukhris O, Trabelsi K, Abdessalem R, Ammar A, Glenn JM, et al. A thirty-five-minute nap improves performance and attention in the 5-m shuttle run test during and outside Ramadan observance. Sports. 2020b;8(7):98.

32. Chennaoui M, Desgorces F, Drogou C, Boudjemaa B, Tomaszewski A, Depiesse F, et al. Effects of Ramadan fasting on physical performance and metabolic, hormonal, and inflammatory parameters in middle-distance runners. Appl Physiol Nutr Metab. 2009;34(4):587–94.
33. Aziz AR, Wahid MF, Png W, Jesuvadian CV. Effects of Ramadan fasting on 60 min of endurance running performance in moderately trained men. Br J Sports Med. 2010;44(7):516–21.
34. Lotfi S, Madani M, Abassi A, Boumahmaza M, Talbi M. CNS activation, reaction time, blood pressure and heart rate variation during ramadan intermittent fasting and exercise. World J Sports. 2010;1:37–43.
35. Aziz AR, Chia M, Singh R, Wahid MF. Effects of Ramadan fasting on perceived exercise intensity during high-intensity interval training in elite youth soccer players. Int J Sports Sci Coach. 2011;6(1):87–98.
36. Güvenç A. Effects of ramadan fasting on body composition, aerobic performance and lactate, heart rate and perceptual responses in young soccer players. J Hum Kinet. 2011;29:79–91.
37. Hammouda O, Chtourou H, Aloui A, Chahed H, Kallel C, Miled A, et al. Concomitant effects of Ramadan fasting and time-of-day on Apolipoprotein AI, B, Lp-a and homocysteine responses during aerobic exercise in Tunisian soccer players. Pasquali R, editor. PLoS One. 2013;8(11):e79873.
38. Hammouda O, Chtourou H, Aloui A, Mejri MA, Chahed H, Miled A, et al. Does Ramadan fasting affect the diurnal variations in metabolic responses and total antioxidant capacity during exercise in young soccer players? Sport Sci Health. 2014;10(2):97–104.
39. Bouhlel H, Latiri I, Zarrouk N, Bigard X, Shephard R, Tabka Z, et al. Effet du jeûne du Ramadan et de l'exercice maximal sur le temps de réaction simple et de choix chez des sujets entraînés. Sci Sports. 2014;29(3):131–7.
40. Aziz AR, Chia MYH, Low CY, Slater GJ, Png W, Teh KC. Conducting an acute intense interval exercise session during the Ramadan fasting month: what is the optimal time of the day? Chronobiol Int. 2012;29(8):1139–50.
41. Trabelsi K, Bragazzi N, Zlitni S, Khacharem A, Boukhris O, El-Abed K, et al. Observing Ramadan and sleep-wake patterns in athletes: a systematic review, meta-analysis and meta-regression. Br J Sports Med. 2020;54(11):674–80.
42. Souissi N, Souissi M, Souissi H, Chamari K, Tabka Z, Dogui M, et al. Effect of time of day and partial sleep deprivation on short-term. High-Power Output Chronobiol Int. 2008;25(6):1062–76.
43. Souissi N, Chtourou H, Aloui A, Hammouda O, Dogui M, Chaouachi A, et al. Effects of time-of-day and partial sleep deprivation on short-term maximal performances of judo competitors. J Strength Cond Res. 2013;27(9):2473–80.
44. Oliver SJ, Costa RJS, Laing SJ, Bilzon JLJ, Walsh NP. One night of sleep deprivation decreases treadmill endurance performance. Eur J Appl Physiol. 2009;107(2):155–61.
45. Jarraya S, Jarraya M, Chtourou H, Souissi N. Effect of time of day and partial sleep deprivation on the reaction time and the attentional capacities of the handball goalkeeper. Biol Rhythm Res. 2014;45(2):183–91.
46. Mah CD, Mah KE, Kezirian EJ, Dement WC. The effects of sleep extension on the athletic performance of collegiate basketball players. Sleep. 2011;34(7):943–50.
47. Kerkeni M, Khaled T, Kerkeni M, Boukhris O, Ammar A, Salem A, et al. Ramadan fasting observance is associated with decreased sleep duration, increased daytime sleepiness and insomnia symptoms among student-athletes. Sleep Med. 2024;122:185.
48. Halson SL. Sleep in elite athletes and nutritional interventions to enhance sleep. Sports Med. 2014;44(S1):13–23.
49. Roky R, Iraki L, HajKhlifa R, Ghazal NL, Hakkou F. Daytime alertness, mood, psychomotor performances, and Oral temperature during Ramadan intermittent fasting. Ann Nutr Metab. 2000;44(3):101–7.
50. Roky R, Houti I, Moussamih S, Qotbi S, Aadil N. Physiological and chronobiological changes during Ramadan intermittent fasting. Ann Nutr Metab. 2004;48(4):296–303.

Chapter 15
Mitigating Physiological and Psychological Challenges During Ramadan: Strategic Recommendations for Athletes

Manel Kerkeni, Mohamed Kerkeni, Omar Boukhris, and Hamdi Chtourou

Abstract During Ramadan, adult Muslims fast from dawn to sunset, abstaining from food and liquids. The fasting duration varies based on location and time of year. Ramadan fasting differs from other regimens as it is total (i.e., no food or fluids) and time-restricted, aligning with the circadian rhythm. This type of fasting can cause hypohydration, disrupted sleep patterns, mood swings, and increased fatigue. Muslim athletes who continue to train and compete during Ramadan face significant challenges. Research shows that the impact of fasting during Ramadan on physical performance varies depending on the intensity of the effort, ranging from no effect to substantial effects. This chapter aims to focus on the possible contributing factors (e.g., circadian rhythm, sleep, nutrition, hydration, and mood states) during the observance of Ramadan fasting that contribute to the decline of athletic performance and provide useful recommendations for athletes, as well as for coaches, healthcare practitioners, sports scientists, and those in sports management roles. The objective is to offer guidance on the implementation of effective behavioral modifications, social support systems, and psychological strategies to overcome these challenges.

M. Kerkeni · M. Kerkeni
High Institute of Sport and Physical Education, University of Sfax, Sfax, Tunisia

Research laboratory, Education, Motricity, Sport and Health (EM2S), LR15JS01, High Institute of Sport and Physical Education, University of Sfax, Sfax, Tunisia

O. Boukhris
Sport, Performance, and Nutrition Research Group, School of Allied Health, Human Services, and Sport, La Trobe University, Melbourne, VIC, Australia

SIESTA Research Group, School of Allied Health, Human Services and Sport, La Trobe University, Melbourne, VIC, Australia

H. Chtourou (✉)
High Institute of Sport and Physical Education, University of Sfax, Sfax, Tunisia

Physical Activity, Sport, and Health, UR18JS01, National Observatory of Sport, Tunis, Tunisia
e-mail: hamdi.chtourou@isseps.usf.tn

© The Author(s), under exclusive license to Springer Nature Singapore Pte Ltd. 2025
M. E. Faris et al. (eds.), *Health and Medical Aspects of Ramadan Intermittent Fasting*, https://doi.org/10.1007/978-981-96-6783-3_15

Keywords Sleep · Nutrition · Hydration · Fasting · Performance

15.1 Introduction

As one of Islam's five fundamental pillars, Ramadan is a month-long period (29–30 days) of daytime fasting, during which Muslims abstain from food, drink, sexual activity, and smoking from dawn to dusk, as highlighted by Trabelsi et al. [1]. The Islamic calendar follows lunar cycles, causing Ramadan to shift approximately 11 days earlier each year, leading to significant variations in fasting conditions depending on the season and geographic location. This means that experiencing Ramadan during a high-altitude summer presents vastly different challenges compared to observing it in a low-altitude winter. For instance, temperate regions can experience fasting durations of up to 18 h during summer months. These durations can even extend further in the polar areas, posing a considerable physiological challenge for those observing the fast.

Ramadan fasting stands out from other dietary restrictions. It is a unique pattern involving complete abstinence from both food and fluids, with a strict time restriction and an intermittent cycle of fasting. Crucially, Ramadan fasting is a "dry" fast, as no fluids are consumed during daylight hours [2]. This makes it particularly challenging, as it can lead to hypohydration, a state of reduced body water.

Ramadan fasting significantly alters the daily routine of Muslims. The shift to two main meals with snacks in between, altered meal timings, and increased religious and social activities created a unique lifestyle during this period [2]. Because physical activity does not warrant breaking the fast, many Muslim athletes and physically active individuals maintain their training and competitions. In addition, international competitions continue as usual, regardless of whether Muslim athletes are observing Ramadan. This puts Muslim athletes in a difficult position, as they may be experiencing hypohydration, sleep disturbances, mood swings, and impaired physical performance [3]. A number of systematic reviews with meta-analyses showed that during Ramadan, athletes who continue training experienced increased fatigue, reduced vigor, decreased carbohydrate and water intake, reduced body mass and body fat, preserved lean mass, shorter sleep duration, impaired sleep quality, and longer daytime naps, but no significant changes in depression, confusion, tension, anger, or daytime sleepiness [1, 4–6]. A recent overview of systematic reviews reported that athletes who continue training during Ramadan may experience negative effects on their mood, sleep, and performance during intense exercise despite maintaining lean mass [7]. Therefore, as it is believed that fasting during Ramadan is not an ideal condition for athletes to train or compete, this chapter reviews the current research on factors affecting athletic performance during Ramadan and offers practical strategies for athletes and coaches to optimize training and competition outcomes.

15.2 Circadian Rhythm

Our sleep-wake patterns are regulated by innate, biological rhythms that operate on an approximately 24-h cycle, known as circadian rhythms [8]. These rhythms are essential for regulating important physiological functions such as sleep, hormone release, and metabolism [8]. One of the key factors contributing to the decrease in physical performance during Ramadan fasting is the alteration of these circadian rhythms.

During Ramadan, the fasting schedule necessitates significant changes in daily routines, particularly in sleep and meal times [9]. The predawn meal (Suhoor) and the post-sunset meal (Iftar) could disrupt the typical sleep pattern, often leading to fragmented sleep and reduced overall sleep duration [10]. In fact, the need to wake up early for Suhoor and stay awake late for Iftar can lead to inadequate sleep duration and poor sleep quality. This disruption in sleep patterns can result in hormonal imbalances, affecting the levels of cortisol and melatonin [8]. These imbalances may have an impact on energy levels, muscle recovery, and overall physical performance. For instance, studies have observed notable shifts in key physiological markers during Ramadan, including a reduction in the amplitude of both body temperature and cortisol secretion, coupled with a two-hour delay in their peak levels [11, 12]. Furthermore, Rocky et al. [13] found a decrease in the amplitude of the melatonin cycle during Ramadan. Melatonin, a key neurohormone, plays a crucial role in sleep-wake regulation, primarily by influencing core body temperature, as explained by Dawson and Encel [14].

Fasting significantly impacts the body's metabolism, resulting in modifications in the utilization of energy substrates [15]. The alteration in meal timing can induce fluctuations in blood glucose levels and glycogen stores, which play a crucial role in maintaining prolonged physical activity. These metabolic shifts, combined with disturbances in circadian rhythms, may undermine endurance and strength.

The alteration of circadian rhythms can also have psychological effects, such as increased feelings of fatigue and decreased motivation, which can further impact physical performance [16].

15.3 Sleep

Sleep is crucial for optimal sports performance and injury prevention [17, 18]. Athletes should prioritize getting sufficient sleep and avoid sleep deficits and chronic sleep deprivation, which often occur due to lifestyle changes during Ramadan [2]. In fact, during Ramadan observance, due to the large amount of food consumed at night as well as nocturnal training, sleep at night is going to be delayed, and its length will be decreased. Thus, night sleep is going to be fragmented or deprived during Ramadan observance. More importantly, the sleep loss or fragmentation observed during Ramadan observance could result in psychological and

physiological perturbations that could have a negative impact on athletic performance. In this context, Trabelsi et al. [6] concluded through a meta-analysis that
sleep duration decreased significantly in athletes who continued to train during
Ramadan fasting. In addition, a recent meta-analysis conducted in 2022 reported a
significant reduction in total sleep time and a deterioration in sleep quality in athletes and moderately trained individuals during the month of Ramadan [5].

Furthermore, it has been shown that total sleep time was reduced significantly by
approximately 1 h per day during Ramadan observance to around 6.4 h [19]. This is not
consistent with the recommended duration of sleep, which is 7–9 h per day [20].
Recently, Trabelsi et al. [7] conducted an overview of a systematic review and found that
maintaining training routines during Ramadan fasting may lead to shorter sleep durations. Therefore, athletes will have insufficient recovery, which obviously could limit
their performance. Moreover, this sleep loss observed during the month of Ramadan
might increase the level of daytime sleepiness [19, 21], which could negatively affect
athletes' physical performance. As a consequence, sleep disruptions, often associated
with Ramadan, may be a contributing factor to reduced athletic performance.

However, athletes often use napping to compensate for sleep loss, and Muslim
athletes during Ramadan are particularly known for this practice. Research showed
that daytime napping significantly increased for these athletes during Ramadan
compared to other times of the year [22, 23]. This adjustment helps them counteract
the sleep disruptions caused by fasting. Studies examining the effects of napping
during Ramadan have found evidence supporting its benefits in maintaining performance and overall well-being of athletes. In one study, Hsouna et al. [24] investigated the effects of a 25-min nap during Ramadan on physical performance,
cognitive performance (attention scores), feelings, and perceived exertion (RPE)
scores. However, this study did not find a significant effect of a 25-min nap during
Ramadan observance.

In contrast, Hsouna et al. [25] reported that a 35-min nap had a beneficial effect on
physical and cognitive performances. The contradiction between these two studies may
be due to the difference in nap duration. In fact, a 25-min nap may be too short to show
significant improvement during Ramadan observance. On the other hand, a 45-min
afternoon nap during Ramadan was found to be more effective than a 25-min nap in
improving performance during the 5-m shuttle run test and reducing RPE scores [26].

Finally, coaches and sports managers must emphasize the strong connection
between sufficient sleep and optimal athletic performance to their athletes. By providing education about healthy sleep habits, especially during Ramadan, they can
empower athletes to prioritize and improve their sleep hygiene throughout the fasting month.

15.4   Nutrition and Hydration

The decrease in nutritional intake and changes in body composition that occur
during Ramadan may have a negative impact on athletic performance. Athletes in
Muslim countries traditionally fast from dawn to sunset for 30 days each year.

This means that all meals are consumed in darkness, which can potentially affect body composition, nutritional intake, and athletic performance (Trabelsi et al. 2021). Since diet plays a significant role in physical performance, fasting during Ramadan can result in dehydration and a lack of energy stores due to the restriction of water and food. This, in turn, can lead to a decrease in body mass. In fact, a meta-analysis by Trabelsi et al. (2021) found that Ramadan fasting led to a reduction in body fat percentage, body mass, carbohydrate intake, and fluid intake among adult athletes. However, a study by Trabelsi et al. [1, 6] demonstrated that body composition, body mass, and food intake were not affected by Ramadan fasting in adolescent athletes.

It is important to consider that these results are specific to teenagers and may not directly translate to adult athletes, who typically experience different training demands and physiological responses. As a result, fasting during Ramadan could limit the energy required for training and competitions among adult athletes, thus affecting their athletic performance (Trabelsi et al. 2021). Therefore, it is important to consider the potential reduction in energy sources that fasting during Ramadan may cause, as they are crucial for optimizing athletic performance.

Furthermore, exercising during daylight hours in Ramadan could lead to a significant loss of fluids, causing dehydration and potentially resulting in body mass loss [22, 27, 28]. This is because fasting restricts fluid intake, making it harder for the body to replenish fluids lost through sweat during exercise. Research has consistently found that lower body mass during Ramadan is directly linked to dehydration [27–29], with studies observing increased urine concentration and decreased body mass [29], along with reduced plasma volume and increased blood cell concentration (i.e., hemoglobin and hematocrit) in athletes [27, 28]. These changes are all indicators of dehydration, which is potentially due to reduced total water intake during Ramadan [27, 28]. In this context, a meta-analysis confirmed a marked decline in daily fluid intake during the month of Ramadan. This supports the conclusion that dehydration is a primary cause of body mass loss during the fasting month [4].

15.5 Mood State

Another reason why Ramadan fasting has a detrimental effect on athletes' performance is facing negative mood states. Indeed, mood states have a direct association with sleep quality [30]. In fact, poor sleep can have wide-ranging negative effects, impacting energy, mood, and cognitive function, ultimately increasing the likelihood of reduced performance across both physical and mental tasks [31]. As the month of Ramadan is characterized by sleep loss, there is a very high probability that athletes will face bad mood states. More importantly, in order to perform better, athletes should be in perfect mood states [30]. Hence, if the well-being of athletes is compromised during Ramadan observance, athletic performance will apparently decline.

In this context, the loss of around 1–2 ours of sleep each night during Ramadan observance could cause chronic sleep deprivation, which provokes mood swings and lethargic feelings, leading to increased tiredness and, as a result, reduced physical performance [32]. Additionally, according to Guedlish et al. [33], there were increases in anxiety, fatigue, and depression measured by the profile of mood states questionnaire during Ramadan fasting compared to before the month of Ramadan. These negative mood states observed during Ramadan observance were responsible for the reduction in athletic performance [33].

Hypohydration associated with Ramadan observance can also negatively impact mood [16]. The timing of training sessions during Ramadan, often coinciding with fasting hours, can contribute to a state of dehydration, with potential cumulative effects throughout the month [3]. This is significant because research outside of a Ramadan context has established a clear link between dehydration and altered mood states [34, 35]. Specifically, studies have shown that even modest levels of dehydration, characterized by a body mass loss of 1.4% or more during rest and exercise, can lead to heightened confusion, reduced energy levels, and increased feelings of fatigue [34, 35]. These findings are further supported by research in real-world athletic settings, such as the study by Moyen et al. [36], which found that dehydration negatively impacted both fatigue and vigor levels in athletes participating in a 161 km ultra-endurance cycling event.

A meta-analysis showed that training during Ramadan (at least three sessions per week) leads to increased fatigue and decreased vigor [16]. However, there was no significant effect on confusion, depression, anger, and tension [16]. The spiritual, religious, and social activities during Ramadan may have helped prevent any decline in certain aspects of athletes' moods. The meta-regression results also revealed that fatigue was influenced by the frequency and length of training sessions per week, as well as the type of physical activity [16]. Meanwhile, anger was only affected by the kind of physical activity [16].

Another explanation for facing negative mood states during the month of Ramadan is restricted food intake, which could lead to low levels of daytime carbohydrates and calories due to fasting [37]. In fact, it has been reported that athletes' negative mood states are correlated with restricted calories and glucides [38]. Therefore, the decline in athletes' performance could be explained by the negative mood states observed during Ramadan observance.

15.6 Practical Recommendations

To limit or reduce the negative effects of potential physiological or psychological factors (i.e., nutrition, hydration, sleep, and mood states) during Ramadan observance, the following recommendations are proposed:

- Athletes observing Ramadan need to manage their nutrition carefully to optimize performance. They should ensure adequate overall nutritional intake, balancing carbohydrates, proteins, and fats. While it is important to maintain total caloric intake, the timing and type of food consumed are crucial. Consuming high-glycemic index foods at the Suhoor meal (predawn) could enhance carbohydrate availability for training later in the day [2]. Athletes can choose either low- or high-glycemic index foods for the Iftar meal (breaking the fast) to manage insulin response and replenish muscle glycogen [2]. However, sports supplements should only be used under the guidance of physicians and nutrition experts.

- Athletes should prioritize optimal hydration between Iftar and Suhoor. They should aim to consume small, frequent amounts of fluids (around 200 ml every 30 min) and add sodium salts to enhance fluid retention and reduce urine loss [2]. It is important to avoid diuretic beverages such as coffee and tea [39]. Athletes should also try to consume Suhoor as close to dawn as possible, especially during long fasting periods (>12 h).
- Training loads should be maintained during Ramadan to prevent detraining effects. To optimize recovery, it is recommended that high-intensity training sessions be scheduled in the early evening hours or, as a secondary option, in the late afternoon. This timing allows players to promptly replenish glycogen stores and rehydrate after training [40].
- Athletes' sleep patterns, including both duration and quality, should be carefully assessed to identify potential interventions. In addition, providing education on sleep hygiene is essential, emphasizing behaviors that promote sleep and avoiding factors that disrupt it. According to O'Donnell and Driller [41], a single one-hour session was found to be effective for elite female athletes, making it a recommended approach for active individuals during Ramadan. Therefore, prioritizing sleep health in athletes involves educating coaches on sleep hygiene and making sleep specialist consultations accessible through sports clubs. Furthermore, scheduling a daily 25- to 45-min nap could enhance alertness and physical performance [25, 26]. It is important to avoid consuming large and late meals before bedtime [42]. The effectiveness of supplements such as tryptophan (1 g/day) or melatonin (5-8 mg) in improving sleep during Ramadan should be verified [43]. Additionally, utilizing a 6-min mindfulness video clip before bedtime can help reduce presleep arousal and enhance sleep quality [43].
- Muslim athletes should consider taking mental preparation courses before Ramadan begins to learn proactive coping skills that will help them navigate the challenges of fasting [44]. In addition, coaches and managers are advised to conduct training rehearsals with athletes who intend to train and compete while fasting prior to the start of Ramadan [2]. This preparation can help reduce negative perceptions and improve the pacing strategies of fasting Muslim athletes during exercise. Another potential way to mitigate declines in physical performance during Ramadan is to listen to music during pre-exercise warm-ups [45]. This strategy has been shown to help maintain exercise performance by distracting fasting athletes from the difficulties associated with Ramadan fasting [45]. Additionally, allowing athletes time for reflection on their religious obligations and ensuring a balance between these commitments and training schedules is crucial for their mental well-being during Ramadan [16].

15.7 Conclusion

Ramadan fasting could significantly impact physiological and psychological well-being, affecting factors such as circadian rhythm, sleep quality, nutrition, hydration, and mood. These changes can, in turn, negatively affect athletes' training and performance. This chapter provides practical recommendations designed to help minimize or avoid these disruptions during Ramadan, allowing athletes to maintain their fitness levels while observing the fast.

Further research is necessary to understand the impacts of athletes observing Ramadan and develop effective strategies. It is recommended that researchers and sports practitioners collaborate closely to ensure scientifically rigorous and practically applicable studies. This collaboration can lead to evidence-based guidelines that optimize athletes' performance and well-being during Ramadan. Additionally, it can facilitate knowledge exchange and the translation of findings into actionable strategies for training, nutrition, hydration, and recovery. By working together, researchers and practitioners can address the unique challenges faced by athletes during Ramadan and contribute to the advancement of sports science in this context.

References

1. Trabelsi K, Ammar A, Boukhris O, Glenn M, et al. Effects of Ramadan observance on dietary intake and body composition of adolescent athletes: systematic review and meta-analysis. Nutrients. 2020a;12(6):1574.
2. Chamari K, Roussi M, Bragazzi NL, Chaouachi A, Abdul RA. Optimizing training and competition during the month of Ramadan: recommendations for a holistic and personalized approach for fasting athletes. Tunis Med. 2019;97(10):1095–103.
3. Trabelsi K, Stannard SR, Chtourou H, Moalla W, Ghozzi H, Jamoussi K, Hakim A. Monitoring athletes' hydration status and sleep patterns during Ramadan observance: methodological and practical considerations. Biol Rhythm Res. 2018;49(3):337–65.
4. Trabelsi K, Ammar A, Boukhris O, Glenn JM, Clark CC, Stannard SR, et al. Dietary intake and body composition during Ramadan in athletes: a systematic review and meta-analysis with meta-regression. J Am Nutr Assoc. 2023;42(1):101–22.
5. Trabelsi K, Ammar A, Glenn JM, Boukhris O, Khacharem A, Bouaziz B, et al. Does observance of Ramadan affect sleep in athletes and physically active individuals? A systematic review and meta-analysis. J Sleep Res. 2022a;31(3):e13503.
6. Trabelsi K, Bragazzi N, Zlitni S, Khacharem A, Boukhris O, El-Abed K, et al. Observing Ramadan and sleep-wake patterns in athletes: a systematic review, meta-analysis, and meta-regression. Br J Sports Med. 2020b;54(11):674–80.
7. Trabelsi K, Ammar A, Boukhris O, Boujelbane MA, Clark C, Romdhani M, et al. Ramadan intermittent fasting and its association with health-related indices and exercise test performance in athletes and physically active individuals: an overview of systematic reviews. Br J Sports Med. 2024;58(3):136–43.
8. Herrera Christopher P, Berrichi H, Chamari K, Davenne D. Circadian rhythm and sleep disturbances during Ramadan: implications on sports performance. Effects of Ramadan fasting on health and athletic performance. Foster City: OMICS Group; 2015.

9. Boukhris O, Hsouna H, Chtourou L, Abdesalem R, BenSalem S, Tahri N, et al. Effect of Ramadan fasting on feelings, dietary intake, rating of perceived exertion, and repeated high intensity short-term maximal performance. Chronobiol Int. 2019a;36(1):1–10.
10. Boukhris O, Trabelsi K, Shephard RJ, Hsouna H, Abdessalem R, Chtourou L, et al. Sleep patterns, alertness, dietary intake, muscle soreness, fatigue, and mental stress were recorded before, during, and after Ramadan observance. Sports. 2019b;7(5):118.
11. Ben Salem L, B'chir S, Bchir F, Bouguerra R, Ben Slama C. Cortisol rhythm during Ramadan. EMHJ. 2003;9(5–6):1093–8.
12. Roky R, Houti I, Moussamih S, Qotbi S, Aadil N. Physiological and chronobiological changes during Ramadan intermittent fasting. Ann Nutr Metab. 2004;48(4):296–303.
13. Roky R, Chapotot F, Hakkou F, Benchekroun MT, Buguet A. Sleep during Ramadan intermittent fasting. J Sleep Res. 2001;10(4):319–27.
14. Dawson D, Encel N. Melatonin and sleep in humans. J Pineal Res. 1993;15(1):1–12.
15. Roky R, Chapotot F, Benchekroun MT, Benaji B, Hakkou F, Elkhalifi H, Buguet A. Daytime sleepiness during Ramadan intermittent fasting: polysomnographic and quantitative waking EEG study. J Sleep Res. 2003;12(2):95–101.
16. Trabelsi K, Ammar A, Boujelbane MA, Khacharem A, Elghoul Y, Boukhris O, et al. Ramadan observance is associated with higher fatigue and lower vigor in athletes: a systematic review and meta-analysis with meta-regression. Int Rev Sport Exerc Psychol. 2022b;18:1–28.
17. Driller MW, Dunican IC, Omond SE, Boukhris O, Stevenson S, Lambing K, Bender AM. Pyjamas, polysomnography and professional athletes: the role of sleep tracking technology in sport. Sports. 2023;11(1):14.
18. Halson SL. Sleep monitoring in athletes: motivation, methods, miscalculations and why it matters. Sports Med. 2019;49(10):1487–97.
19. Faris ME, Jahrami HA, Alhayki FA, Alkhawaja NA, Ali AM, Aljeeb SH, et al. Effect of diurnal fasting on sleep during Ramadan: a systematic review and meta-analysis. Sleep Breathing. 2020;24:771–82.
20. Pujalte GG, Benjamin HJ. Sleep and the athlete. Curr Sports Med Rep. 2018;17(4):109–10.
21. Qasrawi SO, Pandi-Perumal SR, BaHammam AS. The effect of intermittent fasting during Ramadan on sleep, sleepiness, cognitive function, and circadian rhythm. Sleep Breathing. 2017;21(3):577–86.
22. Aziz AR, Che Muhamed AM, Ooi CH, Singh R, Chia MYH. Effects of Ramadan fasting on the physical activity profile of trained Muslim soccer players during a 90-minute match. Sci Med Footb. 2018;2(1):29–38.
23. Tian HH, Aziz AR, Png W, Wahid MF, Yeo D, Png ALC. Effects of fasting during Ramadan month on cognitive function in Muslim athletes. Asian J Sports Med. 2011;2(3):145.
24. Hsouna H, Boukhris O, Trabelsi K, Abdessalem R, Ammar A, Irandoust K, et al. Effects of 25-min nap opportunity during Ramadan observance on the 5-m shuttle run performance and the perception of fatigue in physically active men. Int J Environ Res Public Health. 2020a;17(9):3135.
25. Hsouna H, Boukhris O, Trabelsi K, Abdessalem R, Ammar A, Glenn JM, et al. A thirty-five-minute nap improves performance and attention in the 5-m shuttle run test during and outside Ramadan observance. Sports. 2020b;8(7):98.
26. Boukhris O, Hill DW, Ammar A, Trabelsi K, Hsouna H, Abdessalem R, et al. Longer nap duration during Ramadan observance positively impacts the 5-m shuttle run test performance performed in the afternoon. Front Physiol. 2022;13:811435.
27. Bouhlel E, Salhi Z, Bouhlel H, Mdella S, Amamou A, Zaouali M, et al. Effect of Ramadan fasting on fuel oxidation during exercise in trained male rugby players. Diabetes Metab. 2006;32(6):617–24.
28. Trabelsi K, Rebai H, El-Abed K, Stannard SR, Khannous H, Masmoudi L, et al. Effect of Ramadan fasting on body water status markers after a rugby sevens match. Asian J Sports Med. 2011;2(3):186.

29. Aziz AR, Lim DSL, Sahrom S, Muhamed AC, Ihsan M, Girard O, Chia MYH. Effects of Ramadan fasting on match-related changes in skill performance in elite Muslim badminton players. Sci Sports. 2020;35(5):308–e1.
30. Brandt R, Bevilacqua GG, Andrade A. Perceived sleep quality, mood states, and their relationship with performance among Brazilian elite athletes during a competitive period. J Strength Cond Res. 2017;31(4):1033–9.
31. Andrade A, Bevilacqua G, Casagrande P, Brandt R, Coimbra D. Sleep quality associated with mood in elite athletes. Phys Sportsmed. 2019;47(3):312–7.
32. Singh R, Hwa OC, Roy J, Jin CW, Ismail SM, Lan MF, et al. Subjective perception of sports performance, training, sleep and dietary patterns of Malaysian junior Muslim athletes during Ramadan intermittent fasting. Asian J Sports Med. 2011;2(3):167.
33. Gueldich H, Zghal F, Borji R, Chtourou H, Sahli S, Rebai H. The effects of Ramadan intermittent fasting on the underlying mechanisms of force production capacity during maximal isometric voluntary contraction. Chronobiol Int. 2019;36(5):698–708.
34. Armstrong LE, Ganio MS, Casa DJ, Lee EC, McDermott BP, Klau JF, Lieberman HR. Mild dehydration affects mood in healthy young women. J Nutr. 2012;142(2):382–8.
35. McMorris T, Swain J, Smith M, Corbett J, Delves S, Sale C, et al. Heat stress, plasma concentrations of adrenaline, noradrenaline, 5-hydroxytryptamine, and cortisol, mood state, and cognitive performance. Int J Psychophysiol. 2006;61(2):204–15.
36. Moyen NE, Ganio MS, Wiersma LD, Kavouras SA, Gray M, McDERMOTT BP, et al. Hydration status affects mood state and pain sensation during ultra-endurance cycling. J Sports Sci. 2015;33(18):1962–9.
37. Chtourou H, Hammouda O, Chaouachi A, Chamari K, Souissi N. The effect of time-of-day and Ramadan fasting on anaerobic performances. Int J Sports Med. 2012;33(02):142–7.
38. de Moraes WM, de Almeida FN, Dos Santos LE, Cavalcante KD, Santos HO, Navalta JW, Prestes J. Carbohydrate loading practice in bodybuilders: effects on muscle thickness, photo silhouette scores, mood states, and gastrointestinal symptoms. J Sports Sci Med. 2019;18(4):772.
39. Maughan RJ, Shirreffs SM. Hydration and performance during Ramadan. J Sports Sci. 2012;30(sup1):S33–41.
40. Chaouachi A, Leiper JB, Chtourou H, Aziz AR, Chamari K. The effects of Ramadan intermittent fasting on athletic performance: recommendations for the maintenance of physical fitness. J Sports Sci. 2012;30(sup1):S53–73.
41. O'Donnell S, Driller MW. Sleep hygiene education improves sleep indices in elite female athletes. Int J Exerc Sci. 2017;10(4):522.
42. Bogdan A, Bouchareb B, Touitou Y. Ramadan fasting alters endocrine and neuroendocrine circadian patterns. Meal–time as a synchronizer in humans? Life Sci. 2001;68(14):1607–15.
43. Trabelsi K, Ammar A, Zlitni S, Boukhris O, Khacharem A, El-Abed K, et al. Practical recommendations to improve sleep during Ramadan observance in healthy practitioners of physical activity Recommandations pratiques pour améliorer le sommeil pendant le jeûne de Ramadan chez des pratiquants sains de l'activité physique. Tunis Med. 2019;97(10):1104.
44. Roy J, Hwa OC, Singh R, Aziz AR, Jin CW. Self-generated coping strategies among Muslim athletes during Ramadan fasting. J Sports Sci Med. 2011;10(1):137.
45. Aloui A, Briki W, Baklouti H, Chtourou H, Driss T, Chaouachi A, et al. Listening to music during warming-up counteracts the negative effects of Ramadan observance on short-term maximal performance. PLoS One. 2015;10(8):e0136400.

Part V
Practical and Social Aspects

Chapter 16
Dietary and Lifestyle Changes During Ramadan Fasting Month

Maha H. Alhussain and Meghit Boumediene Khaled

Abstract During the holy month of Ramadan, Muslims worldwide observe fasting—one of the Five Pillars of Islam—by abstaining from all food and fluid from dawn until dusk each day throughout the month. It is reasonable to anticipate that the exclusive eating period during night-time during Ramadan will lead to a noticeable change in normal lifestyle activities. Such changes include dietary and sleep patterns. Meal times shift entirely to the night, with the frequency typically limited to two main meals: one just before dawn and another after sunset. The restrictions on meal timing and frequency may lead to changes in caloric intake, dietary composition, and food selections. However, the extent of these changes can vary widely depending on numerous factors, including geographical location and cultural habits. Ramadan fasting can also influence the regular sleep–wake cycle aligned with the solar day, leading to notable alterations in sleep patterns and quality. These changes manifest as decreased sleep duration, elevated sleep disturbances, modifications in sleep architecture, and overall impacts on sleep quality. Findings regarding lifestyle changes during Ramadan derived from a specific cultural or national context may not be universally applicable, emphasizing the need for cross-cultural research to enhance generalizability.

Keywords Ramadan · Fasting · Lifestyle · Diet · Mealtime · Meal frequency · Sleep pattern

M. H. Alhussain (✉)
Department of Food Sciences and Nutrition, College of Food and Agricultural Sciences, King Saud University, Riyadh, Saudi Arabia
e-mail: mhussien@ksu.edu.sa

M. B. Khaled
Department of Biology, Faculty of Life and Natural Science, Laboratoire de Nutrition, Pathologie, Agrobiotechnologie et Santé (Lab-NuPABS), Djillali Liabes University of Sidi-Bel-Abbès, Sidi Bel Abbès, Algeria

16.1 Introduction

Muslims worldwide observe fasting—one of the Five Pillars of Islam—by abstaining from all food and fluid from dawn until dusk over the full month of Ramadan (Quran, 2:187), which lasts between 29 and 30 consecutive days. Therefore, fasting during Ramadan displaces eating and drinking (including water) during the night-time hours. The duration of fasting hours is substantially affected by the geographical location and the time of the seasonal year in which Ramadan falls, as its start date shifts earlier by approximately 11 days annually and may fall in different seasons. While the average duration of the daily fast is 12 h, it can extend up to 22 h in polar regions in the summer.

It is reasonable to anticipate that the exclusive eating period during night-time hours will lead to profound alterations in everyday lifestyle activities. Indeed, during Ramadan, Islamic societies experience substantial shifts in daily routines, such as adjustments in dietary habits, sleep patterns, and physical activity levels compared with other months. Muslims exhibit special dietary behaviors during Ramadan [1]. Thus, fasting during Ramadan is regarded as one of the main factors that influence dietary patterns. Ramadan fasting can also affect the regular sleep–wake cycle aligned with the solar day, [2, 3]. In addition, the propensity to engage in exercise is likely to be impaired, even if the exercise period is deliberately moved to after dusk. This chapter highlights global lifestyle changes observed during Ramadan, focusing on changes in dietary and sleep patterns and sedentary behaviors.

16.2 Dietary Pattern

16.2.1 Meal Timing and Frequency

Ramadan fasting is regarded as a type of "time-restricted feeding," where food and fluid are restricted to a specified time daily with no calorie restriction. It involves consistent diurnal abstinence from food and fluid. Accordingly, the eating period during Ramadan is shifted to the night-time hours. The daily fasting and eating periods are highly dependent upon the time of year and the geographical location. During the eating period, Muslims are allowed to eat and drink freely without restriction on the amount or type of food. Despite the sudden shift in mealtime seen during Ramadan, the favorable impacts of Ramadan fasting on general health have been consistently reported [4–6]. It should be recognized that the unique features of Ramadan fasting, which involve a long duration of the practice for 1 month, may allow physiological and chronological adaptations to the new pattern. Maintaining a consistent meal schedule can contribute to better health outcomes [7, 8] and can promote energy balance [9, 10].

Besides mealtime, the potential health benefits obtained during Ramadan fasting can be associated with meal frequency. Studies exploring acute metabolic responses to various meal frequencies might support the advantages of reducing meal frequency [11]. Moreover, in a prospective analysis, increasing the frequency of daily meals beyond three meals was linked to a higher risk of weight gain [12]. Due to time-restricted feeding, meal frequency is expected to decrease, and several studies have confirmed this reduction in daily meal frequency during Ramadan [13, 14]. The common eating habit during Ramadan is to eat two main meals: one large meal to break the fast at sunset (Iftar) and a smaller meal nearly 30 min before dawn (Suhoor) [15, 16]. Some individuals also eat an additional meal or snack between Iftar and Suhoor [17]. Suhoor is considered an important meal in Islamic traditions. Skipping this meal is a critical violation that many Muslims do in favor of more sleep. This practice would be expected to promote metabolic abnormalities.

As meal frequency is reduced to two or three meals per day during Ramadan, the variety and quantity of food consumed are altered. This, in turn, would be expected to influence caloric and nutrient intake.

16.2.2 Caloric and Nutrient Intake

Theoretically, time-restricted feeding and skipping meals (e.g., Ramadan fasting) would lead to a reduction in caloric intake. Yet, in reality, this is not the case for most cultures observing Ramadan. Caloric and nutrient intake is variable according to the variations in eating and social habits practiced by Muslims in different countries. The length of fasting duration (i.e., during the summer months when people typically increase fluid intake to manage thirst) can also have an impact on daily caloric and nutrient intake. The changes in caloric intake during Ramadan are inconsistent across different studies. Some studies have revealed a reduction in caloric intake [18–20], while others have shown an increase in caloric intake instead [21–23]. A lack of significant differences between caloric intake during and before Ramadan fasting has also been reported [24–27]. Results of the changes in caloric intake during Ramadan in varied countries are summarized in Table 16.1.

Despite the inconsistency of daily caloric intake findings, accumulating evidence shows that Ramadan fasting is associated with a reduction in body mass, BMI, and fat mass [23, 24, 34, 35]. This observation may propose an application in weight loss strategies among individuals with overweight or obesity.

Aside from caloric intake, fasting during Ramadan can result in notable modifications in the composition of the diet and macronutrients, and contradictory findings have been reported in this matter (Table 16.1). Such inconsistency might be attributed to several factors, including cultural habits and dietary norms of the populations.

With regard to vitamins, the changes in their intake during Ramadan are not consistent between studies. Some studies reported no changes in vitamin B complex [36], vitamin C [37], and vitamin E [18, 37] during Ramadan. By contrast, a significant decrease in vitamin C and vitamin E during Ramadan was observed [18]. Another study showed that vitamin C and folate were significantly higher in

Table 16.1 Summarized results of the changes in daily caloric and macronutrient intake during Ramadan in varied countries

Reference	Country	N	Caloric intake	Macronutrient		
				Carbohydrate	Protein	Fat
Alzhrani et al. [23]	Saudi Arabia	115	↑	↔	↓	↔
Shatila et al. [28]	Lebanon	62	↔	↔	↔	↔
Barakat et al. [29]	Morocco	340	↑	↑	↓	↓
Kocaaga et al. [20]	Turkey	33	↓	↓	↓	↔
Nachvak et al. [19]	Iran	160	↓	↑	↓	↓
Yeoh et al. [30]	Singapore	29	↔	↔	↔	↑
Khattak et al. [25]	Malaysia	30	↔	↔	↔	↔
Vasan et al. [31]	India	70	↑	↑	↑	↑
Sadiya et al. [32]	UAE	19	↔	↔	↓	↑
Lamri-Senhadji et al. [22]	Algeria	46	↑	↑	↔	↔
Maughan et al. [33]	Tunisia	59	↔	↓	↑	↔
Al-Hourani and Atoum [24]	Jordan	57	↔	↔	↔	↔

Note: ↑: increase; ↓: decrease; ↔: no change

Ramadan [28]. In terms of minerals, a previous study showed no changes in calcium intake [36]. However, it has been reported that calcium was the most inadequately consumed nutrient during Ramadan [38]. Another study found a significant increase in calcium intake during Ramadan [29]. Maughan and colleagues reported a reduction in sodium and iron intake during Ramadan [33]. On the other hand, Shatila et al. indicated that sodium and iron intake were similar between Ramadan and ordinary days [28]. Barakat et al. showed an increase in sodium intake during Ramadan [29].

A factor contributing to discrepant findings across studies investigating changes in nutrient intake is the variation in dietary assessment methods. Furthermore, the variations in the findings reflect differences in meal composition and food selection between countries and cultures.

16.2.3 Food Selections

It should be recognized that food selections during Ramadan can vary greatly between different cultures and countries. They are tightly linked to social norms and traditions, with specific dishes eaten only during Ramadan. Economic status and individual dietary behavior also have major impacts on food selections. In general, Muslims traditionally start the Iftar meal with dates, following the example of Prophet Muhammad, who reportedly broke his fast with dates. Prophet Mohammed also said, "The best Suhoor for the believer is dates," so Muslims often incorporate dates into Suhoor. Dates have many great health and nutrition benefits that make them worthy of this sunnah superfood status. They provide readily available carbohydrates, mainly fructose and glucose, for a quick boost after a long day of fasting, as well as fiber for slower digestion [39].

Although Suhoor comprised types of food that were normally eaten at breakfast on regular days, Iftar consisted of a great variety of foods [38]. Fasting people consume a greater variety of foods [14, 16] as Ramadan meals usually become communal gatherings with family members. Several new dishes are included in daily food intake during Ramadan, while some foods are eliminated. Reduced intake of fast foods, as well as the frequency of restaurant visits during Ramadan, has been observed [14, 23]. Fried food and sugar-containing foods are consumed more frequently during Ramadan [16, 32]. This behavior might be explained by the change in food selections when people fast. Furthermore, it is closely tied to the traditions of consuming certain sweets that are specific to Ramadan (e.g., Arabic sweets, pastries, and sugar-sweetened beverages). Beverages, in general, are common in Ramadan to alleviate the dehydration symptoms associated with fasting.

16.3   Sleep Pattern and Sedentary Behavior

It is widely recognized that the allocation of time to daily activities, including sleep, sedentary behavior, and physical activity, has significant implications for an individual's health and overall well-being. Inadequate sleep, prolonged sedentary behavior, and limited physical activity are recognized as prevalent contributors to weight gain and obesity. Such suboptimal patterns of daily movement also elevate the risk of various noncommunicable diseases [40–43].

Fasting during Ramadan can cause disruptions in sleep patterns. Alterations in food and fluid intake disrupt the sleep–wake cycle, potentially resulting in reduced sleep duration, increased sleep disturbances, changes in sleep architecture, and impacts on sleep quality. These disturbances mirror those caused by time-zone transitions, rotating shift work, and sleep deprivation [44].

The extended intervals between Ramadan's main meals (Suhoor and Iftar) during Ramadan may result in a reduction in daytime physical activity and exercise. Conversely, there is typically an increase in night-time activity during this period, while post-Ramadan sees a return to more daytime-oriented activity. Lessan et al. noted a common tendency for individuals to remain awake during the night and sleep after the Suhoor meal, with bedtimes around midnight and waking early in the morning [44]. A reduction in sleep duration could offset decreases in energy expenditure due to diminished physical activity and a lower resting metabolic rate, thereby exerting minimal influence on overall energy expenditure.

Ramadan fasting shifts mealtimes to the night-time hours, partially altering the usual circadian pattern of eating and drinking. In the customary daily activities of Muslims, the morning call to prayer marks the beginning of the day and, along with physical and social activities, food consumption, and light exposure, helps align the body clock with the solar day.

Studies on sleep patterns during Ramadan fasting are limited and primarily rely on questionnaires assessing individuals working or studying during daytime fasting. Data on sleep duration during Ramadan vary by country and appear to be influenced by differences in lifestyle and culture [45]. Changes in mealtimes can disrupt circadian rhythm and sleep patterns. Ramadan fasting is associated with disruptions in circadian rhythms and alterations in sleep–wake cycles, alongside hormonal fluctuations involving leptin, adiponectin, ghrelin, cortisol, and melatonin [46, 47]. Research indicates substantial delays in both bedtime and waketime, coupled with a significant decrease in total sleep duration during Ramadan [3, 48]. These changes could contribute to weight gain, though a corresponding reduction in food intake may mitigate this. The effect of Ramadan fasting on both the duration and quality of sleep is mixed, with some studies indicating negative effects [3, 44] and others finding no impact [49, 50]. Impairments in sleep quantity and quality, as well as excessive daytime sleepiness, may result from physiological and behavioral changes during Ramadan, such as waking up for Suhoor and dawn prayers and increased nocturnal activities like social gatherings, shopping, and prayers such as Attarawih [3, 50, 51]. A recent systematic review suggests that maintaining moderate physical activity during Ramadan may help mitigate its negative effects on sleep quality [40].

Modifications in meal timings during Ramadan, including eating solely at night, have been proposed to alter circadian rhythms and disrupt standard biological clocks. Changes in eating and sleeping schedules during fasting periods have been found to lower morning cortisol levels and raise evening levels. Adrenal sensitivity to corticotrophin stimulation was not negatively affected during Ramadan [52]. Recent systematic reviews and meta-analyses [3] indicated a reduction in sleep duration and a concurrent increase in Epworth Sleepiness Scale (ESS) scores during Ramadan. Shifts in circadian rhythm resulting from the prolonged practice of altered meal and sleep timings could lead to changing sleep patterns during Ramadan [3].

The impact of fasting during Ramadan on sleep patterns and other physiological parameters has been subject to varying interpretations in the literature. Changes in lifestyle, such as postponed start times for educational and work commitments, increased nocturnal activity, late-night social interactions, and night-time prayer practices, may contribute to shifts in circadian rhythms [45]. Employing validated portable devices to assess skin temperature, sleep patterns, and energy expenditure during Ramadan has demonstrated considerable delays in bedtime and wake-up time, as well as alterations in circadian rhythms. These outcomes suggest that factors beyond fasting and mealtimes may exert an influence on sleep patterns and circadian rhythms during Ramadan [53].

Nugraha et al. evaluated daytime sleepiness utilizing the ESS and showed that fasting during Ramadan did not adversely affect fatigue, sleepiness, mood, health-related quality of life, or body composition-related metrics [54]. A prospective observational study by Çelik et al. [55] investigated the impact of Ramadan fasting on sleep quality using the Pittsburgh Sleep Quality Index (PSQI) in 32 healthy Turkish adults. The authors concluded that fasting during Ramadan did not impact sleep quality, which aligns with the findings of Boukhris et al. [50] and Al-Barha and Aljaloud [56].

In a prospective study conducted in Saudi Arabia, Alzhrani et al. [23] found an association between Ramadan and fasting. They increased caloric and carbohydrate intake, as well as alterations in chronotype and daytime sleepiness. The study reported a notable shift in participants' ESS scores before and during Ramadan, with a higher proportion of participants exhibiting normal sleepiness levels during Ramadan than before. Sleep duration remained stable between the two study periods, with mean daily sleep duration falling within the recommended range for overall health (7–9 h for adults) [57]. However, certain studies [17, 58] present contrasting findings, noting a decrease in total sleep duration during Ramadan. The augmented practice of additional worship activities, such as Taraweeh prayers at night, may account for the reduced sleep duration observed in previous investigations.

A study in Tunisia [59] explored the impact of Ramadan fasting on cognitive performance, sleep quality, daytime sleepiness, and insomnia among 58 elderly participants categorized as either physically active or sedentary. Employing global scores from the PSQI, Insomnia Severity Index (ISI), and ESS, the study discovered that both groups experienced excessive daytime sleepiness and poor sleep quality. The sedentary group experienced notably more adverse effects from Ramadan fasting, including a considerable reduction in sleep duration from before to during the fasting period. In contrast, the active group did not exhibit significant changes in sleep duration.

A multinational cross-sectional study across 27 countries and diverse ethnic and racial backgrounds examined sleep duration, disturbance, and quality in 24,541 participants during the COVID-19 period [60]. Structural equation modeling (SEM) was employed to explore the impact of dietary and lifestyle factors on these sleep parameters. The study identified significant associations between modified food patterns, sufficient plant-based protein consumption, and regular physical activity with optimal sleep duration (7–9 h). While smoking was linked to lower self-evaluated sleep quality and increased sleep disturbance, improved intake of vegetables, fruits, and plant-based proteins was deemed essential for enhancing sleep quality during Ramadan fasting. Regular physical activity and avoiding smoking were also highlighted as crucial factors for improving sleep quality during Ramadan [60].

Studies assessing the sleep–wake pattern in various Muslim countries exhibited a notable and sudden delay in bedtime and waketime during Ramadan among those practicing diurnal intermittent fasting. Contradictory findings regarding the effects of Ramadan fasting on sleep duration may reflect cultural and lifestyle differences between countries or the variations in the assessment tools used [2, 60].

The influence of diurnal intermittent fasting on circadian rhythm, sleep, and daytime sleepiness presents an intriguing area for further investigation. Given the relatively small sample size in current studies, future research would benefit from larger cohorts to more accurately identify potential predictors of circadian rhythm alterations during Ramadan. Additionally, findings regarding lifestyle changes from a specific cultural or national context may not be universally applicable, emphasizing the need for cross-cultural research to enhance generalizability.

16.4 Conclusion

In conclusion, fasting during Ramadan profoundly impacts various aspects of lifestyle, particularly dietary patterns, sleep behaviors, and physical activity. The shift to a time-restricted eating model results in significant alterations in meal timing and frequency, which—while potentially beneficial—can also lead to inconsistencies in caloric and nutrient intake across different cultures. Although some evidence suggests that Ramadan fasting can promote weight loss and favorable health outcomes, variations in dietary habits and regional practices introduce complexities that warrant further investigation. Additionally, the effects of fasting during Ramadan on sleep patterns are multifaceted, with studies showing both disruptions and stabilizations in sleep duration and quality. These discrepancies highlight the need for more robust research employing standardized assessment methods to understand the full impact of Ramadan fasting on circadian rhythms, sleep, and overall well-being. As Ramadan practices may differ significantly among Muslim communities worldwide, future studies should aim to explore these lifestyle changes across diverse populations, enabling a more nuanced understanding of the health implications of fasting. Overall, Ramadan fasting presents both challenges and opportunities for health promotion, emphasizing the importance of mindful dietary choices and maintaining physical activity to optimize benefits during this holy month.

References

1. Osman F, Haldar S, Henry CJ. Effects of time-restricted feeding during Ramadan on dietary intake, body composition and metabolic outcomes. Nutrients. 2020;12(8):2478.
2. BaHammam AS, Almeneessier AS. Recent evidence on the impact of Ramadan diurnal intermittent fasting, mealtime, and circadian rhythm on cardiometabolic risk: a review. Front Nutr. 2020;7:28.
3. Faris MAIE, Jahrami HA, Alhayki FA, Alkhawaja NA, Ali AM, Aljeeb SH, et al. Effect of diurnal fasting on sleep during Ramadan: a systematic review and meta-analysis. Sleep Breath. 2020;24:771–82.
4. Fernando HA, Zibellini J, Harris RA, Seimon RV, Sainsbury A. Effect of Ramadan fasting on weight and body composition in healthy non-athlete adults: a systematic review and meta-analysis. Nutrients. 2019;11(2):478.
5. Jahrami HA, Alsibai J, Obaideen AA. Impact of Ramadan diurnal intermittent fasting on the metabolic syndrome components in healthy, non-athletic Muslim people aged over 15 years: a systematic review and meta-analysis. Br J Nutr. 2020;123(1):1–22.
6. Madkour MI, Obaideen AK, Dalah EZ, Hasan HA, Radwan H, Jahrami HA, et al. Effect of Ramadan diurnal fasting on visceral adiposity and serum adipokines in overweight and obese individuals. Diabetes Res Clin Pract. 2019;153:166–75.

7. St-Onge M-P, Ard J, Baskin ML, Chiuve SE, Johnson HM, Kris-Etherton P, et al. Meal timing and frequency: implications for cardiovascular disease prevention: a scientific statement from the American Heart Association. Circulation. 2017;135(9):e96–e121.
8. Ahola AJ, Mutter S, Forsblom C, Harjutsalo V, Groop P-H. Meal timing, meal frequency, and breakfast skipping in adult individuals with type 1 diabetes–associations with glycaemic control. Sci Rep. 2019;9(1):20063.
9. Alhussain MH, Macdonald IA, Taylor MA. Impact of isoenergetic intake of irregular meal patterns on thermogenesis, glucose metabolism, and appetite: a randomized controlled trial. Am J Clin Nutr. 2022;115(1):284–97.
10. BaHammam AS, Pirzada A. Timing matters: the interplay between early mealtime, circadian rhythms, gene expression, circadian hormones, and metabolism-a narrative review. Clocks Sleep. 2023;5(3):507–35. https://doi.org/10.3390/clockssleep5030034.
11. Paoli A, Tinsley G, Bianco A, Moro T. The influence of meal frequency and timing on health in humans: the role of fasting. Nutrients. 2019;11(4):719.
12. Van Der Heijden AA, Hu FB, Rimm EB, Van Dam RM. A prospective study of breakfast consumption and weight gain among US men. Obesity. 2007;15(10):2463–9.
13. Frost G, Pirani S. Meal frequency and nutritional intake during Ramadan: a pilot study. Hum Nutr Appl Nutr. 1987;41(1):47–50.
14. Ali Z, Abizari A-R. Ramadan fasting alters food patterns, dietary diversity, and body weight among Ghanaian adolescents. Nutr J. 2018;17:1–14.
15. Azizi F. Islamic fasting and health. Ann Nutr Metab. 2010;56(4):273–82.
16. Trepanowski JF, Bloomer RJ. The impact of religious fasting on human health. Nutr J. 2010;9:1–9.
17. Roky R, Chapotot F, Hakkou F, Benchekroun MT, Buguet A. Sleep during Ramadan intermittent fasting. J Sleep Res. 2001;10(4):319–27.
18. Sajjadi SF, Hassanpour K, Assadi M, Yousefi F, Ostovar A, Nabipour I, et al. Effect of Ramadan fasting on macronutrients & micronutrients intake: an essential lesson for healthcare professionals. J Nutr Fasting Health. 2018;6(4):205–12.
19. Nachvak SM, Pasdar Y, Pirsaheb S, Darbandi M, Niazi P, Mostafai R, et al. Effects of Ramadan on food intake, glucose homeostasis, lipid profiles, and body composition. Eur J Clin Nutr. 2019;73(4):594–600.
20. Kocaaga T, Tamer K, Karli U, Yarar H. Effects of Ramadan fasting on physical activity level and body composition in young males. Int J Appl Exerc Physiol. 2019;8:2322–3537.
21. Benli Aksungar F, Eren A, Ure S, Teskin O, Ates G. Effects of intermittent fasting on serum lipid levels, coagulation status, and plasma homocysteine levels. Ann Nutr Metab. 2005;49(2):77–82.
22. Lamri-Senhadji M, El Kebir B, Belleville J, Bouchenak M. Assessment of dietary consumption and time-course of changes in serum lipids and lipoproteins before, during and after Ramadan in young Algerian adults. Singapore Med J. 2009;50(3):288.
23. Alzhrani A, Alhussain MH, BaHammam AS. Changes in dietary intake, chronotype and sleep pattern upon Ramadan among healthy adults in Jeddah, Saudi Arabia: a prospective study. Front Nutr. 2022;9:966861.
24. Al-Hourani H, Atoum M. Body composition, nutrient intake and physical activity patterns in young women during Ramadan. Singapore Med J. 2007;48(10):906.
25. Khattak MMAK, Mamat NM, Bakar WAMA, Shaharuddin MFN. Does religious fasting affect energy and macro-nutrients intakes? J Nutr Food Sci. 2013;43(3):254–60.
26. Harder-Lauridsen NM, Rosenberg A, Benatti FB, Damm JA, Thomsen C, Mortensen EL, et al. Ramadan model of intermittent fasting for 28 d had no major effect on body composition, glucose metabolism, or cognitive functions in healthy lean men. Nutrition. 2017;37:92–103.
27. Sana'a AA, Ismail M, Baker A, Blair J, Adebayo A, Kelly L, et al. The effects of diurnal Ramadan fasting on energy expenditure and substrate oxidation in healthy men. Br J Nutr. 2017;118(12):1023–30.

28. Shatila H, Baroudi M, El Sayed AR, Chehab R, Forman MR, Abbas N, et al. Impact of Ramadan fasting on dietary intakes among healthy adults: a year-round comparative study. Front Nutr. 2021;8:689788.
29. Barakat I, Chamlal H, Elayachi M, Belahsen R. Food expenditure and food consumption before and during Ramadan in Moroccan households. J Nutr Metab. 2020;2020:1.
30. Yeoh E, Zainudin SB, Loh WN, Chua CL, Fun S, Subramaniam T, et al. Fasting during Ramadan and associated changes in glycemia, caloric intake, and body composition with gender differences in Singapore. Ann Acad Med Singap. 2015;44(6):202–6.
31. Vasan SK, Karol R, Mahendri N, Arulappan N, Jacob JJ, Thomas N. A prospective assessment of dietary patterns in Muslim subjects with type 2 diabetes who undertake fasting during Ramadan. Indian J Endocrinol Metab. 2012;16(4):552–7.
32. Sadiya A, Ahmed S, Siddieg HH, Babas IJ, Carlsson M. Effect of Ramadan fasting on metabolic markers, body composition, and dietary intake in Emiratis of Ajman (UAE) with metabolic syndrome. In: Diabetes, metabolic syndrome, and obesity: targets and therapy, vol. 4; 2011. p. 409–16.
33. Maughan RJ, Bartagi Z, Dvorak J, Zerguini Y. Dietary intake and body composition of football players during the holy month of Ramadan. J Sports Sci. 2008;26(S3):S29–38.
34. Sadeghirad B, Motaghipisheh S, Kolahdooz F, Zahedi MJ, Haghdoost AA. Islamic fasting and weight loss: a systematic review and meta-analysis. Public Health Nutr. 2014;17(2):396–406.
35. Mazidi M, Rezaie P, Chaudhri O, Karimi E, Nematy M. The effect of Ramadan fasting on cardiometabolic risk factors and anthropometrics parameters: a systematic review. Pak J Med Sci. 2015;31(5):1250.
36. Rakicioğlu N, Samur G, Topcu A, Topcu AA. The effect of Ramadan on maternal nutrition and composition of breast milk. Pediatr Int. 2006;48(3):278–83.
37. Ibrahim WH, Habib HM, Jarrar AH, Al Baz SA. Effect of Ramadan fasting on markers of oxidative stress and serum biochemical markers of cellular damage in healthy subjects. Ann Nutr Metab. 2009;53(3–4):175–81.
38. Yucecan NK, Sevinc. Some behavioral changes were observed among fasting subjects, as well as their nutritional habits and energy expenditure during Ramadan. Int J Food Sci Nutr. 2000;51(2):125–34.
39. Al-Farsi MA, Lee CY. Nutritional and functional properties of dates: a review. CRC Crit Rev Food Sci Nutr. 2008;48(10):877–87.
40. Wang F, Boros S. The effect of physical activity on sleep quality: a systematic review. Eur J Phys. 2021;23(1):11–8.
41. Chattu VK, Manzar MD, Kumary S, Burman D, Spence DW, Pandi-Perumal SR. The global problem of insufficient sleep and its serious public health implications. Healthcare. 2018;7:1.
42. Romieu I, Dossus L, Barquera S, Blottière HM, Franks PW, Gunter M, et al. Energy balance and obesity: what are the main drivers? Cancer Causes Control. 2017;28:247–58.
43. Amagasa S, Machida M, Fukushima N, Kikuchi H, Takamiya T, Odagiri Y, et al. Is objectively measured light-intensity physical activity associated with health outcomes after adjustment for moderate-to-vigorous physical activity in adults? A systematic review. Int J Behav Nutr Phys Act. 2018;15:1–13.
44. Lessan N, Saadane I, Alkaf B, Hambly C, Buckley AJ, Finer N, et al. The effects of Ramadan fasting on activity and energy expenditure. Am J Clin Nutr. 2018;107(1):54–61.
45. Bahammam A. Does Ramadan fasting affect sleep? Int J Clin Pract. 2006;60(12):1631–7.
46. Jahrami HA, Alsibai J, Clark CC, Faris MAIE. A systematic review, meta-analysis, and meta-regression of the impact of diurnal intermittent fasting during Ramadan on body weight in healthy subjects aged 16 years and above. Eur J Nutr. 2020;59(6):2291–316.
47. Al-Rawi N, Madkour M, Jahrami H, Salahat D, Alhasan F, BaHammam A, et al. Effect of diurnal intermittent fasting during Ramadan on ghrelin, leptin, melatonin, and cortisol levels among overweight and obese subjects: a prospective observational study. PLoS One. 2020;15(8):e0237922.

48. Almeneessier AS, Bahammam AS, Sharif MM, Bahammam SA, Nashwan SZ, Perumal SRP, et al. The influence of intermittent fasting on the circadian pattern of melatonin while controlling for caloric intake, energy expenditure, light exposure, and sleep schedules: a preliminary report. Ann Thorac Med. 2017;12(3):183–90.
49. BaHammam AS, Almushailhi K, Pandi-Perumal SR, Sharif MM. Intermittent fasting during R amadan: does it affect sleep? J Sleep Res. 2014;23(1):35–43.
50. Boukhris O, Trabelsi K, Shephard RJ, Hsouna H, Abdessalem R, Chtourou L, et al. Sleep patterns, alertness, dietary intake, muscle soreness, fatigue, and mental stress were recorded before, during, and after Ramadan observance. Sports. 2019;7(5):118.
51. Trabelsi K, Ammar A, Glenn JM, Boukhris O, Khacharem A, Bouaziz B, et al. Does observance of Ramadan affect sleep in athletes and physically active individuals? A systematic review and meta-analysis. J Sleep Res. 2022;31(3):e13503.
52. Bahijri S, Borai A, Ajabnoor G, Abdul Khaliq A, AlQassas I, Al-Shehri D, et al. Relative metabolic stability, but disrupted circadian cortisol secretion during the fasting month of Ramadan. PLoS One. 2013;8(4):e60917.
53. Qasrawi SO, Pandi-Perumal SR, BaHammam AS. The effect of intermittent fasting during Ramadan on sleep, sleepiness, cognitive function, and circadian rhythm. Sleep Breath. 2017;21:577–86.
54. Nugraha B, Ghashang SK, Hamdan I, Gutenbrunner C. Effect of Ramadan fasting on fatigue, mood, sleepiness, and health-related quality of life of healthy young men in summer time in Germany: a prospective controlled study. Appetite. 2017;111:38–45.
55. Mengi Çelik Ö, Koçak T, Köksal E. Effects of diurnal Ramadan intermittent fasting on cardiometabolic risk factors and sleep quality in healthy Turkish adults. Ecol Food Nutr. 2022;61(5):595–607.
56. Al-Barha NS, Aljaloud KS. The effect of Ramadan fasting on body composition and metabolic syndrome in apparently healthy men. Am J Mens Health. 2019;13(1):1557988318816925.
57. Alfawaz RA, Aljuraiban GS, AlMarzooqi MA, Alghannam AF, BaHammam AS, Dobia AM, et al. The recommended amount of physical activity, sedentary behavior, and sleep duration for healthy Saudis: a joint consensus statement of the Saudi Public Health Authority. Ann Thorac Med. 2021;16(3):239–44.
58. Alghamdi AS, Alghamdi KA, Jenkins RO, Alghamdi MN, Haris PI. Impact of Ramadan on physical activity and sleeping patterns in individuals with type 2 diabetes: the first study using Fitbit device. Diabet Ther. 2020;11:1331–46.
59. Boujelbane MA, Trabelsi K, Jahrami HA, Masmoudi L, Ammar A, Khacharem A, et al. Time-restricted feeding and cognitive function in sedentary and physically active elderly individuals: Ramadan diurnal intermittent fasting as a model. Front Nutr. 2022;9:1041216.
60. Khan MA, BaHammam AS, Amanatullah A, Obaideen K, Arora T, Ali H, et al. Examination of sleep in relation to dietary and lifestyle behaviors during Ramadan: A multi-national study using structural equation modeling among 24,500 adults amid COVID-19. Front Nutr. 2023;10:1040355.

Chapter 17
Food Safety Practices, Food-Borne Diseases, and Food Waste During Ramadan Fasting Month

Murad A. Al-Holy and Amin N. Olaimat

Abstract Ramadan is a holy month for Muslims worldwide; fasting during Ramadan is one of the five pillars of Islam. The types of food, dietary habits, and the amount of food usually prepared and served this month are quite different from those in other months of the year. This chapter explores the effect of dietary habits and food-handling practices during Ramadan on the prevalence of food-borne diseases (FBD) and the best ways to reduce food waste. Thirty-one viral and bacterial food-borne pathogens are thought to be implicated in most of the reported cases of FBD. Several factors could contribute to increasing the prevalence of FBD during Ramadan. These include the preparation of meals ahead of time before the onset of the sunset meal (*iftar*) or predawn meal (*suhoor*), keeping the food at room temperature for a long time, the increased dependence on buying ready-to-eat (RTE) meals from unreliable sources, using improper cooking temperatures, and the preparation of food for large gatherings of family and friends. Additionally, increased consumption of animal-based food, such as poultry, meat, and eggs, during Ramadan is more frequently implicated in causing FBD. During Ramadan, foods prepared for the *iftar* are often extravagant, resulting in unnecessary overeating and wasting lavish foods. Hence, proper meal planning, preserving and using leftovers, and donating extra food are some measures that could be implemented to reduce food waste during Ramadan.

Keywords Ramadan fasting · Food-borne disease · Food waste · Prevalence · Animal-based food

M. A. Al-Holy (✉)
Faculty of Applied Medical Sciences, Department of Clinical Nutrition and Dietetic, The Hashemite University, Zarqa, Jordan

Faculty of Allied Medical Sciences, Department of Nutrition and Integrative Health, Middle East University, Amman, Jordan
e-mail: murad@hu.edu.jo

A. N. Olaimat
Faculty of Applied Medical Sciences, Department of Clinical Nutrition and Dietetic, The Hashemite University, Zarqa, Jordan

M. E. Faris et al. (eds.), *Health and Medical Aspects of Ramadan Intermittent Fasting*, https://doi.org/10.1007/978-981-96-6783-3_17

17.1   Introduction

Ramadan is a holy month for Muslims worldwide. During Ramadan, gatherings for extended family and friends and giving money and food to poor people massively increase. Profound changes in daily dietary practices, sleep schedules, and physical activity are common during Ramadan. Adult Muslims refrain from eating and drinking during Ramadan days, from sunrise to sunset [1]. Also, the types of food and the amounts usually prepared and served this month are quite different from those in other months. These practices during Ramadan may have some consequences on the extent of food poisoning episodes and the amounts of food waste.

Food-borne diseases (FBD) are a major health threat and are considered a major cause of disease and fatalities. It is believed that 600 million people around the world are affected by FBD, which results in huge public health and economic burdens. FBD result from consuming foods contaminated by disease-causing agents or their by-products. Foods of animal sources, such as milk, poultry, meat, fish, and eggs, are most frequently associated with FBD [2]. The symptoms of FBD may range from mild abdominal discomfort to fatal neural signs and death. Some people are more vulnerable to FBD than others. For example, individuals with immunosuppressed systems, such as those suffering from diabetes, liver or kidney disease, and cancer; infants; older people; and pregnant women are more susceptible to FBD compared to healthy adults [3]. Thirty-one viral and bacterial food-borne pathogens are thought to be implicated in most of the reported cases of FBD. However, the most widely known agents are norovirus, *Campylobacter jejuni*, *Escherichia coli* O157:H7, *Salmonella* spp., *Listeria monocytogenes,* and *Clostridium perfringens*. These pathogens are associated with significant hospitalization, morbidity, and mortality. Serious consequences could result from FBD, especially for highly vulnerable groups.

17.1.1   Salmonella spp.

According to the World Health Organization, *Salmonella* spp. is considered the most important cause of diarrhea worldwide [4]. Also, it is estimated that about 1.35 million people in the United States are infected with *Salmonella,* and it results in approximately 420 fatalities every year. It is believed that for every confirmed case of salmonellosis, there are about 30 more people with *Salmonella* illnesses that are *not* reported [5]. The economic burden caused by *Salmonella* ranks third among a list of 14 food-borne pathogens, with an annual cost of about $3.3 billion [6]. Worldwide, the most prevalent *Salmonella* implicated in human food poisoning outbreaks are *Salmonella* Enteritidis and S*almonella* Typhimurium, with poultry products being the principal source of transmission [7].

Salmonella is widely prevalent in the environment. The microbes usually emanate from foods of animal origin, such as eggs, milk, chicken, and meats, which are foods that are consumed frequently during Ramadan. However, food items such as sprouts, cantaloupe, and fruits may also serve as a source of salmonellosis transmission. The primary mode for *Salmonella* infection in humans is through the fecal–oral route or through ingesting contaminated food products [8]. Salmonellosis is a zoonotic disease that can be easily transmitted from animals to humans and from humans to humans. Therefore, strict personal hygiene, such as handwashing and sanitization of equipment and food contact surfaces and equipment used in food production, are necessary practices to prohibit the disease's spread. *Salmonella* spreading is more common in hot climates and summer because it can increase easily at warm temperatures. Therefore, it is crucial to keep perishable food items and leftovers refrigerated or frozen [5, 13]. Additionally, adequate heat processing and prevention of cross-contamination between cooked and raw food items and keeping ready-to-eat (RTE) foods away from the danger zone (5–60 °C) are crucial to prevent the transmission of *Salmonella* [5].

A salmonellosis outbreak in Riyadh, Saudi Arabia, was reported among attendees at a public gathering. Of the foods and drinks served at the gathering, rice, meat, and sweets were primarily linked to the outbreak. Stool samples were obtained, and non-typhoidal *Salmonella* was isolated from 62 individuals who were involved in the outbreak. *Salmonella* Typhimurium was also isolated in stool samples of some of the restaurant employees. Food inspection revealed that food items were contaminated by carrier food handlers, which were held at high ambient temperatures due to the lack of air conditioning [9]. In another study conducted in Makkah, Saudi Arabia, in Ramadan 2014, RTE food samples were collected and tested for *Salmonella* spp. and *E. coli* presence. The study revealed that 31% and 22% of the samples were contaminated by *E. coli* and *Salmonella* spp., respectively [10].

17.1.2 Campylobacter jejuni

Campylobacter is an enteric bacterial pathogen associated with food of animal origin, particularly poultry as reservoirs. *Campylobacter* is one of the most prevalent food-borne pathogens (FBPs) worldwide. *Campylobacter jejuni* is believed to be responsible for approximately 90% of cases of campylobacteriosis. *C. jejuni* is predominantly transmitted to humans by contaminated poultry, raw milk, and untreated water. The WHO recognizes food-borne zoonosis, including those caused by *C. jejuni*, as an important cause of human illness [2]. It is estimated that *C. jejuni* is implicated in causing >95 million cases of food poisoning and > 20,000 fatalities worldwide [11]. In the United States, the CDC reported that about 1.5 million individuals become ill from *C. jejuni* yearly [12].

Campylobacter spp. are considered part of the nonpathogenic microbiota, indigenous to the intestinal tract of birds and livestock such as cattle, sheep, and pigs. However, poultry is deemed a unique and primary reservoir of *C. jejuni* [13]. Most of the cases of campylobacteriosis are reported during the summer months; this is particularly because *C. jejuni* strains grow optimally at 37–42 °C. Birds are a major reservoir for *C. jejuni* since the microbe is used to birds' body temperature (41–42 °C) and can carry *C. jejuni* in the gastrointestinal tract of birds without exhibiting an immune reaction. It is believed that the number of illnesses caused by *C. jejuni* greatly outnumbers the number of reported outbreaks [12]. People may develop *C. jejuni* infection upon eating underheated or raw poultry or other foods that have been cross-contaminated with undercooked or raw poultry products [12]. Outbreaks have also been associated with contaminated water, unpasteurized dairy products, and fresh produce [12].

In different governorates in Egypt, it was reported that the detection rates for *C. jejuni* ranged from 4.1 to 48% in patients with gastroenteritis, and the source of infection was attributed to the consumption of undercooked and contaminated poultry [14, 15]. In Oman, it was reported that *C. jejuni* came in second place after *Salmonella* spp. as the most dominant causative agent of bacterial food-borne poisoning [16]. In Lebanon, a study was conducted between 2016 and 2017 and included 1000 patients with diarrhea. *C. jejuni* was reported as a principal bacterial causative agent of gastroenteritis with a detection rate of 21.5% [17]. On the other hand, in the United Arab Emirates (2017–2019), *C. jejuni* contributed only to about 1.9% of the cases of diarrhea among children under the age of 5 years [18]. *C. jejuni* infection is most frequently associated with diarrhea, occasional bloody diarrhea, abdominal cramps, nausea, fever, and occasional vomiting.

C. jejuni is sensitive to heating, freezing, and drying. Chilling and freezing can remarkably diminish the microbial load of *C. jejuni* on raw chicken and meat. Adequate cooking of chicken and meat products is important to completely eradicate *C. jejuni* from food. Additionally, it is recommended to avoid washing raw chicken in the kitchen sink to avoid the possibility of transmitting the microbe to ready-to-eat (RTE) foods, plates, and other kitchen utensils through cross-contamination [12].

17.1.3   Clostridium perfringens

Clostridium perfringens is one of the prevalent causes of bacterial food-borne toxico-infection. According to the CDC, it is estimated that this bacterium causes approximately one million cases of food poisoning annually [19]. In England, 8–13% of gastrointestinal food-borne outbreaks are estimated to be linked to *C. perfringens* [20]. Most *C. perfringens* cases of food poisoning are undiagnosed because it is a self-limiting disease, where the symptoms usually vanish 24 h after their appearance. Further, clinical and public health laboratories do not routinely test for *C. perfringens*, which is generally detected when it is implicated in causing an overwhelmingly large outbreak [19]. Food poisoning caused by *C. perfringens* is usually transmitted through cooked meat and poultry [21]. These food items are commonly used to prepare dishes served during Ramadan. Such foods could act as a vehicle for transmission of *C. perfringens*, especially when meat and poultry are cooked and held at room temperature for a long time without adequate reheating or refrigeration. Outbreaks of *C. perfringens* food poisoning mostly happen when large groups of individuals are served while food is kept at improper temperatures. These conditions are more likely to occur during family and friends gatherings like the *iftar* feast during Ramadan.

Holding dishes rich in proteins of animal origin, such as poultry, fish, meat, and gravy, for a protracted time at room temperature longer than an hour could provide sufficient time for spores of *C. perfringens* to germinate and proliferate rapidly in food [22]. Warm temperatures (12–54 °C) stimulate the outgrowth of *C. perfringens*. This temperature range could be provided by keeping food hot prior to serving and during the cooling and reheating processes of cooked foods [23]. The spores of *C. perfringens* usually occur in small numbers in poultry, raw meat, dehydrated soups, raw vegetables, sauces, and spices [22]. The spores of *C. perfringens* exhibit outstanding resistance to heating at high temperatures (100 °C) for more than 1 h, and their presence in foods may be inevitable. Spores of *C. perfringens* that endure cooking temperatures could germinate and grow rapidly in inadequately refrigerated foods after cooking. Upon ingesting contaminated food, the organisms may sporulate in the intestine and release the enterotoxins that inflict the disease. The disease may typically occur 8–15 h after ingesting the contaminated food [24]. The poisoning caused by *C. perfringens* is manifested by abdominal cramps, diarrhea, and gases [19]. In an outbreak of FBD reported in Greece, cooked minced beef that was not reheated was implicated in the *C. perfringens* outbreak. The organism was isolated from minced beef and the stools of suspected cases [25]. Since *C. perfringens* is ubiquitous in the environment, it is unavoidable that the spores of *C. perfringens* will appear in raw foods. Hence, to avoid food poisoning with *C. perfringens*, cooking meat and poultry to a safe internal temperature of no less than 70 °C is important. The cooked food should not be held long after cooking and should always be kept out of the danger zone (5–60 °C). Leftovers should be refrigerated immediately after eating at 4 °C and reheated to a temperature of no less than 70 °C in the cold spot of food [26].

17.1.4   Staphylococcus aureus

Staphylococcus aureus food-borne poisoning is an acute intoxication that occurs when ingesting food contaminated with enterotoxin of the bacterium. Intoxication caused by *Staph. aureus* is regarded as one of the most dominant causes of FBD worldwide [27]. Certain types of *Staph. aureus* are capable of producing heat-stable enterotoxin. Humans frequently carry *Staph. aureus* naturally on their skin, nasal cavity, throat, fingernails, or hair. Infected wounds may also be a source of large counts of *Staph. aureus* [27]. It is estimated that 20–30% of people carry *Staph. aureus* on their skin and nasal cavity [28]. Therefore, outbreaks of poor personal hygiene, improper and frequent food handling, and inappropriate temperatures can also occur [29]. Several foods have been recurrently implicated in staphylococcal intoxication, including chicken, meat and meat products, eggs, milk and dairy products, bakery products, and salads [29]. Salted food products, such as cured meat products, have also been involved as a vehicle of *Staph. aureus* FBD [30]. Such foods are lavishly consumed during Ramadan, and a lack of hygienic food handling and abusive holding temperatures for a long time before serving may trigger *Staph. aureus* outgrowth and enterotoxin production, eliciting gastroenteritis.

The food poisoning caused by *Staph. aureus* has a rapid onset (2–8 h) and includes abdominal cramps with or without diarrhea, nausea, and violent vomiting [31]. The disease is ordinarily self-limiting and usually vanishes within 24–48 h after the onset of the disease. However, symptoms could be severe and necessitate hospitalization, particularly when people with suppressed immune systems are affected, such as debilitated people, infants, and older people [32]. A food poisoning outbreak occurred in June 2017 among participants at the Ramadan buffet in a canteen in a training institute in Rabat, Morocco. The onset of symptoms among suspected cases occurred 2–17 h after *iftar* consumption. Fifty cases developed dizziness, diarrhea, and abdominal cramps, with only two of the cases developing bloody diarrhea. Out of the 50 cases, 43 were hospitalized. *Staph. aureus* and its enterotoxin were detected in briwates (thin dough stuffed with chicken) [33]. To avoid contamination with *Staph. aureus*, good food hygiene measures should be implemented, such as thorough and frequent handwashing, wearing gloves whenever working in food preparation areas, and handling raw and cooked foods in separate areas [34].

17.1.5   Listeria monocytogenes

Listeria monocytogenes is a ubiquitous food-borne bacterium that can be isolated from soil, water, and animal digestive tracts. Therefore, its presence in food is not unusual [35]. RTE foods are of particular concern for food and health authorities because such foods may become contaminated during handling, processing, and serving, and *L. monocytogenes* can multiply to dangerous levels during distribution and storage. A study conducted in Malaysia revealed that the prevalence of *L. monocytogenes* in food and environmental samples was 16%, and in RTE vegetable products and raw food of animal origin, it was 21% [36]. This reflects the wide-spreading nature of the organism and the high possibility of its transmission through RTE foods [37]. In the United Kingdom, between 1999 and 2011, the majority of listeriosis outbreaks that occurred at the home level were attributed to cold sandwich consumption [38]. In 2021, 2268 confirmed cases of listeriosis were reported among 30 European Union member states. Most of the cases were reported among individuals older than 64 years, and 94 of the reported cases were pregnancy-associated, some of which resulted in miscarriages and neonatal death [39]. Fish, meat products, chicken, and cheese are the foods most frequently associated with listeriosis outbreaks [40].

L. monocytogenes could result in a disease that varies in symptoms from mild to a life-threatening condition known as listeriosis, and it is one of the FBD that results in high hospitalization and mortality rates. The condition ranges in symptoms from self-limiting influenza-like symptoms in some individuals to meningitis, brain infection, severe blood infection, and death. *L. monocytogenes* infections are associated with a higher mortality rate than other food-borne pathogens. The mortality rate of food-borne listeriosis may reach 20–30% of the susceptible individuals [36]. Moreover, adults with suppressed immunity are more prone to septicemia and meningitis compared to other individuals [36]. A study has concluded that intermittent fasting may protect mice from infectious and noninfectious diseases such as cancer, diabetes, and neurodegeneration [41]. Another study indicated that short-term fasting (24 h fasting with water provided) mice showed enhanced survival against *L. monocytogenes* infection compared with ad libitum mice [42]. It was indicated that short-term fasting could alter and improve the composition of innate immune cells, with increased intestinal dendritic cells, and hence provide protection against *L. monocytogenes*.

Notably, *L. monocytogenes* could grow over a wide range of food storage temperatures (1–48 °C) and thrive under refrigeration conditions, in contrast to many other FBPs. This unique capability of *L. monocytogenes* makes it especially difficult to control by cold storage [43]. The prevention and eradication of *L. monocytogenes* in RTE foods is crucial in protecting consumers against listeriosis. As *L. monocytogenes* is of particular concern and threat to vulnerable individuals, consumers of this group must take strict precautionary measures in proper handling of food to prevent RTE foods from contamination and growth of *L. monocytogenes*. Adequate and frequent handwashing and storing RTE foods at low temperatures are crucial to prevent listeriosis. Also, cleaning and sanitation of food contact surfaces is pivotal to avoiding colonization and biofilm formation of *L. monocytogenes* [44]. Street vending of RTE foods is popular during the holy month of Ramadan. The safety of such foods is questionable, as they may not be processed or handled appropriately. Therefore, obtaining raw and RTE foods from reliable sources is recommended [36].

17.1.6 Escherichia coli

Escherichia coli is a group of Gram-negative bacteria, and most of its types are harmless. As *E. coli* mostly originates from the intestinal tract of humans and warm-blooded animals, it is used as an indicator for monitoring water and food safety and the appropriateness of food handling and processing. Yet, some strains of *E. coli* are very virulent, such as Shiga toxin-producing *E. coli* (STEC), which can cause severe FBD by producing toxins known as Shiga toxins similar to the toxins produced by *Shigella dysenteriae,* especially among the most vulnerable groups to FBD [45]. In addition to *E. coli* O157:H7, which results in bloody diarrhea and hemolytic uremic syndrome (HUS), other non-O157:H7 strains (O26, O145, O111, O121, and O45) might result in severe and life-threatening food poisoning [46]. STEC has a growth temperature range of 7–50 °C [47].

Symptoms caused by STEC infection include abdominal cramps and diarrhea, and sometimes, it progresses into bloody diarrhea (hemorrhagic colitis). Fever and vomiting may also occur. In people with weak immune systems (particularly children and the elderly), the infection may lead to a life-threatening condition, such as hemolytic uremic syndrome. It may progress to hemolytic anemia, acute renal failure, and thrombocytopenia [48].

The main reservoir of *E. coli* O157:H7 is the intestinal tract of cattle. However, the intestinal tract of other animals, such as sheep, goats, pigs, and poultry, could also serve as a source of pathogen contamination. Therefore, consuming contaminated foods, particularly undercooked or raw meat from such animals, could elicit the disease. Using contaminated water or vegetables irrigated with contaminated water or untreated animal dung as fertilizer and cross-contamination with raw meats and animal feces could also serve as a source of contamination of the food chain and produce contaminated raw vegetables and sprouts [45]. Undercooked hamburgers, cured salami, unpasteurized apple juice, cheese, and raw milk are examples of foods involved in outbreaks of *E. coli* O157:H7 [47]. Fruits and vegetables, including sprouts, spinach, and salads, were also associated with outbreaks of *E. coli* O157:H7 [48]. Another mode of transmission of *E. coli* is the fecal–oral route via person-to-person contact, especially when infected individuals are in the asymptomatic carrier state [47].

Appropriate cooking of meat and milk products until all parts of the food reach a temperature of 70 °C or higher will destroy STEC. Adequate cooking of meat cuts and preventing cross-contamination of raw and cooked food products, or the contamination of meat products with RTE foods such as fruits and vegetables, is vitally important. This is particularly important when preparing food for large gatherings of people who meet to break their fast at the end of a Ramadan day. Frequent handwashing, especially before and after dealing with food and after toilet contact, is highly recommended for food handlers and those who care for children, older people, and immunosuppressed individuals [47].

17.2 Viruses

Food-borne viruses cannot multiply in food but are linked with many food-borne cases and outbreaks. It was estimated that food-borne viral infections represent 59% (5.5 million) of total FBD (9.4 million) that happened in the United States every year, with noroviruses being the leading cause of viral and bacterial FBD, with a total of 5.46 million cases occurring every year. Further, noroviruses are the second leading cause of hospitalizations and the fourth leading cause of death among food-borne pathogens in the United States [49, 50]. In addition to norovirus, astrovirus, hepatitis A virus, rotavirus, and sapovirus were categorized among the 31 main pathogens responsible for FBD in the United States [51]. However, other viruses, including adenovirus and hepatitis E virus, are also linked to food-borne outbreaks [52].

These viruses can be transmitted to humans via the fecal–oral route, directly by person-to-person contact, or indirectly by ingesting contaminated food or water [53]. Therefore, raw and cooked foods, including fresh produce, salads, bakery, and delicatessen items that are extensively handled, are often implicated in FBD. Food handlers are considered the most substantial source of viral food-borne illnesses. Food handlers can spread the virus when touching RTE foods with their bare, inadequately washed hands. Therefore, personal protective equipment and disinfection should be used appropriately [53]. In 2021, an outbreak of hepatitis A virus was linked to eating Medjool dates from Jordan, including 30 illnesses in different parts of England and one person in Wales. This outbreak was reported before the start of Ramadan, which allowed action to be taken to reduce the number of people affected since date consumption is likely to increase during Ramadan, particularly because dates are consumed first at *iftar* to break fasting [54]. It is necessary to identify the sources of viral contamination and determine appropriate risk prevention measures, including avoiding food contaminated with viruses during Ramadan. Therefore, routine surveillance of viral food-borne outbreaks can provide valuable insight to develop effective proactive control measures. However, the prevention and control strategies for food contamination with food-borne viruses are more practical. These strategies include cleaning and disinfection of food contact surfaces, proper washing of fresh produce before consumption, use of potable water in food processing, increasing awareness and educating food handlers and Muslim consumers about food-borne viruses, encouraging handwashing with soap and disinfectants, and applying strict personal hygiene for all individuals, mainly in large gatherings during Ramadan [53].

17.3   Food Waste During Ramadan

Fasting during the holy month of Ramadan is supposed to bring multiple health benefits to fasting people. Nonetheless, the perceived health benefits are compromised by unhealthy eating practices and extravagant ceremonial eating behaviors in many Muslim countries.

A study conducted in Rabat, Morocco, in 2018 at the household level revealed a remarkable increase in household expenditure on food during Ramadan. Compared to other months of the year, an estimated increase of more than 50% in food spending was reported regardless of the household standard of living [1]. The food products that contributed most to the increment in food expenditure during Ramadan include meat, chicken, milk and milk products, fruits, and cereals.

A remarkable increase in daily energy intake during Ramadan was reported, which exceeded the recommended nutrient intake (RNI) by 18%. Total carbohydrates, saturated fats, and sodium intake increased significantly compared to the RNI. Although calcium intake increased during Ramadan compared to other months of the year, it was still lower than the RNI. The increase in energy intake is attributed to the consumption of high-energy-density foods. High energy intake and insufficient physical activity during Ramadan may increase the problems of overweight and obesity. On the other hand, the improvement in calcium intake is linked to increased consumption of dairy products, which become one of the main food items served at *iftar* and *suhoor* meals. Likewise, the increased sodium intake during Ramadan particularly comes from the increased consumption of bread and other food items such as briks/burek, salted briwates, stuffed bread, and quiches [55].

Another study revealed that Muslim consumers in Bangladesh spent 40.6% more on food and drinks during Ramadan than they would have otherwise [56]. The festive spirit of eating and drinking at the end of each fasting day contributed to the increased spending among Muslims. The extravagant spending practice during Ramadan was associated with increased demand for food and price hikes in food commodities. Hence, an adequate goods supply is required to regulate market prices.

Although good deeds, charity, donations, and giving and feeding people in need are common practices in Ramadan, foods prepared for the *iftar* are often extravagant, resulting in unnecessary overeating and wasting huge amounts of food, resources, and money. Hence, proper meal planning, preserving and using leftovers, and donating extra food are some measures that could be taken to reduce food waste during Ramadan.

17.4   Conclusions

Microbes can grow over a wide temperature range of 5–60 °C, called the danger zone. Therefore, RTE foods and perishable food products should be kept out of the danger zone. Necessary measures should be implemented to prevent the entry of food-borne pathogens into the food system and preclude the proliferation of pathogens in food, especially RTE foods. These include proper handling and chilling of food in the market and at home or restaurant levels, appropriate storage and cooking temperatures, prevention of cross-contamination, and applying appropriate personal hygienic practices. Obtaining RTE foods and raw materials from reliable sources is also important. Although good deeds, charity, donations, and giving and feeding people in need are common practices during Ramadan, foods prepared for the *iftar* are often extravagant, resulting in unnecessary overeating and wasting lavish amounts of food, resources, and money. Hence, proper meal planning, preserving and using leftovers, and donating extra food are some measures that could be taken to reduce food waste during Ramadan. More research is warranted to address the effect of dietary practices during Ramadan on the spread of FBD and the magnitude of food waste. It was reported that Ramadan intermittent fasting research was relevant to Sustainable Development Goal 3 (SDG 3) (Good health and well-being), especially to target 3.4 (noncommunicable diseases) such as diabetes, pregnancy, metabolic diseases, and obesity, but not FBD and food waste [57].

References

1. Barakat I, Chamlal H, El Jamal S, Elayachi M, Belahsen R. Food expenditure and food consumption before and during Ramadan in Moroccan households. J Nutr Metab. 2020:1–7.

2. Havelaar AH, Kirk MD, Torgerson PR, Gibb HJ, Hald T, Lake RJ, et al. World Health Organization global estimates and regional comparisons of the burden of food-borne disease in 2010. PLoS Med. 2015;12:e1001923.
3. Rezaeigolestani M, Hashemi M, Nematy M. Risk factors for food-borne bacterial illnesses during Ramadan. J Nutr Fasting Health. 2017;5(4):138–43.
4. Balasubramanian R, Im J, Lee J-S, Jeon HJ, Mogeni OD, Kim JH, et al. The global burden and epidemiology of invasive non-typhoidal salmonella infections. Hum Vaccin Immunother. 2018;15:1421–6.
5. Centers for Disease Control and Prevention (CDC). Campylobacteriosis. 2024a. https://www.cdc.gov/campylobacter/technical.html#print. Accessed 25 Mar 2024.
6. Hoffmann S, Batz MB, Morris JG. Annual cost of illness and quality-adjusted life year losses in the United States due to 14 food-borne pathogens. J Food Prot. 2012;75:1292–302.
7. Mkangara M. Prevention and control of human Salmonella enterica infections: an implication in food safety. Int J Food Sci. 2023;2023:1–26.
8. Pui CF, Wong WC, Chai LC, Nillian E, Ghazali FM, Cheah YK, et al. Simultaneous detection of Salmonella spp., Salmonella Typhi, and Salmonella Typhimurium in sliced fruits using multiplex PCR. Food Control. 2011;22:337–42.
9. Aljoudi A, Al-Mazam A, Choudhry A. Outbreak of foodborne Salmonella among guests of a wedding ceremony: the role of cultural factors. J Fam Community Med. 2010;17:29.
10. Ahmad OB, Asghar A, Abd El-Rahim IH. The use of PCR for the detection of Escherichia. coli and Salmonella in food samples collected from Makkah Restaurants during Ramadan 1434. The 14th Scientific Forum for the Hajj, Umrah, and Visit Research, Umm Alqura University. 2014.
11. Thomas KM, de Glanville WA, Barker GC, Benschop J, Buza JJ, Cleaveland S, et al. Prevalence of Campylobacter and Salmonella in African food animals and meat: a systematic review and meta-analysis. Int J Food Microbiol. 2020;315:108382.
12. Skarp CPA, Hänninen M-L, Rautelin HIK. Campylobacteriosis: the role of poultry meat. Clin Microbiol Infect. 2016;22:103–9.
13. Centers for Disease Control and Prevention (CDC). Salmonella. 2024b. https://www.cdc.gov/salmonella/general/prevention.html. Accessed 26 Mar 2024.
14. Ghoneim NH, Abdel-Moein KA, Barakat A, Hegazi AG, El-Razik KA, Sadek SA. Isolation and molecular characterization of Campylobacter jejuni from chicken and human stool samples in Egypt. Food Sci Technol. 2021;41:195–202. https://doi.org/10.1590/fst.01620.
15. Zeinhom MA, Abdel-Latef GK, Corke H. Prevalence, characterization, and control of campylobacter jejuni isolated from raw milk, cheese, and human stool samples in Beni-Suef governorate, Egypt. Foodborne Pathog Dis. 2021;18:322–30.
16. Isalmi AS, Al-Busafi SA, AL-Lamki RNA, Mabruk M. The ecology and antibiotic resistance patterns of gastrointestinal tract infections in a tertiary care hospital in Oman. J Pure Appl Microbiol. 2021;15:1634–42.
17. Ibrahim JN, Eghnatios E, El Roz A, Fardoun T, Ghssein G. Prevalence, antimicrobial resistance and risk factors for campylobacteriosis in Lebanon. J Infect Dev Ctries. 2019;13:11–20.
18. Alsuwaidi AR, Al Dhaheri K, Al Hamad S, George J, Ibrahim J, Ghatasheh G, et al. Etiology of diarrhea by multiplex polymerase chain reaction among young children in The United Arab Emirates: a case-control study. BMC Infect Dis. 2021;21. https://doi.org/10.1186/s12879-020-05693-1.
19. Centers for Disease Control and Prevention CDC. Clsotridium perfringens food poisoning. 2024c. https://www.cdc.gov/foodsafety/diseases/clostridium-perfringens.html.
20. Gormley FJ, Little CL, Rawal N, Gillespie IA, Lebaigue GK, Adak GK. A 17-year review of food-borne outbreaks: describing the continuing decline in England and Wales (1992–2008). Epidemiol Infect. 2011;139:688–99.
21. Wen Q, McClane BA. Detection of Enterotoxigenic Clostridium perfringens type A isolates in American retail foods. Appl Environ Microbiol. 2004;70:2685–91.
22. Grass JE, Gould LH, Mahon BE. Epidemiology of food-borne disease outbreaks caused by Clostridium perfringens, United States, 1998–2010. Foodborne Pathog Dis. 2013;10:131–6.

23. Dolan GP, Foster K, Lawer J, Amar C, Swift C, Aird H, et al. An epidemiological review of gastrointestinal outbreaks associated with Clostridium perfringens, North East of England, 2012–2014. Epidemiol Infect. 2015;144:1386–93.
24. Liu F, Lee SA, Xue J, Riordan SM, Zhang L. Global epidemiology of campylobacteriosis and the impact of COVID-19. Front Cell Infect Microbiol. 2022;12 https://doi.org/10.3389/fcimb.2022.979055.
25. Mellou K, Kyritsi M, Chrysostomou A, Sideroglou T, Georgakopoulou T, Hadjichristodoulou C. Clostridium perfringens food-borne outbreak during an athletic event in Northern Greece, June 2019. Int J Environ Res Public Health. 2019;16:3967.
26. Miyamoto K, Nagahama M. Clostridium: food poisoning by Clostridium perfringens. In: Caballero B, Finglas PM, Toldrá F, editors. Encyclopedia of food and health. Academic Press; 2016.
27. Sergelidis D, Angelidis AS. Methicillin-resistant Staphylococcus aureus: a controversial food-borne pathogen. Lett Appl Microbiol. 2017;64:409–18.
28. Kluytmans JA, Wertheim HF. Nasal carriage of Staphylococcus aureus and prevention of noso-comial infections. Infection. 2005;2005(33):3–8.
29. Bergdoll MS, Wong AL. Staphylococcus food poisoning. In: Encyclopedia of food sciences and nutrition; 2003. p. 5556–61. https://doi.org/10.1016/B0-12-227055-X/01140-8.
30. Qi Y, Miller KJ. Effect of low water activity on staphylococcal enterotoxin A and B biosynthe-sis. J Food Prot. 2000;63:473–8.
31. Balaban N, Rasooly A. Staphylococcal enterotoxins. Int J Food Microbiol. 2000;2000(61):1–10.
32. Murray RJ. Recognition and management of Staphylococcus aureus toxin-mediated disease. Intern Med J. 2005;35 https://doi.org/10.1111/j.1444-0903.2005.00984.x.
33. Moumni Abdou H, Dahbi I, Akrim M, Meski FZ, Khader Y, Lakranbi M, et al. Outbreak investigation of a multi pathogen food-borne disease in a training institute in Rabat, Morocco: a case-control study. JMIR Public Health Surveill. 2019;5:e14227.
34. Savini F, Romano A, Giacometti F, Indio V, Pitti M, Decastelli L, et al. Investigation of a Staphylococcus aureus sequence type 72 food poisoning outbreak associated with food-handler contamination in Italy. Zoonoses Public Health. 2023;70:411–9.
35. Roberts BN, Chakravarty D, Gardner JC, Ricke SC, Donaldson JR. Listeria monocytogenes response to anaerobic environments. Pathogens. 2020;9:210.
36. Jibo GG, Raji YE, Salawudeen A, Amin-Nordin S, Mansor R, Jamaluddin TZMT. A system-atic review and meta-analysis of the prevalence of Listeria monocytogenes in South-East Asia; a one-health approach of human-animal-food-environment. One Health. 2022;15:100417.
37. Tabit FT. Contamination, prevention and control of Listeria monocytogenes in food process-ing and food service environments. In: Listeria monocytogenes; 2018. https://doi.org/10.5772/intechopen.76132.
38. Little CL, Amar CFL, Awoisayo A, Grant KA. Hospital-acquired listeriosis associated with sandwiches in the UK: a cause for concern. J Hosp Infect. 2012;82(1):13–8.
39. Disease surveillance in England and Wales, January 2021. Vet Rec. 2021;188:97–101. https://doi.org/10.2807/1560-7917.ES.2021.26.20.2100432.
40. The European Union one health 2022 Zoonoses report. EFSA J. 2023:21. https://doi.org/10.2903/j.efsa.2023.8442. Available at: https://www.efsa.europa.eu/en/efsajournal/pub/7666
41. Farache J, Koren I, Milo I, Gurevich I, Kim K-W, Zigmond E, et al. Luminal bacteria recruit CD103+ dendritic cells into the intestinal epithelium to sample bacterial antigens for presenta-tion. Immunity. 2013;38:581–95. https://doi.org/10.1016/j.immuni.2013.01.009.
42. Ju Y-J, Lee K-M, Kim G, Kye Y-C, Kim HW, Chu H, et al. Change of dendritic cell subsets involved in protection against Listeria monocytogenes infection in short-term-fasted mice. Immune Netw. 2022;22. https://doi.org/10.4110/in.2022.22.e16.
43. Capita R, Felices-Mercado A, García-Fernández C, Alonso-Calleja C. Characterization of listeria monocytogenes originating from the Spanish meat-processing chain. Food Secur. 2019;8:542.

44. Codex Alimentarius: Guidelines on the application of general principles of food hygiene to the control of Listeria monocytogenes in foods, CAC/GL 61–2007 [Internet]. 2007. Available from: http://www.fao.org/input/download/standards/10740/CXG_061e.pdf. Accessed: 29 Mar 2024.
45. Hariri S. Detection of Escherichia coli in food samples using culture and polymerase chain reaction methods. Cureus. 2022;14(12):e32808. https://doi.org/10.7759/cureus.32808.
46. Bosilevac JM, Koohmaraie M. Predicting the presence of non-O157 Shiga toxin-producing Escherichia coli in ground beef by using molecular tests for Shiga toxins, Intimin, and O Serogroups. Appl Environ Microbiol. 2012;78:7152–5.
47. World Health Organization (WHO). WHO Fact sheet on Enterohaemorrhagic Escherichia coli (EHEC) 2018. 2018. https://www.who.int/news-room/fact-sheets/detail/e-coli
48. Kintz E, Byrne L, Jenkins C, McCarthy N, Vivancos R, Hunter P. Outbreaks of Shiga toxin–producing Escherichia coli linked to sprouted seeds, salad, and leafy greens: a systematic review. J Food Prot. 2019;82:1950–8.
49. Centers for Disease Control and Prevention (CDC). Burden of food-borne illness: findings | estimates of food-borne illness | CDC. https://www.cdc.gov/foodborneburden/2018-foodborne-estimates.html.2018. Accessed 30 Mar 2024.
50. Velebit B, Djordjevic V, Milojevic L, Babic M, Grkovic N, Jankovic V, et al. The common food-borne viruses: a review. IOP Conf Ser Earth Environ Sci. 2019;333:012110.
51. Scallan E, Hoekstra RM, Angulo FJ, Tauxe RV, Widdowson M-A, Roy SL, et al. Food-borne illness acquired in the United States – major pathogens. Emerg Infect Dis. 2011;17:7–15.
52. Soares VM, dos Santos EAR, Tadielo LE, Cerqueira-Cézar CK, da Cruz Encide Sampaio AN, Eisen AKA, et al. Detection of adenovirus, rotavirus, and hepatitis E virus in meat cuts marketed in Uruguaiana, Rio Grande do Sul, Brazil. One Health. 2022;14:100377.
53. Olaimat AN, Taybeh AO, Al-Nabulsi A, Al-Holy M, Hatmal MM, Alzyoud J, et al. Common and potential emerging food-borne viruses: a comprehensive review. Life. 2024;14:190.
54. Garcia Vilaplana T, Leeman D, Balogun K, Ngui SL, Phipps E, Khan WM, et al. Hepatitis A outbreak is associated with the consumption of dates in England and Wales from January 2021 to April 2021. Eur Secur. 2021, 26 https://doi.org/10.2807/1560-7917.es.2021.26.20.2100432.
55. Jafri A, El Kardi Y, Derouiche A. Sodium chloride composition of commercial white bread in Morocco. East Mediterr Health J. 2017;23:708–10.
56. Hosen MZ. Effect of Ramadan on purchasing behavior: a panel data analysis. Int Rev Econ. 2024; https://doi.org/10.1007/s12232-024-00445-y.
57. AbuShihab KH, Obaideen K, Alameddine M, Alkurd R, Khraiwesh HM, Mohammad Y, Abdelrahim DN, Madkour M, Faris ME. Reflection on Ramadan fasting research related to sustainable development goal 3 (good health and well-being): a bibliometric analysis. J Relig Health. 2023; https://doi.org/10.1007/s10943-023-01955-9.

.

Chapter 18
The Impact of Ramadan Fasting on Patient Medication Practices and Management

Yasser Bustanji

Abstract This chapter thoroughly investigates the impact of Ramadan fasting on medication utilization and administration among individuals with chronic illnesses. It underscores the crucial role of healthcare practitioners in formulating individualized healthcare plans to meet the requirements of fasting patients. Understanding the impact of fasting on medication pharmacokinetics and pharmacodynamics is essential for optimizing treatment efficacy and safety. The chapter emphasizes the physiological and pharmacological factors to consider when fasting, such as drug metabolism and absorption alterations. It explores common health issues, including cardiovascular diseases, diabetes, asthma, gastrointestinal disorders, chronic renal disease, mental health disorders, and epilepsy, and their respective management strategies during Ramadan fasting. Healthcare providers are vital in assisting fasting patients by providing education, personalized medication management strategies, and fostering interdisciplinary collaboration. Ethical and religious considerations are also addressed, highlighting the significance of keeping patients' values while safeguarding their health and welfare.

Keywords Diabetes · Epilepsy · Cardiovascular disease · Patient education · Health applications

18.1 Introduction

Ramadan, an integral component of the Islamic faith, is a designated timeframe characterized by deep self-reflection and abstaining from food and drink from daybreak to sunset, emphasizing personal restraint, worship, and communal engagement. It mandates that all capable adult Muslims fast, exempting those who have

Y. Bustanji (✉)
College of Medicine, University of Sharjah, Sharjah, United Arab Emirates

School of Pharmacy, The University of Jordan, Amman, Jordan
e-mail: ybustanji@sharjah.ac.ae

© The Author(s), under exclusive license to Springer Nature Singapore Pte Ltd. 2025
M. E. Faris et al. (eds.), *Health and Medical Aspects of Ramadan Intermittent Fasting*, https://doi.org/10.1007/978-981-96-6783-3_18

legitimate reasons such as illness or travel. This period entails more than just refraining from consuming food and beverages; it also involves comprehensive spiritual refinement, promoting individual development, heightened dedication, and ethical behavior. Ramadan encourages acts of kindness, compassion, and a heightened communal spirit through communal dining and intensified religious observances, concluding in the commemoration of Eid al-Fitr.

This chapter provides an overview of the diverse effects of Ramadan fasting on medication utilization and administration, emphasizing the importance of modifying healthcare approaches to meet the spiritual and physical welfare of individuals undergoing fasting.

18.1.1   The Importance of Understanding the Impact of Fasting on Medication Use and Management

Healthcare providers and patients need to comprehend and handle medication use during Ramadan. Fasting can impact medication pharmacokinetics and pharmacodynamics due to alteration of food consumption, fluid intake, and metabolism [1]. This may necessitate drug dosage and timing adjustments to ensure effectiveness and safety [2, 3]. Individuals with conditions such as diabetes, hypertension, and cardiovascular diseases may find it challenging to adhere to medication schedules while fasting [4]. Healthcare providers should offer personalized guidance, such as modifying schedules or exploring different treatments, to improve adherence and avoid complications. Educating patients, particularly those with chronic illnesses, on fasting exemptions, medication use behavior, and the significance of engaging with healthcare providers to ensure safe fasting is crucial. However, counseling before Ramadan about medication adjustments is essential to get the desired results.

Educating patients about the effects of fasting on their medication and health empowers them to make informed decisions regarding their care [5]. Healthcare providers are essential in guiding patients toward safe fasting practices and emphasizing potential health risks. This educational approach improves patient autonomy and adherence to treatment plans and emphasizes the importance of respecting individual beliefs in patient care. Enhancing the patient–provider relationship can lead to increased patient satisfaction [5].

An integrated, team-based approach is essential for effectively managing medications during Ramadan, requiring collaboration among physicians, pharmacists, and dietitians to develop comprehensive care strategies. Pharmacists play a crucial role in supporting patients by recommending medication options, modifying doses, and offering nutritional guidance to help maintain their health during fasting [6]. Risk stratification guides healthcare professionals and patients in making informed fasting decisions for individuals with chronic illnesses. For managing medications during Ramadan, it is crucial to collaborate and focus on the patient's needs, balancing religious practices with health priorities [7].

18.2   Physiological and Pharmacological Considerations During Fasting

Ramadan fasting has a significant effect on physiological changes, which in turn have an impact on the pharmacokinetics and pharmacodynamics of medications. Fasting can substantially affect the body's processes for drug distribution, metabolism, excretion, and absorption. Hence, modifying how drugs are administered to fasting patients may be necessary. Understanding these modifications is crucial for healthcare providers to guarantee safe and effective drug administration, emphasizing the need for customized pharmaceutical care [3].

18.2.1   Physiological Effects of Fasting on Metabolism

During Ramadan fasting, the body undergoes notable physiological changes due to prolonged periods without food or drink. These changes affect various aspects of metabolism, including glucose regulation, lipid metabolism, and the circadian rhythm of hormonal secretion. It is essential to understand these metabolic changes to optimize drug treatment during fasting. The body shifts to using fatty acids and ketone bodies for energy during fasting, which impacts hepatic enzyme-mediated drug metabolism pathways [8–10]. Moreover, changes in eating and sleeping habits during Ramadan impact circadian rhythms. This disrupts the synchronization between the body's internal clocks and the central clock in the brain [11]. Such misalignment can affect drug pharmacokinetics through changes in absorption, distribution, metabolism, and elimination processes. Modifications in the liver's detoxification schedule, influenced by circadian rhythms, can impact drug effectiveness and safety. This highlights the need to adapt medication schedules during Ramadan to synchronize with these biological changes [11].

18.2.2   Pharmacokinetic Changes During Fasting

Ramadan fasting results in notable changes in how drugs are absorbed, distributed, metabolized, and eliminated. The alterations stem from changes in dietary habits during fasting, which influence the gastrointestinal environment's pH, gastric motility, and secretions, subsequently affecting the efficacy of medications [12]. This is significant for medications with distinct gastrointestinal absorption timeframes. Delayed gastric emptying and altered gastric pH due to fasting may impact drug absorption, potentially reducing the efficacy [13]. Many drug classes are known to be affected by food status and gastric motility changes, like antibiotics (doxycycline, erythromycin), antifungal agents (ketoconazole), cardiovascular drugs (digoxin, beta-blockers), NSAIDs (ibuprofen, naproxen), psychotropic drugs (lithium), osteoporosis medications (alendronate), and levothyroxine for treatment of thyroid dysfunction [3, 14–16].

In addition, fasting impacts liver enzyme activity, which is essential for drug metabolism. This activity, linked to circadian rhythms, is altered during fasting, impacting drug metabolism rates and plasma concentrations. Moreover, fluctuations in plasma volume and body composition while fasting may impact drug distribution, especially for medications with high protein binding, affecting their effectiveness and potential harm [2, 3].

Medications such as warfarin, diazepam, ibuprofen, furosemide, diclofenac, sulfamethoxazole, citalopram, glipizide, lorazepam, and simvastatin have high protein binding, affecting their distribution and interaction potential. Alterations in plasma protein levels during fasting can modify the distribution of medications, leading to a potential increase in the free fraction of drugs such as warfarin [17, 18]. This, in turn, might enhance the pharmacological effects of these medications, at the same time increasing the risk of toxicity. The drug-protein binding characteristics necessitate careful monitoring to manage interactions and ensure safety and efficacy, emphasizing the importance of understanding protein binding in pharmacology. During fasting, the switch from utilizing glucose to lipids can alter the function of cytochrome P450 enzymes in the liver [19], potentially influencing the metabolic clearance of drugs. Examples of drugs metabolized by the cytochrome P450 system include warfarin (anticoagulant), omeprazole (proton pump inhibitor (PPI)), clopidogrel (antiplatelet agent), simvastatin (statin for cholesterol management), diazepam (benzodiazepine), and immunosuppressant (cyclosporine). The cytochrome P450 system plays a crucial role in drug metabolism, affecting the efficacy and safety of these medications [3, 20].

It should be emphasized that changes in renal blood flow and urine pH can lead to variations in renal function and medication excretion rates. The potential influence of hydration status on renal medication clearance throughout Ramadan is a notable aspect that warrants attention. Medications such as lithium, furosemide, methotrexate, digoxin, and gentamicin, which are excreted through the kidneys, are influenced by the body's hydration status. Adequate hydration is necessary when taking these drugs to ensure their safe and effective elimination. The reduction in the excretion of these drugs poses an elevated risk of toxicity [21].

Patient compliance adds a layer of complexity to these all-encompassing pharmacokinetic and pharmacological factors. Patients who want to fast may change or skip their medication without consulting healthcare providers, which could result in suboptimal treatment of their conditions. To preserve the drug's effectiveness and minimize side effects throughout Ramadan, healthcare professionals frequently need to adjust medication schedules or shift to new formulations, such as going from immediate- to extended-release formulations [18]. The lack of tailored advice for fasting patients causes confusion and possible medication nonadherence. Patients and healthcare professionals must work together to overcome these problems.

18.3 Common Health Conditions and Medication Management During Ramadan

Handling chronic illnesses during Ramadan necessitates a thorough and customized strategy to guarantee the safety and effectiveness of drug regimens while fulfilling patients' fasting practices. Medication regimen adjustments are necessary for various health conditions throughout Ramadan. This encompasses, but is not limited to, cardiovascular disease, the use of anticoagulants like warfarin, diabetes, asthma and chronic obstructive pulmonary disease (COPD), gastrointestinal disorders, and chronic kidney disease (CKD). It also includes mental health disorders and epilepsy. Ensuring the safety and efficacy of treatment protocols requires a thorough comprehension of each illness and the potential consequences of fasting, emphasizing the significance of a comprehensive and personalized healthcare treatment during this month.

Managing cardiovascular conditions and anticoagulant drugs, including warfarin, must be carefully adjusted throughout Ramadan to align with fasting patterns and maintain patient safety and treatment effectiveness [4, 17]. When managing elevated blood pressure or cholesterol conditions, the focus is on scheduling and selecting antihypertensives and statins for the evening hours after Iftar, using long-acting formulations for long-term control, and coordinating the administration of statins with the body's increased production of cholesterol at night. In this example, rosuvastatin and atorvastatin are preferred over simvastatin, as their long half-lives extend to 18 h [22]. A sustained-release antihypertensive formulation can replace the immediate-release ones as they offer an improved plasma concentration-time profile for a prolonged time. The timing of diuretic administration should be tailored to align with the patient's routine and lifestyle throughout Ramadan nights. Pre-Ramadan health consultations catered to each person's unique needs are an additional component of this strategy. At the same time, warfarin management demands careful international normalized ratio (INR) monitoring and dose adjustment in response to dietary modifications. Furthermore, significant emphasis should be placed on educating patients about maintaining a consistent diet, recognizing symptoms, and the importance of regular monitoring [23, 24]. This integrated approach emphasizes how crucial it is to provide patients with individualized care and ongoing monitoring throughout Ramadan to preserve their cardiovascular health and efficiently control their warfarin without endangering their safety [4].

Managing diabetes during Ramadan requires careful adjustment of insulin and oral hypoglycemic agents to prevent low or high blood sugar levels. Timing and dosing of insulin, particularly long-acting, are crucial for maintaining stable blood sugar levels. Choosing oral medications such as metformin decreases the chances of hypoglycemia [25]. Dosing modifications should be determined by pre-Ramadan glucose management following Suhoor and Iftar meals. Continuous glucose monitoring during fasting enables prompt adjustments, enhancing glucose management and minimizing complications [25].

It is essential for those with asthma or COPD observing Ramadan to modify their medication regimen to manage their condition effectively during fasting. Inhalers such as corticosteroids and bronchodilators are permissible, as they do not affect fasting since they are nonnutritive.

Long-acting inhalers administered around Suhoor or Iftar are recommended to maintain consistent management of symptoms. Long-acting inhalers could be beta-2 agonists, such as salmeterol, formoterol, and indacaterol, or antimuscarinic inhalers, such as tiotropium, glycopyrronium, and aclidinium. A clearly defined plan for managing acute flare-ups is essential, as it may require breaking the fast for health reasons. Healthcare providers must educate patients on correct inhaler use and the importance of seeking immediate medical help for severe symptoms to manage diseases effectively while fasting [26].

Effective management of gastrointestinal disorders during Ramadan requires adjusting the timing of antacids and proton pump inhibitors (PPIs). For optimal benefit, it is recommended to take PPIs (lansoprazole, dexlansoprazole, esomeprazole, and pantoprazole) just before Suhoor to align with the natural peak in acid production and enhance the medication's effectiveness [12]. Antacids can be used after breaking fast and before daybreak to alleviate symptoms such as acidity and heartburn. These modifications promote gastrointestinal health and enable individuals to fast comfortably while maintaining the effectiveness of their medication [27].

Chronic kidney disease (CKD) patients fasting during Ramadan need to carefully manage their fluid intake and medication dosing to fast safely. Maintaining proper hydration outside of fasting periods is crucial to avoid dehydration and regulate electrolyte levels, especially for individuals taking diuretics. It is essential to modify medication classes and timing to coincide with Suhoor and Iftar and consider potential dosage adjustments to uphold therapeutic levels while safeguarding renal function. It is crucial to closely monitor kidney function and collaborate with healthcare providers to create personalized care plans during Ramadan [28].

Effectively managing mental health conditions or epilepsy during Ramadan necessitates a careful balance to maintain treatment effectiveness and safety while fasting [1]. It is crucial to synchronize the timing of psychotropic medications with Suhoor and Iftar for patients to ensure therapeutic plasma levels, which may involve dose adjustments or choosing long-acting formulations. In managing epilepsy, it is essential to maintain consistent plasma levels of antiepileptic drugs to avoid seizures [29]. This may involve transitioning to extended-release formulations, i.e., Depakine chrono®, extended-release sodium valproate used for epilepsy management. However, modifying the timing of medication is another valid option. In mental health conditions and epilepsy, it is important to stay well hydrated, get enough sleep, and closely follow healthcare providers' guidance to adjust treatment strategies. This integrated strategy enables patients to safely observe Ramadan while balancing their religious obligations with their health requirements [11].

18.4   Role of Healthcare Providers in Supporting Fasting Patients

18.4.1   The Importance of Patient Education and Pre-Ramadan Medical Assessment

Healthcare providers are responsible for guaranteeing the safety and welfare of fasting patients during Ramadan, particularly those with chronic medical conditions. Thorough patient education and pre-Ramadan assessments are crucial for patients to maintain their health during fasting. Healthcare professionals educate patients, enabling them to comprehend how to modify their diet and medication and identify symptoms that may necessitate medical intervention. This collaborative effort promotes a relationship that helps patients feel supported in making health management decisions [30].

Medical assessments before Ramadan are essential for healthcare providers to assess patients' ability to fast safely, considering their health status and potential risks. These evaluations enable the categorization of patients based on risk level, facilitating tailored recommendations that correspond to each patient's health requirements. For instance, diabetic patients may need to monitor blood glucose levels and adjust medication dosages. At the same time, individuals with cardiovascular conditions could be advised to consider their diet and manage medication schedules [5–7].

The healthcare team, consisting of physicians, dietitians, and pharmacists, offers support beyond clinical guidance. They emphasize patient education and promote a comprehensive health approach during Ramadan. Engaging with the community and working with religious leaders to provide precise health information enhances a well-rounded strategy for fasting and healthcare [5–7].

18.4.2   The Critical Role of Healthcare Providers in Developing Personalized Medication Management Plans

Healthcare providers are essential in supporting fasting patients during Ramadan through personalized medication management strategies. Understanding how fasting affects the body's processes and medication pharmacokinetics is crucial for ensuring patient safety and adherence during this process. Customizing these plans requires analyzing the patient's existing medication regimen and modifying medications impacted by fasting-induced alterations in circadian rhythms or those necessitating food consumption. Aligning dosing times with Suhoor or Iftar can help maintain medication efficacy and minimize side effects, ensuring optimal support for fasting patients' health and well-being [2].

Healthcare professionals need to assess the potential for dehydration during Ramadan, as it can have a substantial impact on the concentration of medication and renal function. This may necessitate the implementation of dosage modifications or the adoption of alternative, safer drugs to mitigate potential complications such as hypoglycemia in diabetes or dehydration resulting from diuretics [31]. In addition, it is crucial to instruct patients on monitoring adverse reactions, timing medications correctly with meals, and implementing proper hydration and nutrition strategies during nonfasting periods. Written guidelines or digital reminders can greatly enhance adherence and safety [32].

Effective management of fasting patients requires collaboration between the healthcare team and patients. Open communication enables the modification of medication regimens according to patient input and the continuous evaluation of health results. Implementing this dynamic approach guarantees individualized care and enhances health outcomes by monitoring and adjusting treatment plans.

18.4.3   Monitoring and Follow-up During Ramadan

Comprehensive monitoring and subsequent evaluation to modify drug regimens as required and deal with any potential health concerns that may emerge. By establishing effective channels of communication, patients can rapidly report any symptoms or concerns they may have, such as dehydration, hypoglycemia, elevated blood pressure, hypotension, asthmatic attack, or any adverse effects associated with their medications [33, 34]. In addition, educating patients on self-monitoring procedures enables them to control their health better while fasting, thus decreasing the likelihood of complications. Regular face-to-face, telephonic, or digital engagements are essential for timely adjustments to treatment approaches, ensuring a safe fasting experience [35]. Regularly assessing the effectiveness of medication regimens for chronic illnesses is crucial, particularly for medications requiring precise dosing to ensure medical safety, efficacy, and religious adherence.

18.4.4   Interdisciplinary Approach Involving Physicians, Pharmacists, and Dietitians

An interdisciplinary approach involving physicians, pharmacists, and dietitians is essential for optimal medication management and the overall well-being of patients observing fasting during Ramadan. This collaborative model aims to address the diverse needs of individuals who fast, particularly those with chronic conditions that necessitate medication. Its primary goal is to improve patient care and outcomes.

Physicians have a crucial role in the team, conducting initial assessments and continuously monitoring patients to determine if they are suitable for fasting. They also adjust medication regimens to prevent potential complications [33, 34]. The efforts are backed by pharmacists who offer crucial medication counseling, adapt dosing schedules to match fasting hours, and guide suitable medication formulations to ensure effective treatment and reduce side effects [35]. Dietitians play a crucial role in providing nutritional advice to enhance the effectiveness of medications and promote patient well-being. They prioritize balanced nutrition and hydration to maintain energy levels and minimize the potential risks associated with fasting [30]. During Ramadan, it is crucial to implement an integrated care approach that encompasses nutritional and medication management to ensure optimal patient care. Studies have demonstrated that conducting pre-Ramadan assessments, providing personalized medication counseling, and offering dietary advice positively impact patient outcomes, adherence, and satisfaction [7]. The joint efforts of healthcare professionals underline the need for interdisciplinary care in making religious fasting safer for patients [30].

18.5   Enhancing Adherence and Patient-Centered Care

18.5.1   Empowering Patients Through Education on Medication Timing and Dietary Advice

Educating patients about medication timing and diet during Ramadan is critical, especially for individuals with chronic diseases such as diabetes. Specialized care plans that include personalized guidance on hydration, blood glucose monitoring, and medication adjustments are critical. This education fills the knowledge gap for healthcare professionals regarding fasting management by incorporating medical and religious issues. Collaboration among healthcare providers, religious leaders, and initiatives such as pre-Ramadan counseling campaigns improves patient empowerment and promotes safe fasting practices [30, 36].

Pharmacists are crucial in assisting patients with healthy fasting practices throughout Ramadan, highlighting the necessity for specialized training programs to improve their advisory skills. The increasing utilization of digital resources to manage fasting also indicates a need for educational materials from pharmacists and patients [18, 35].

A comprehensive patient-centered approach that emphasizes self-management and incorporates perspectives from religious leaders, healthcare professionals, and pharmacists is critical for educating patients about safe fasting, medication, and nutrition. Initiatives such as launching educational campaigns to educate patients on correct medication use and diet during fasting are crucial for increasing patient engagement and empowerment in managing their health [37].

18.5.2 Use of Technology and Mobile Apps for Reminders and Tracking

Technology and smartphone apps significantly enhance self-management and patient care, particularly during Ramadan. Digital technologies, encompassing functionalities such as blood glucose monitoring, blood pressure and heart rate measures, and prescription reminders, are imperative for effectively managing chronic illnesses. However, to achieve their maximum capabilities, it is widely recognized that these applications must align more closely with existing health guidelines. Research emphasizes mobile apps' efficacy in managing chronic illnesses, wherein culturally customized versions enhance patient involvement. Barriers to using eHealth applications must be removed to increase their prevalence among patients and providers. Developing applications that are quickly used, culturally aware, and compliant with health protocols is crucial for improving healthcare. Implementing this strategy can significantly enhance health results and the overall welfare of patients [38].

18.6 Ethical and Religious Considerations

Ethical and religious considerations are crucial in managing patient care throughout the holy month of Ramadan, particularly for patients suffering from chronic illnesses. Islam offers exemptions for individuals whose health may deteriorate due to fasting, but several patients, motivated by their religious duties and personal convictions, choose to fast [39].

Healthcare providers must carefully balance adhering to medical best practices and respecting the patient's religious beliefs and practices. This involves a deep understanding of the patient's religious commitments, clear communication, and collaborative decision-making to ensure that health interventions do not inadvertently compromise religious observance. It emphasizes the importance of informed consent, patient autonomy, and sensitivity and adaptability in care plans to safely and effectively accommodate fasting practices [40]. The literature also highlights the importance of risk stratification for patients and the provision of suitable counseling to manage their health during fasting periods correctly [7]. These insights promote a collaborative approach that integrates medical guidance with religious considerations, ensuring patients can observe Ramadan without compromising their health.

18.7 Conclusion

This chapter emphasizes the value of integrating medical and religious concerns into healthcare plans during Ramadan, stressing the need for individualized treatment for those who are fasting during Ramadan and have chronic illnesses. It addresses the necessity of modifying medication dosages and schedules and providing patient education on self-care practices. Joint efforts among healthcare professionals and religious figures are essential for formulating care plans that respect religious practices while promoting health. Medication safety is guaranteed by ongoing monitoring and adaptable treatment programs. The chapter promotes a respectful, patient-centered approach, supporting fasting patients' health and stressing interdisciplinary teamwork and ethical behavior.

References

1. Shah JA, Rahman MU, Abdikaxarovich SA, Sikandar P, Yerjan AD. Impact of fasting on human health during Ramadan. Int J Publ Health Sci. 2023;12(4):1611–25. https://doi.org/10.11591/ijphs.v12i4.23062.
2. Aadil N, Houti IE, Moussamih S. Drug intake during Ramadan. Br Med J. 2004;329(7469):778–82. https://doi.org/10.1136/bmj.329.7469.778.
3. Bauer LA. From applied clinical pharmacokinetics. In: Applied clinical pharmacokinetics, 3e. 2nd ed. New York: McGraw-Hill Medical; 2015.
4. Akhtar AM, Ghouri N, Chahal CAA, Patel R, Ricci F, Sattar N, et al. Ramadan fasting: recommendations for patients with cardiovascular disease. Heart. 2022;108(4):258–65. https://doi.org/10.1136/heartjnl-2021-319273.
5. Shaltout I, Zakaria A, Abdelwahab AM, Hamed AK, Elsaid NH, Attia MA. Culturally based pre-Ramadan education increased benefits and reduced hazards of Ramadan fasting for type 2 diabetic patients. J Diabetes Metab Disord. 2020;19(1):179–86. https://doi.org/10.1007/s40200-020-00489-1.
6. Mahmood A, Dar S, Dabhad A, Aksi B, Chowdhury TA. Advising patients with existing conditions about fasting during Ramadan. BMJ. 2022;376. https://doi.org/10.1136/bmj-2020-063613.
7. Alam AY. Pre-Ramadan diabetes risk stratification and patient education. J Pak Med Assoc. 2023;73(3):641–5. https://doi.org/10.47391/JPMA.17-23.
8. Madkour M, Giddey AD, Soares NC, Semreen MH, Bustanji Y, Zeb F, et al. Ramadan diurnal intermittent fasting is associated with significant plasma metabolomics changes in subjects with overweight and obesity: a prospective cohort study. Front Nutr. 2023;9. https://doi.org/10.3389/fnut.2022.1008730.
9. Faris MAIE, Kacimi S, Al-Kurd RA, Fararjeh MA, Bustanji YK, Mohammad MK, et al. Intermittent fasting during Ramadan attenuates proinflammatory cytokines and immune cells in healthy subjects. Nutr Res. 2012;32(12):947–55. https://doi.org/10.1016/j.nutres.2012.06.021.
10. Faris MAIE, Hussein RN, Al-Kurd RA, Al-Fararjeh MA, Bustanji YK, Mohammad MK. Impact of Ramadan intermittent fasting on oxidative stress measured by urinary 15- F 2t -isoprostane. J Nutr Metab. 2012;2012. https://doi.org/10.1155/2012/802924.
11. Qasrawi SO, Pandi-Perumal SR, BaHammam AS. The effect of intermittent fasting during Ramadan on sleep, sleepiness, cognitive function, and circadian rhythm. Sleep Breath. 2017;21(3):577–86. https://doi.org/10.1007/s11325-017-1473-x.
12. Jiang Y, Sonu I, Garcia P, Fernandez-Becker NQ, Kamal AN, Zikos TA, et al. The impact of intermittent fasting on patients with suspected gastroesophageal reflux disease. J Clin Gastroenterol. 2023;57(10):1001–6. https://doi.org/10.1097/MCG.0000000000001788.
13. Courtney R, Radwanski E, Lim J, Laughlin M. Pharmacokinetics of posaconazole coadministered with antacid in fasting or nonfasting healthy men. Antimicrob Agents Chemother. 2004;48(3):804–8. https://doi.org/10.1128/AAC.48.3.804-808.2004.

14. Liu H, Lu M, Hu J, Fu G, Feng Q, Sun S, et al. Medications and food interfering with the bioavailability of levothyroxine: a systematic review. Ther Clin Risk Manag. 2023;19:503–23. https://doi.org/10.2147/TCRM.S414460.

15. Kambayashi A, Shirasaka Y. Food effects on gastrointestinal physiology and drug absorption. Drug Metab Pharmacokinet. 2023;48. https://doi.org/10.1016/j.dmpk.2022.100488.

16. Zou P. Does food affect the pharmacokinetics of non-orally delivered drugs? A review of currently available evidence. AAPS J. 2022;24(3):59. https://doi.org/10.1208/s12248-022-00714-0.

17. Rabea EM, Abbas KS, Awad DM, Elgoweini NH, El-Sakka AA, Mahmoud NH, et al. Does Ramadan fasting affect the therapeutic and clinical outcomes of warfarin? A systematic review and meta-analysis. Eur J Clin Pharmacol. 2022;78(5):755–63. https://doi.org/10.1007/s00228-022-03281-7.

18. Grindrod K, Alsabbagh W. Managing medications during Ramadan fasting. Can Pharm J. 2017;150(3):146–9. https://doi.org/10.1177/1715163517700840.

19. Lammers LA, Achterbergh R, Romijn JA, Mathôt RAA. Short-term fasting alters pharmacokinetics of cytochrome P450 probe drugs: does protein binding play a role? Eur J Drug Metab Pharmacokinet. 2018;43(2):251–7. https://doi.org/10.1007/s13318-017-0437-7.

20. Emara MH, Soliman H, Elnadry M, Mohamed Said E, Abd-Elsalam S, Elbatae HE, et al. Ramadan fasting and liver diseases: a review with practice advices and recommendations. Liver Int. 2021;41(3):436–48. https://doi.org/10.1111/liv.14775.

21. Farooq S, Nazar Z, Akhter J, Irafn M, Subhan F, Ahmed Z, et al. Effect of fasting during Ramadan on serum lithium level and mental state in bipolar affective disorder. Int Clin Psychopharmacol. 2010;25(6):323–7. https://doi.org/10.1097/YIC.0b013e32833d18b2.

22. Dabhad A, Akbar A, Shah S, Ghouri N. Case-based learning: medicines management during Ramadan. Pharm J. 2022;308(7959). https://doi.org/10.1211/PJ.2022.1.135985.

23. Alwhaibi A, Alenazi M, Alwagh F, Al-Ghayhab A, Alghadeer S, Bablghaith S, et al. Does Ramadan fasting disrupt international normalised ratio control in warfarin-treated medically stable patients? Int J Clin Pract. 2021;75(11):e14796. https://doi.org/10.1111/ijcp.14796.

24. López-Bueno M, Fernández-Aparicio Á, González-Jiménez E, Montero-Alonso MÁ, Schmidt-Riovalle J. Self-care by Muslim women during Ramadan fasting to protect nutritional and cardiovascular health. Int J Environ Res Public Health. 2021;18(23). https://doi.org/10.3390/ijerph182312393.

25. Rashid F, Abdelgadir E. A systematic review on efficacy and safety of the current hypoglycemic agents in patients with diabetes during Ramadan fasting. Diabetes Metab Syndr Clin Res Rev. 2019;13(2):1413–29. https://doi.org/10.1016/j.dsx.2019.02.005.

26. Khan MH, Al-Lehebi R. Respiratory disease and Ramadan. Lancet Respir Med. 2020;8(5):449–50. https://doi.org/10.1016/S2213-2600(20)30112-0.

27. Rimmani HH, Rustom LBO, Rahal MA, Shayto RH, Chaar H, Sharara AI. Dexlansoprazole is effective in relieving heartburn during the fasting month of Ramadan. Dig Dis. 2019;37(3):188–93. https://doi.org/10.1159/000496091.

28. Ansari F, Latief M, Manuel S, Shashikiran K, Dwivedi R, Prasad D, et al. Impact of fasting during Ramadan on renal functions in patients with chronic kidney disease. Indian J Nephrol. 2022;32(3):262–5. https://doi.org/10.4103/ijn.IJN_521_20.

29. Ebrahimi Meimand HA, Jahani Moghaddam MK. Evaluation of the effects of fasting during the holy month of Ramadan on patients with epileptic attacks who visited the emergency room. J Kerman Univ Med Sci. 2023;30(5):267–70. https://doi.org/10.34172/jkmu.2023.45.

30. Sugiharto S, Natalya W, Otok BW. Healthcare providers' knowledge, attitude, and perspective regarding diabetes self-management during Ramadan fasting: a cross-sectional study. Nurse Media J Nurs. 2021;11(1):124–32. https://doi.org/10.14710/NMJN.V11I1.33926.

31. Gameil MA, Marzouk RE, El-Sebaie AH, Eldeeb AAA. Influence of sodium-glucose Co-transporter 2 inhibitors on clinical and biochemical markers of dehydration during the Holy Ramadan. Diabetes Metab Syndr Clin Res Rev. 2022;16(9):102606. https://doi.org/10.1016/j.dsx.2022.102606.

32. Hassanein M, Afandi B, Yakoob Ahmedani M, Mohammad Alamoudi R, Alawadi F, Bajaj HS, et al. Diabetes and Ramadan: practical guidelines 2021. Diabetes Res Clin Pract. 2022;185. https://doi.org/10.1016/j.diabres.2021.109185.
33. Amin MEK, Abdelmageed A. Clinicians' perspectives on caring for Muslim patients considering fasting during Ramadan. J Relig Health. 2020;59(3):1370–87. https://doi.org/10.1007/s10943-019-00820-y.
34. Amin MEK, Abdelmageed A, Farhat MJ. Communicating with clinicians on fasting during Ramadan: the patients' perspective. J Relig Health. 2021;60(2):922–40. https://doi.org/10.1007/s10943-019-00910-x.
35. Amin MEK, Chewning B. Pharmacist–patient communication about medication regimen adjustment during Ramadan. Int J Pharm Pract. 2016;24(6):419–27. https://doi.org/10.1111/ijpp.12282.
36. Alom J. Empowering Islamic leaders to help patients practise a safe Ramadan. BMJ. 2022;376. https://doi.org/10.1136/bmj.o624.
37. Kalra B, Kalra S, Jawad F. Ramadan fasting during pregnancy: obstetric risk stratification. J Pak Med Assoc. 2018;68(4):666–8.
38. Fernández C, Vicente MA, Guilabert M, Carrillo I, Mira JJ. Developing a mobile health app for chronic illness management: insights from focus groups. Digit Health. 2023;9. https://doi.org/10.1177/20552076231210662.
39. Khoshniat Nikoo M, Shadman Z. Ethical considerations of Ramadan fasting in diabetic patients according to Shiite school of thought. Int J Diabetes Dev Ctries. 2014;34(4):180–7. https://doi.org/10.1007/s13410-013-0184-5.
40. Ahmed S, Khokhar N, Shubrook JH. Fasting during Ramadan: a comprehensive review for primary care providers. Diabetology. 2022;3(2):276–91. https://doi.org/10.3390/diabetology3020019.

Chapter 19
On the Contribution of Ramadan Fasting Month to the United Nations' Sustainable Development Goals (SDGs)

Khaled Obaideen, Mohamed Alameddine, Nivine Hanach, Dana N. Abdelrahim, and MoezAlIslam E. Faris

Abstract Ramadan, the ninth month of the Islamic lunar calendar, is a period of profound spiritual significance for Muslims worldwide and is marked by fasting, prayer, reflection, and community. Beyond its religious dimensions, Ramadan offers a unique lens through which to explore the intersection of faith, culture, and global development challenges. This chapter examines how Ramadan's observance aligns with and promotes the United Nations Sustainable Development Goals (SDGs). Through practices embedded in the observance of Ramadan, Muslims contribute to poverty alleviation, food security, health and well-being, quality education, gender equality, sustainable water and energy management, economic growth, resilient infrastructure, reduced inequalities, sustainable cities, responsible consumption, climate action, marine and terrestrial conservation, peaceful and inclusive societies, and global partnerships. This chapter demonstrates the potent influence of cultural and religious practices in achieving global

K. Obaideen (✉)
Sustainable Engineering Asset, Management Research Group, University of Sharjah, Sharjah, UAE

M. Alameddine
Department of Health Care Management, College of Health Sciences, University of Sharjah, Sharjah, UAE

Research Institute for Medical and Health Sciences, University of Sharjah, Sharjah, UAE

N. Hanach
Research Institute for Medical and Health Sciences, University of Sharjah, Sharjah, UAE

Faculty of Health, Medicine and Life Sciences, Health Promotion, Care and Public Health Research Institute, Maastricht University, Maastricht, Netherlands

D. N. Abdelrahim
Research Institute for Medical and Health Sciences, University of Sharjah, Sharjah, UAE

M. E. Faris
Department of Clinical Nutrition and Dietetics, Faculty of Allied Medical Sciences, Applied Science Private University, Amman, Jordan

309

development agendas. It underscores the potential for cultural and religious observances to aid in achieving these global objectives.

Keywords Ramadan · Sustainable Development Goals (SDGs) · Community engagement · Environmental stewardship · Sustainable development

19.1 Introduction

Ramadan, the ninth month of the Islamic lunar calendar, holds profound spiritual significance for Muslims worldwide, marked by fasting, prayer, reflection, and community. Beyond its religious dimensions, Ramadan offers a unique lens through which to explore the intersection of faith, culture, and global development challenges. Sustainable Development Goals (SDGs) are a universal call to action to end poverty, protect the planet, and ensure peace and prosperity by 2030 [1]. Understanding the role of Ramadan in achieving the SDGs is important because it highlights the intersection of cultural and religious practices with global development objectives [2]. Through its emphasis on charity, community, and ethical behavior, Ramadan naturally aligns with many SDGs, demonstrating how religious observances can contribute to sustainable development. Recognizing these connections can inspire more inclusive and culturally sensitive approaches to achieving these critical global goals, as shown in Fig. 19.1. This chapter delves into how the observance of Ramadan aligns with and promotes the United Nations' SDGs, demonstrating the potent influence of cultural and religious practices in achieving global development agendas.

Environment

•**Synergy:** Can inspire community initiatives for environmental protection.
•**Trade-off:** Higher energy use for night-time activities and gatherings.

•**Synergy:** Encourages responsible consumption patterns that can benefit marine life (e.g., reduced overfishing).
•**Trade-off:** Increased use of water and potential for waste generation during Ramadan could affect waterways and marine environments indirectly.

•**Synergy:** Promotes initiatives for better water management and sanitation.
•**Trade-off:** Higher water usage for religious practices.

•**Synergy:** Can inspire community initiatives for environmental protection.
•**Trade-off:** Higher energy use for night-time activities and gatherings.

Social

•**Synergy:** Enhances community support systems and local economies.
•**Trade-off:** Potential for dependency on charity rather than sustainable development solutions.

Synergy: Promotes sustainable consumption.
Trade-off: Potential increase in waste.

•**Synergy:** Encourages a holistic approach to health and well-being.
•**Trade-off:** Health risks for some individuals due to fasting.

•**Synergy:** Fosters intercultural understanding and respect.
•**Trade-off:** Potential distractions from academic studies.

•**Synergy:** Encourages the adoption of energy-saving practices and technologies in homes, mosques, and businesses during Ramadan nights.
•**Trade-off:** The potential increase in energy use for lighting and cooking during night hours may counteract efforts towards energy conservation.

•**Synergy:** Supports efforts towards building inclusive and peaceful communities.
•**Trade-off:** Large gatherings may pose challenges to public order and safety.

•**Synergy:** Can empower women through leadership in community activities.
•**Trade-off:** Increased domestic burdens for women during Ramadan.

•**Synergy:** Raises awareness and mobilizes resources for food security.
•**Trade-off:** Seasonal focus may not address long-term hunger solutions.

Economy

•**Synergy:** Creates temporary employment opportunities.
•**Trade-off:** Possible disruptions to regular **work patterns due to fasting.**

•**Synergy:** Can drive demand for sustainable infrastructure and innovative solutions in resource management, energy efficiency, and waste reduction.
•**Trade-off:** Increased consumer demand may stress existing infrastructure and lead to overexploitation of resources without sustainable practices.

•**Synergy:** Builds solidarity and social cohesion.
•**Trade-off:** Short-term relief may not address root causes of inequality.

•**Synergy:** Raises awareness about food waste and sustainable consumption.
•**Trade-off:** Potential for increased food waste and consumption during night hours.

Fig. 19.1 Contribution of Ramadan fasting month to the UN SDGs

19.1.1   SDG 1: No Poverty

When considering its role in achieving SDG 1, which focuses on ending poverty in all forms worldwide, Ramadan contributes in several meaningful ways. Zakat (obligatory charitable giving), one of the five pillars of Islam, holds deep significance and plays a vital role during this holy Ramadan month. Muslims are required to give *Zakat*, which is typically 2.5% of their savings, to those in need [3]. This act of giving helps redistribute wealth within the community, ensuring that the less fortunate receive a share to help alleviate their poverty. Additionally, the practice of giving *Zakat al-Fitr* (charity given at the end of Ramadan) before the *Eid* prayer is specifically aimed at providing for the poor so that they can also celebrate the festival [4, 5]. Ramadan fosters a sense of solidarity and community among Muslims. Communal prayers (*Taraweeh*), the breaking of the fast together (*Iftar*), and shared charitable activities strengthen communal ties and encourage a societal model where people look out for each other. This heightened sense of community can lead to more organized collective efforts to tackle poverty and support those in need. The fast during Ramadan serves as a practical way to develop empathy toward the less fortunate, who may often experience hunger and thirst. This empathy can inspire further action to help alleviate poverty.

The increased demand for various goods and services during Ramadan, such as food, clothing, and *Eid* decorations, can boost local businesses and markets. This economic stimulation can be particularly beneficial to small traders and local artisans, potentially lifting them out of poverty. Ramadan teaches about a balance between materialism and spirituality, reminding individuals of the importance of not being overly attached to material wealth. This perspective can shift societal values toward greater equality and fairness in the distribution of resources, indirectly supporting poverty reduction efforts. Ramadan has a multifaceted impact on efforts to achieve SDG 1. Through practices embedded in the observance of Ramadan, Muslims contribute to poverty alleviation by redistributing wealth, enhancing community cohesion, fostering empathy, stimulating local economies, and promoting a balanced approach to material wealth. These actions are intrinsic to the ethos of Ramadan and align closely with the objectives of SDG 1, showcasing how cultural and religious practices can intertwine with global development goals.

19.1.2   SDG 2: Zero Hunger

SDG 2 aims to "end hunger, achieve food security and improved nutrition, and promote sustainable agriculture." The observance of Ramadan, through its unique practices and spiritual lessons, can also support and enhance efforts toward achieving this goal. During Ramadan, Muslims are encouraged to donate more generously to those in need. This includes providing food to those who cannot afford it and ensuring that no one in the community goes hungry. Initiatives such as community *Iftar*s are common, where food is shared with everyone, especially those in need [6]. This practice not only helps feed the hungry but also raises awareness about the importance of community support in achieving food security. Ramadan's attention shifts toward moderation, health, and the nutritional quality of the food consumed during *Suhoor* and *Iftar*. The practice of fasting can teach the dietary discipline and benefits of balanced eating. In many communities, there is an emphasis on including a diverse range of foods in the meals that break the fast, which can contribute to better nutrition. The ethos of Ramadan stresses the importance of not being wasteful. This is particularly relevant to food consumption. Additionally, fasting is supposed to lead to reduced personal consumption and a re-evaluation of needs versus wants, promoting more sustainable lifestyles. Though the philosophy of Ramadan fasting emphasizes self-esteem and self-control, particularly in food consumption, the current popular practice often contradicts this philosophy. Recent studies indicate that Ramadan observance is associated with increased food purchases and waste, which completely contradicts Ramadan's ethics and morals. This trend undermines the positive effects of Ramadan on reducing food waste and conflicts with the SDG of poverty alleviation and combating hunger [7].

Fasting teaches self-control and appreciation for the food one has, encouraging more mindful eating practices and potentially reducing food waste, a significant issue in global food security. Although less direct, the spirit of stewardship and responsibility advocated during Ramadan can extend to how communities perceive agriculture and sustainability. The emphasis on simplicity and moderation can lead to supporting more sustainable agricultural practices, such as buying local produce or choosing products that are less harmful to the environment, thereby promoting sustainable agriculture. Community initiatives during Ramadan often aim to create more resilient local food systems. For instance, mosques and charities may organize local food drives or support local farmers and producers by purchasing their goods for charitable distribution. Such activities can strengthen local food systems and economies, making them more resilient when faced with challenges. Ramadan provides a meaningful opportunity to advance the goals of SDG 2 through its emphasis on charity, community engagement, and sustainable practices. While the primary focus of Ramadan is spiritual renewal, the month also promotes actions and values that can significantly contribute to ending hunger, improving nutrition, promoting sustainable agriculture, and building resilient food systems. These contributions demonstrate the profound impact that cultural and religious practices can have on addressing global challenges such as hunger and food security.

19.1.3 SDG 3: Good Health and Well-Being

SDG 3 aims to "ensure healthy lives and promote well-being for all at all ages." Through its spiritual and communal practices, Ramadan significantly contributes to this goal [2]. Fasting during Ramadan can improve blood sugar control, heart health, and weight management when balanced, nutritious meals are consumed. It encourages disciplined eating habits, helping to prevent obesity and diabetes. The sense of community and spiritual reflection during Ramadan fosters mental well-being and reduces loneliness and stress. Abstaining from smoking and other poor habits during Ramadan promotes better health, as well as encourages better sleep discipline. Health and nutrition education during Ramadan is emphasized through programs in mosques and community centers, which discuss best practices for fasting, hydration, and meal preparation. These efforts improve dietary habits and promote a healthier lifestyle. Many mosques and Islamic organizations take the opportunity to launch health-related initiatives such as health screenings, blood donation camps, and seminars, increasing awareness and access to health services, which are crucial for preventive health care. Overall, Ramadan aligns with the objectives of SDG 3 by promoting both physical and mental health, encouraging healthy lifestyles, and catalyzing community health initiatives. Through fasting, community bonding, educational efforts, and health campaigns, Ramadan demonstrates the power of religious observances in supporting global health goals and enhancing the quality of life of individuals and communities alike.

19.1.4   SDG 4: Quality Education

SDG 4 aims to "ensure inclusive and equitable quality education and promote lifelong learning opportunities for all." Ramadan, a period marked by reflection, community engagement, and personal development, can significantly contribute to achieving these educational objectives. Ramadan is a time when Muslims are encouraged to engage in increased learning and reflection, particularly through the reading and study of the Quran. This emphasis on learning fosters a culture of intellectual curiosity and personal growth, aligning with the lifelong learning aspect of SDG 4. Many mosques and community centers host special classes and lectures during Ramadan to facilitate this learning, which is accessible to people of all ages. During Ramadan, educational programs in mosques and community centers are often open to all, regardless of one's level of prior knowledge or education. This inclusive approach ensures that everyone has the opportunity to learn about religion, health, or social issues. Such inclusivity is fundamental to SDG 4, which aims to provide equal educational opportunities for all members of society. Ramadan offers the opportunity to deepen our understanding of Islamic teachings and history, contributing to the preservation and transmission of cultural and religious heritage. This type of education is critical to fostering social cohesion and mutual respect among diverse populations [8]. By encouraging an appreciation of cultural diversity within educational contexts, Ramadan supports the broader goals of SDG 4. The communal activities associated with Ramadan, such as shared *Iftars* and collective prayers, also serve as educational experiences that teach important social skills such as cooperation, empathy, and respect for others. These are essential competencies in any well-rounded educational system and are crucial for personal development. The discipline required to fast and engage in additional religious practices during Ramadan teaches both children and adults values of commitment, perseverance, and responsibility. These qualities are vital in educational settings and beneficial for personal development and success in lifelong learning. In recent years, many organizations have started using digital platforms to deliver educational content during Ramadan, making learning more accessible to a wider audience. This use of technology not only helps reach people who may not be able to attend in-person sessions but also aligns with the SDG 4 focus on enhancing the use of enabling technology to promote education [9]. Ramadan actively supports the aims of SDG 4 through its promotion of a learning culture that extends beyond traditional educational systems. By fostering a spirit of lifelong learning, inclusivity, and the development of personal and social skills, Ramadan contributes to the creation of more equitable and comprehensive educational opportunities. This holistic approach to learning during Ramadan demonstrates how cultural practices can play a pivotal role in achieving global educational goals.

19.1.5   SDG 5: Gender Equality

SDG 5 aims to "achieve equality and empower all women and girls." Ramadan offers unique opportunities to advance this goal through community engagement, spiritual growth, and social practices [3, 8]. Ramadan encourages increased participation in religious practices among both men and women. In many communities, there has been a growing emphasis on ensuring that women have equal access to mosques and prayer spaces during Ramadan [10]. This includes providing adequate facilities for women to pray and participate in religious activities, such as lectures and Quran study sessions. Empowering women in their religious communities can help elevate their status and voice in broader community affairs. During Ramadan, women often take on leadership roles, organizing *Iftar*s, educational programs, and community outreach initiatives. These roles not only highlight the capacity and leadership of women in managing community affairs but also provide platforms for demonstrating their skills and contributions, which are crucial for challenging traditional sex-related roles and stereotypes. Ramadan is a time when many organizations focus on social issues, including equality, through talks, seminars, and discussions. These programs can help educate communities about the importance of women's rights and equality. By aligning these discussions with the spiritual and ethical considerations emphasized during Ramadan, the messages can have a more profound impact on the community. Many communities see an increase in charitable activities during Ramadan. This includes support for vulnerable groups, such as women at risk of domestic violence, single mothers, and widows. Providing targeted support and resources for women during this month can help address specific related challenges and empower women at the grassroots level. Ramadan often stimulates local economies through an increased demand for goods and services.

Further, the sympathy and merciful behavior that fasting individuals should embody during Ramadan are expected to influence the reduction of violence against women positively. Islamic regulations emphasize compassion and mercy throughout the year, with these principles being particularly underscored during Ramadan, especially toward women.

Women entrepreneurs and business owners can benefit from these economic activities. Markets, craft fairs, and online sales see a boost during the holy month, providing women with opportunities to showcase their businesses and crafts and contributing to their economic independence and empowerment. The communal and inclusive nature of Ramadan activities can foster a supportive environment that promotes equality. As communities come together to pray, have breakfast, and share communal activities, there are opportunities to practice inclusivity and equality in these settings, setting precedents for behavior outside of Ramadan. Ramadan supports SDG 5 by providing opportunities for women to actively participate in the religious, social, and economic spheres. By fostering an environment in which women can demonstrate leadership, gain financial independence, and receive community support, Ramadan significantly contributes to advancing equality and empowering women and girls. The holy month's focus on community, spirituality, and social justice makes it a potent time to address and promote equality issues.

19.1.6   SDG 6: Clean Water and Sanitation

SDG 6 aims to "ensure availability and sustainable management of water and sanitation for all." Ramadan, a period marked by an emphasis on discipline and reflection, offers unique opportunities to contribute to the realization of this goal. During Ramadan, Muslims fast from dawn until sunset, abstaining from consuming any food or water. This practice inherently promotes mindfulness in water usage [11]. The discipline learned from fasting can extend to more conscious water use during non-fasting hours and beyond the month of Ramadan. Community leaders often use Ramadan as a time to educate people about the importance of conserving water, given its significance in daily rituals and its scarcity in many parts of the Muslim world. Mosques and community centers frequently organize educational programs during Ramadan that focus on various aspects of sustainability, including water conservation. These programs can effectively raise awareness about the critical state of water resources globally and locally and educate attendees on practical steps to reduce water waste. Increased attendance at mosques during Ramadan often leads to higher demand for ablution facilities. This can drive improvements in water infrastructure, such as the installation of water-saving taps and the repair of leaks. Some mosques implement rainwater harvesting systems to manage water more sustainably, serving as community models for water stewardship [12]. Charity (*Zakat* and *Sadaqah*) is significantly emphasized during Ramadan. Many charitable projects focus on improving water access and sanitation in underprivileged areas. Muslims are encouraged to donate to causes that construct wells, install sanitation facilities, and provide clean drinking water to communities suffering from water scarcity. This not only helps address immediate needs but also contributes to long-term sustainability goals. Ramadan brings together Muslims from diverse backgrounds, fostering a sense of global community and shared responsibility. This solidarity can be powerful in mobilizing support for international water and sanitation projects. A month-long focus on communal well-being and charity can inspire collective actions that extend support beyond local communities to global scales. The teachings during Ramadan often encourage a lifestyle that is not just about abstaining from food and drink but also about overall moderation and sustainability. This ethos can inspire individuals and communities to adopt sustainable practices in their daily lives, including those related to water use and sanitation. Ramadan inherently supports SDG 6's aims through its emphasis on conservation, education, community improvement, and charitable giving. By promoting more sustainable water usage practices, improving water infrastructure, and supporting global water-related initiatives, the observance of Ramadan can significantly contribute to ensuring the availability and sustainable management of water and sanitation for all. This alignment of spiritual practice with sustainability goals underscores the potential of cultural and religious practices to aid in achieving global development objectives.

19.1.7   SDG 7: Affordable and Clean Energy

SDG 7 aims to "ensure access to affordable, reliable, sustainable, and modern energy for all." While Ramadan is primarily a spiritual observance, its practices can indirectly support this goal. During Ramadan, many people adopt simpler lifestyles and reduce their consumption of goods and services, including energy [5]. Fasting limits cooking to once a day, thereby reducing the use of kitchen appliances and energy consumption. Additionally, communities often turn off lights and electronic devices during the day and gather after sunset to break their fasts, which helps reduce individual energy use. Community *Iftar*s held in mosques or community centers are more energy-efficient than separate family meals, as large-scale cooking optimizes energy use and reduces the carbon footprint. Ramadan also provides an opportunity for community leaders to promote sustainability by adopting energy-efficient technologies and encouraging the community to do the same. Charitable giving during Ramadan often focuses on long-term, sustainable projects, such as solar-powered water pumps and solar panels for community buildings, aligning with the spirit of Ramadan and contributing to SDG 7. Educational campaigns during Ramadan also raise awareness about energy conservation and sustainability. Increased economic activity during Ramadan can support the energy sector by encouraging businesses to invest in sustainable operations and technologies. Thus, Ramadan's observance supports SDG 7 by promoting reduced energy consumption, fostering sustainable practices, facilitating renewable energy investments, and educating the public about sustainability.

19.1.8   SDG 8: Decent Work and Economic Growth

SDG 8 aims to "promote sustained, inclusive, and sustainable economic growth, full and productive employment, and decent work for all." Ramadan, a period of heightened spiritual and community activities, can indirectly contribute to achieving these objectives in several ways. Ramadan can significantly boost local economies [13]. The demand for food products, clothing, and other goods typically increases as families prepare for the month of fasting and subsequent *Eid* celebrations. This increased demand can lead to higher sales volumes for small- and medium-sized enterprises (SMEs), artisans, and vendors, potentially supporting economic growth and sustaining local jobs. Community *Iftars* and charity events during Ramadan provide opportunities for small businesses and local vendors to participate in a larger marketplace. These events can help include marginalized groups, such as small-scale farmers, craftspeople, and other informal workers, who might gain access to new markets and customers. Efforts to source products and services from a diverse range of providers can promote the inclusivity of economic opportunities. The spirit of generosity and community support during Ramadan can also inspire and facilitate entrepreneurship, particularly among young people and women. Many communities see a surge in start-up endeavors related to food, craft, and service industries during Ramadan, supported by increased community spending and the festive atmosphere leading up to *Eid*. During Ramadan, there is a significant increase in *Zakat* and *Sadaqah*, much of which is directed toward poverty alleviation and supporting social enterprises. These funds can help create jobs and provide services in underserved areas, thereby contributing to economic development and social well-being. Many mosques and community organizations offer workshops and seminars during Ramadan, including skill development and professional training. These learning opportunities can improve the employability and productivity of individuals, particularly youth and women, thus aligning them with the goals of decent work and economic growth. The ethical teachings emphasized during Ramadan encourage fair treatment and justice, including in the workplace. This can lead to heightened awareness and advocacy for labor rights, better working conditions, and fair pay, especially in regions where labor injustices are prevalent. The focus on spiritual reflection and family during Ramadan encourages a re-evaluation of work-life balance, which can lead to more sustainable work practices. Employers might be more inclined to accommodate flexible working hours or work-from-home arrangements during the month and practices that could have lasting benefits for employee well-being and productivity. Ramadan supports SDG 8 by stimulating economic activity, promoting inclusive economic opportunities, encouraging entrepreneurship, supporting charitable efforts, enhancing skills development, advocating for decent work, and fostering a better work-life balance. Through its unique combination of spiritual depth, community focus, and shift in daily routines, Ramadan provides a platform for economic and social practices that can contribute significantly to sustainable development and economic growth.

19.1.9   SDG 9: Industry, Innovation, and Infrastructure

SDG 9 aims to "build resilient infrastructure, promote inclusive and sustainable industrialization, and foster innovation." With its unique social dynamics and focus on the community, Ramadan can indirectly support these objectives through various avenues. During Ramadan, mosques and community centers often see increased attendance and activities, leading to improvements in the local infrastructure. Efforts to accommodate larger crowds, such as upgrading facilities, enhancing accessibility, and improving utilities (such as water and energy systems), contribute to resilient community infrastructure, benefiting the community year-round. The emphasis on sustainability and reduced consumption during Ramadan provides a platform for promoting sustainable industrial practices. Many communities initiate efforts to minimize waste and increase recycling, inspiring local businesses to adopt environmentally friendly practices that align with sustainable industrialization goals. Technology plays a crucial role in observing Ramadan, especially through virtual communal prayers, online charity platforms, and mobile apps for prayer times and Quran reading. This reliance on technology fosters innovation and the development of new tools that enhance the communal and spiritual experiences of Ramadan, thus contributing to broader technological advancement. The economic activity generated during Ramadan boosts local industries, from food production to retail and services, stimulating economic growth and supporting small and medium enterprises, which are crucial for sustainable industrialization. Ramadan creates opportunities for entrepreneurial ventures in sectors such as food services, e-commerce, and event management by incorporating innovative business models and technologies. Supporting these initiatives fosters innovation and economic diversification. Social enterprises receive significant funding during Ramadan through *Zakat* and *Sadaqah*, often developing creative solutions to social, environmental, and financial challenges and contributing to sustainable industrialization and innovation. Ramadan brings together diverse groups, facilitating networking and collaboration and sharing ideas and best practices across sectors, leading to innovative projects and collaborations that contribute to industrial and infrastructural development. Through its communal activities and the ethos of sustainability and charity, Ramadan fosters environments that enhance community infrastructure, promote sustainable industrial practices, stimulate innovation, and encourage economic growth and entrepreneurship, demonstrating how cultural practices can support global development objectives.

19.1.10   *SDG 10: Reduced Inequality*

SDG 10 aims to "reduce inequality within and among countries." Ramadan, as a period of spiritual reflection, community engagement, and charitable giving, uniquely addresses various aspects of inequality. The increased emphasis on charity (*Zakat* and *Sadaqah*) during Ramadan plays a significant role in redistributing wealth, alleviating poverty, and reducing economic disparities within communities. Zakat, one of the five pillars of Islam, requires financially capable Muslims to give a portion of their wealth to those in need, amplifying these efforts during Ramadan to reach more beneficiaries and address the economic roots of inequality. Ramadan fosters unity and brotherhood among participants, bridging the social divide. Community *Iftar*s and collective prayers bring together people from various socioeconomic backgrounds, promoting interactions across social strata and fostering understanding and solidarity among diverse groups. Charitable initiatives during Ramadan target marginalized groups, including people experiencing poverty, orphans, refugees, and migrant workers, providing them with food, clothing, and financial assistance, thereby alleviating immediate inequalities. The global observance of Ramadan encourages solidarity within local communities and across borders. Many Muslims donate to international aid projects, reducing disparities in less developed countries by funding education, healthcare, water, sanitation, and emergency relief. Educational and cultural activities during Ramadan are made available to all community members, helping to reduce educational inequalities and empowering individuals with knowledge and skills. Sermons and talks address issues of justice, equity, and support for the vulnerable, raising awareness about broader issues of inequality and the roles individuals can play locally and globally. Ramadan increases opportunities for volunteerism, building networks, and social capital, particularly for disadvantaged individuals, leveling the playing field to access opportunities and resources. Through charitable giving, community solidarity, support for marginalized groups, global aid, and educational empowerment, Ramadan actively supports SDG 10, demonstrating how religious and cultural practices can reduce inequalities and promote a more just and inclusive society.

19.1.11   SDG 11: Sustainable Cities and Communities

SDG 11 aims to "make cities and human settlements inclusive, safe, resilient, and sustainable." Ramadan, through its community-centric activities and emphasis on inclusivity, can play a significant role in advancing this goal. During Ramadan, mosques and community centers often become focal points for gathering and transcending socioeconomic and cultural boundaries. These spaces are used not only for prayer but also for communal *Iftars*, social gatherings, and charity events, making them inclusive venues that welcome diverse populations. Enhancing these spaces to improve accessibility and safety can contribute to more inclusive cities. The increased community activities during Ramadan can lead to enhanced safety measures in urban areas. Nighttime prayers (Tarawih) mean that more people are out in the evenings, often resulting in better-lit streets and increased community vigilance, which can help reduce crime rates and improve overall neighborhood safety. Charity initiatives during Ramadan usually address issues such as homelessness and inadequate housing by providing shelter and meals to those in need. These efforts can be part of broader strategies to deal with urban poverty and homelessness, thus enhancing the resilience of cities against social issues. Islamic traditions generally emphasize the importance of living a simple, low-cost life. Still, specifically during Ramadan, a reduction in consumption and mindfulness in resource use is highly encouraged, which can align with sustainable urban practices. Efforts to reduce waste during community meals, promote recycling, and minimize energy use during Ramadan can serve as models for sustainable practices during other city events and activities. Ramadan plays a significant role in cultural preservation and fostering a strong community identity, which are important aspects of sustainable human settlements. The traditions practiced during Ramadan, including the arts, food, and music associated with it, enrich the cultural tapestry of cities and promote a sense of belonging and community pride. In many cities, public transport systems adjust their schedules to accommodate the increased activity during Ramadan nights, particularly for Tarawih prayers. These adjustments can lead to improved public transport services that benefit all urban dwellers and contribute to a more sustainable and accessible city. Ramadan encourages active community participation in both planning and executing various activities. This active engagement can be a model for participatory governance practices, in which community members are more involved in decision-making processes about urban development and management. Ramadan contributes to SDG 11 by fostering inclusivity, enhancing safety, promoting sustainable urban practices, and preserving cultural identities within urban settings. Through its community-centric practices and ethos of care and sharing, Ramadan demonstrates how cultural and religious observances can positively influence the development of cities and human settlements, making them more inclusive, safe, resilient, and sustainable.

19.1.12 SDG 12: Responsible Consumption and Production

SDG 12 aims to "ensure sustainable consumption and production patterns." Ramadan, with its emphasis on moderation, mindfulness, and community responsibility, significantly contributes to this goal. Ramadan teaches moderation in consumption, making individuals more conscious of their eating habits and discouraging overconsumption and waste. This awareness extends to other areas, encouraging critical thinking about overall consumption patterns and the adoption of sustainable options. The daily fasts from dawn to sunset heighten the value of food, leading to more thoughtful food preparation and reduced waste. Communities often organize *Iftar*s to minimize waste by using shared dishes and donating excess food. Spiritual reflection during Ramadan encourages individuals to reconsider their environmental impact, fostering sustainable practices, such as reducing energy use, increasing recycling, and choosing sustainable transportation. Ramadan inspires community-based sustainability initiatives, including but not limited to clean-up days, recycling drives, and educational programs on environmental responsibility, improving local environments, and building community cohesion. Increased demand for local produce and products during Ramadan supports local farmers and small businesses, reducing the carbon footprint associated with transportation and promoting sustainable production. The culture of donation during Ramadan, including clothes, electronics, and other goods, reduces waste, supports reuse, and is central to sustainable consumption patterns. Emphasizing ethical and sustainable food production during Ramadan encourages food producers to adopt more sustainable and humane farming practices. Ramadan supports SDG 12 by promoting responsible consumption, reducing waste, encouraging sustainable lifestyles, and fostering community-based sustainability initiatives, highlighting how cultural and religious practices can contribute to the SDGs.

19.1.13   SDG 13: Climate Action

SDG 13 aims to "take urgent action to combat climate change and its impacts." Although Ramadan is primarily a religious observance, its practices can indirectly support climate action in several ways. During Ramadan, many community leaders and organizations use the opportunity to educate about various social and ethical issues, including climate change. This can involve discussions during sermons, workshops, and community meetings that focus on the importance of environmental stewardship and the actions individuals and communities can take to mitigate climate change. The practice of fasting from sunrise to sunset leads to a natural reduction in daily consumption patterns. This can extend beyond food to include less energy use and fewer travel activities, which collectively reduce carbon footprints. The discipline learned in Ramadan about the moderation and consideration of resources can inspire continued environmentally friendly practices. Many mosques and Islamic organizations implement more sustainable practices during Ramadan, such as using renewable energy for nighttime lighting, reducing water usage for ablutions, and encouraging carpooling to nightly prayers. These practices not only serve the immediate community during Ramadan but also set examples for sustainability that can be adopted year-round. Charitable giving spikes during Ramadan, and many donors look for ways to make a lasting impact. Investing in reforestation projects, green technology, and other environmentally beneficial initiatives can be particularly appealing. Such projects not only help offset carbon emissions but also improve local environments and biodiversity. With a heightened focus on the significance of sustenance due to fasting, Ramadan encourages minimizing food waste, which is a significant contributor to methane emissions in landfills. Communities often organize collective *Iftar*s where food consumption can be more carefully controlled, and leftovers are distributed to those in need, reducing waste. The increased demand for food and goods during Ramadan often benefits local producers and markets, which can have a lower carbon footprint than imported goods. Promoting regional and sustainable shopping can help reduce transportation emissions and support more sustainable production practices. The spirit of community and solidarity during Ramadan can inspire collective action on environmental issues. This could include community-based initiatives like clean-up drives, planting trees, or campaigns aimed at reducing single-use plastics within the community. While not directly focused on climate change, Ramadan provides a framework within which sustainable practices are encouraged and can flourish. By promoting a culture of moderation, awareness, and community action, Ramadan can contribute significantly to global efforts to combat climate change, highlighting how cultural observances can intersect with environmental stewardship.

19.1.14 SDG 14: Life Below Water and SDG 15: Life on Land

SDG 14 and SDG 15 focus on conserving marine resources and promoting sustainable use of terrestrial ecosystems, respectively. Although it is primarily a spiritual observance, Ramadan can indirectly support these goals. During Ramadan, seafood consumption often increases, presenting opportunities to promote sustainable fishing practices. Community leaders and environmental groups can educate about responsibly sourced seafood, reducing its impact on marine ecosystems. The heightened awareness of waste reduction during Ramadan encourages the minimization of single-use plastics in large *Iftars*, which helps reduce ocean pollution. Charitable giving during Ramadan, such as *Zakat* and *Sadaqah*, can fund marine conservation projects, such as coral reef restoration and marine wildlife protection. Educational programs during Ramadan can highlight the importance of marine conservation and environmental stewardship, raise awareness about the broader impacts of pollution, and encourage community-driven clean-up efforts.

Similarly, Ramadan supports SDG 15 by fostering environmental stewardship and promoting sustainable land use. Emphasizing the Islamic principles of stewardship ('Khalifa') [14], Ramadan encourages actions to protect terrestrial ecosystems. Charitable funds can support reforestation projects and green initiatives, enhancing local and global environmental efforts. The focus on moderation and avoiding excess reduces waste and minimizes the impact of landfills and terrestrial pollution. Ramadan also serves as a platform for education about land degradation and conservation through sermons and workshops. Community-driven clean-up events during Ramadan targeted local parks and forests, fostering responsibility for local environments. In agricultural regions, Ramadan promotes sustainable practices, such as using less harmful pesticides and better water management. The communal spirit of Ramadan empowers communities to advocate for policies that protect natural habitats, sustainably manage forests, and combat land degradation. While not directly focused on conservation, Ramadan's practices and ethos significantly support SDGs 14 and 15 by promoting sustainable consumption, environmental education, and community-driven conservation efforts, demonstrating the potential of religious observances to enhance SDGs.

19.1.15 SDG 16: Peace, Justice, and Strong Institutions

SDG 16 aims to "promote peaceful and inclusive societies for sustainable development, provide access to justice for all, and build effective, accountable, and inclusive institutions at all levels." Ramadan, with its focus on community, reflection, and ethical conduct, can indirectly support the objectives of this goal in several ways. Ramadan fosters a sense of unity and peace within communities. The shared experiences of fasting, prayer, and communal *Iftars* (meals to break the fast) bring people together, often bridging the social and economic divides. This enhanced social cohesion is fundamental to building peaceful societies. During Ramadan, mosques and community centers typically open their doors wider, welcoming diverse members of the community to participate in Ramadan activities. This inclusivity is crucial for fostering a sense of belonging among all societal groups, including marginalized and minority populations, thus contributing to social harmony and peace. The spiritual reflection encouraged during Ramadan promotes ethical behavior and personal accountability. Sermons and teachings often focus on virtues such as honesty, integrity, and justice, which are critical for the development of just and accountable institutions. Ramadan provides community leaders with an opportunity to address local issues of justice and reform. For example, many communities use this time to organize legal aid clinics or forums to discuss community grievances and find solutions, promoting access to justice for all. The principles of forgiveness and reconciliation are emphasized during Ramadan, which can help resolve conflicts at both personal and community levels. This focus can extend to broader peacebuilding efforts, where communities work together to address and resolve longstanding disputes. Ramadan inspires a surge in charitable giving, which often supports not only people in need but also funds community projects and initiatives that strengthen local institutions. For instance, funding during Ramadan can help improve educational institutions, healthcare facilities, and other community services, thus making them more effective and accessible.

Global observation of Ramadan fosters a sense of solidarity among Muslims worldwide, which can be leveraged to support international initiatives aimed at promoting peace, justice, and strong institutions. This includes support for global campaigns against corruption, violence, and injustice. Ramadan activities often engage youth, providing them with roles in organizing events, leading community service projects, and participating in discussions. This involvement can be instrumental in nurturing the next generation of leaders committed to promoting peaceful and inclusive societies. While the primary focus of Ramadan is spiritual renewal, the month-long observance also supports the goals of SDG 16 by promoting peace, inclusivity, and ethical conduct. Through community cohesion, ethical reflection, support for institutional strengthening, and conflict resolution, Ramadan contributes to building the foundations of peaceful, just, and inclusive societies.

19.1.16 SDG 17: Partnerships for the Goals

SDG 17 aims to "strengthen the means of implementation and revitalize the Global Partnership for Sustainable Development." Ramadan, with its global observance and emphasis on solidarity, generosity, and community, can play a vital role in promoting these partnerships and supporting the broader framework of the SDGs. Muslims worldwide observe Ramadan, creating a unique opportunity to foster global partnerships. This month can serve as a platform for international cooperation in various development projects as communities around the world come together in spirit and action. Collaborations can be formed between different countries, NGOs, and faith-based organizations to address common challenges, such as poverty, health, and education. During Ramadan, the level of giving and charity increases significantly. This mobilization of financial resources can support a wide range of sustainable development projects globally. *Zakat* (mandatory alms-giving) and *Sadaqah* (voluntary charity) can be strategically directed toward funding initiatives that support the SDGs, from building schools and hospitals to supporting clean water projects and renewable energy solutions. Ramadan provides opportunities for cross-cultural and interfaith dialogue, where knowledge and expertise about sustainable development practices can be shared. Workshops, seminars, and conferences held during Ramadan can address topics related to the SDGs and explore ways to implement best practices globally. The spirit of cooperation during Ramadan can encourage the transfer of technologies that promote sustainable development. This can include technologies for clean energy, water purification, and sustainable agriculture.

Faith-based initiatives can play a role in facilitating these transfers, especially to underserved and less developed regions. Ramadan encourages the involvement of various stakeholders in community activities, including businesses, nonprofit organizations, government agencies, and religious groups. These multi-stakeholder partnerships are critical for achieving the SDGs, as they bring diverse resources and perspectives to the table. The global and inclusive nature of Ramadan can help promote policy coherence for sustainable development. By aligning religious practices and teachings with the goals of the SDGs, policymakers can create synergies and reduce policy conflicts. This alignment can be particularly powerful in countries in which religion plays a significant role in social and political life. Ramadan is a period when many people are motivated to volunteer and engage in community services. This can be leveraged to enhance capacity building in critical areas related to sustainable development, such as healthcare, education, and environmental protection. The training and skill development offered during Ramadan can empower individuals and communities to contribute more effectively to the SDGs. Ramadan actively supports SDG 17 by fostering global partnerships, mobilizing resources, sharing knowledge, encouraging technology transfer, and promoting multi-stakeholder partnerships. These contributions highlight how cultural and religious practices can be integral to global efforts aimed at achieving the SDGs, demonstrating the powerful role that faith and community can play in this global endeavor.

19.2 Conclusion

The observance of Ramadan significantly contributes to the United Nations SDGs through its spiritual, ethical, and community-oriented practices. By promoting charity and redistribution of wealth, enhancing community cohesion, fostering empathy, and stimulating local economies, Ramadan supports efforts to end poverty (SDG 1) and hunger (SDG 2). The health benefits of fasting, mental well-being from community bonding, and educational programs promote good health and well-being

(SDG 3) and quality education (SDG 4). Ramadan also advances gender equality (SDG 5) by encouraging women's participation in religious and community activities and supports sustainable management of water (SDG 6) and energy (SDG 7) through mindfulness and conservation practices. Economic growth and decent work (SDG 8) are stimulated through increased demand for goods and services, inclusive economic opportunities, and charitable investments in social enterprises. The emphasis on sustainable practices and innovation during Ramadan contributes to resilient infrastructure and sustainable industrialization (SDG 9), while efforts to redistribute wealth and support marginalized groups address inequalities (SDG 10). Ramadan's community-centric activities enhance the inclusivity, safety, and sustainability of cities (SDG 11) and promote responsible consumption and production (SDG 12). The month-long focus on moderation and environmental stewardship supports climate action (SDG 13) and marine and terrestrial conservation (SDGs 14 and 15). Ramadan fosters peaceful and inclusive societies (SDG 16) through ethical behavior, conflict resolution, and support for institutional strengthening. Finally, the global observance of Ramadan strengthens partnerships (SDG 17) by mobilizing resources, sharing knowledge, and encouraging multi-stakeholder collaboration. Through its unique combination of spiritual depth, community focus, and practical actions, Ramadan provides a powerful example of how cultural and religious practices can significantly contribute to global development objectives, highlighting the potential for cultural and religious observances to play an integral role in achieving the SDGs.

Declaration of generative AI and AI-assisted technologies in the writing process.

During the preparation of this work, the authors used ChatGPT to proofread. After using this tool/service, the authors reviewed and edited the content as needed and took full responsibility for the content of the publication.

References

1. Obaideen K, et al. Wireless power transfer: applications, challenges, barriers, and the role of AI in achieving sustainable development goals – a bibliometric analysis. Energ Strat Rev. 2024;53:101376. 05/01/2024
2. AbuShihab K, et al. Reflection on Ramadan fasting research related to sustainable development goal 3 (good health and Well-being): a bibliometric analysis. J Relig Health. 2023:1–31.
3. Gazi AK. The social impacts of the holy fast of Ramadan in the context of Bangladesh: a content analysis. J Halal Stud. 2020;1:27–33.
4. Olanipekun WD, et al. The role of zakat as a poverty alleviation strategy and a tool for sustainable development: insights from the perspectives of the holy prophet (PBUH). Arabian J Business Manag Rev (Oman Chapter). 2015;5:8.
5. Mohammed MO, et al. Zakat on wealth and asset: lessons for SDGs. In: Islamic Wealth and the SDGs: Global Strategies for Socio-economic Impact. Springer; 2021. p. 375–92.
6. Siddiqi MH. Practicing Islam in the United States. The Oxford handbook of American Islam. 2014:159–73.
7. Sobian A. Household food waste reduction: an Islamic perspective. TAFHIM: IKIM J Islam Contemporary WORLD. 2022;15

8. Shalihin N, Sholihin M. Ramadan: the month of fasting for muslim and social cohesion—mapping the unexplored effect. Heliyon. 2022;8:e10977. 10/01/ 2022
9. Trabelsi K, Chtourou H. Teaching physical education during Ramadan observance: practical recommendations. Int J Sport Stud Health. 2019;2:1–6.
10. Alghafli Z, et al. A qualitative study of Ramadan: a month of fasting, family, and faith. Religions. 2019;10:123.
11. Othman A, et al. Assessment of supplied water quality during mass gatherings in arid environments. J King Saud Unive-Sci. 2022;34:101918.
12. Kapli FWA, et al. Feasibility studies of rainwater harvesting system for ablution purposes. Water. 2023;15:1686.
13. Eyerci C, et al. Ramadan effect on prices and production: case of Turkey. Statistika Statistics Economy J. 2021;101
14. Hossain M. Exploring the Muslim Canadian environmental philanthropy narrative. J Muslim Philanthropy Civil Soc. 2022;6